ORAL-PATHOLOGY
MEDICINE *and* RADIOLOGY

ORAL-PATHOLOGY
MEDICINE *and* RADIOLOGY

By
TARGET EDUCARE

Dr. Ambika Gupta
MDS (Oral Medicine and Radiology),
Asstt. Professor
Government Dental College, Rohtak

Foreword by
Dr. Ashok Dhoble

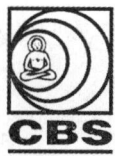

CBS

CBS PUBLISHERS & DISTRIBUTORS
NEW DELHI · BANGALORE · PUNE (INDIA)

ISBN : 978-81-239-1639-2

First Edition : 2008

Publishing Director : Vinod K. Jain

Published by :
Satish Kumar Jain for CBS Publishers & Distributors,
4819/XI, 24 Ansari Road, Darya Ganj, New Delhi - 110 002 (India)
E-mail: cbspubs@vsnl.com • Website: www.cbspd.com

Branch Office :
2975, 17th Cross, K.R. Road, Bansankari 2nd Stage, Bangalore-70
Fax : 080-26771680 • E-mail : cbsbng@vsnl.net

Design & Layout by :
Limited Colors, Delhi-110092

Printed at :
India Binding House, Noida (UP)

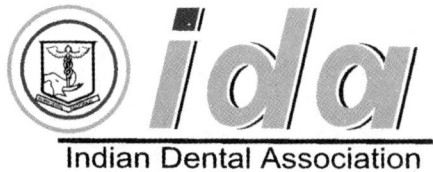

Dr. ASHOK DHOBLE
Hon. Secretary General
Bombay Mutual Terrace, 2nd Floor,
534, Sandhurst Bridge, Opera House,
Mumbai 400 007
Tel: 91-22-2364-3344/2363 6655
ashokdhoble@ida.org.in

Indian Dental Association

Foreword

It gives me great pleasure and satisfaction to write this foreword of **Oral Pathology, Oral Medicine and Radiology by Target Educare** compiled and edited by **Dr. Ambika Gupta.** The hallmark of this book is that the entire book has been written by the person specializing in this branch of dentistry. The design and presentation of this book is clear, lucid and precise. The entire book is divided into chapters to ease assimilation of all important facts and MCQs on that particular topic, discussing the oral medicine, pathology and radiology part simultaneously, so that there is no need to refer to three different books while studying a particular topic. Another excellent feature of this book is that each MCQ has been explained with rationale for the right answer.

In the present scenario, when the MCQs are no longer repeated time and again from the MCQs books available in the market, this compendium shall serve the need for quick revision of the entire subject and help the students seeking admission to postgraduate courses. This book is also valuable for the undergraduate and postgraduate students to prepare for the viva. The author deserves hearty congratulations for her excellent contribution.

Dr. ASHOK DHOBLE
Hon. Secretary General
Indian Dental Association, Head Office

Preface

To begin with, I earnestly regard the power and mercy of Almighty who has showered this endeavor and acquainted me with this humble piece of work.

The subjects of Oral Medicine, Pathology and Radiology, on the whole are poorly learned and ignored at the undergraduate level. The foremost reason being the recent recognition of these branches as a specialty in dentistry. So, the students appearing for PG entrance examination usually face difficulty, answering the frequently asked questions from this subject.

This book has been prepared to present the entire subject in a nutshell in a simple and easy manner. We have taken care to design the book in such a manner that it meets the needs of students. All topics have received considerable attention with special emphasis on certain important aspects.

I wish to express my gratitude to all those who were directly or indirectly involved in writing of this book. My highest esteems and regards to my teachers Dr. F. R. Karjodkar and Dr K.P.Sansare for their valuable suggestions, constant encouragement, kind-heartedness, critical appraisals and practical solutions that helped me tremendously. A very genuine thanks to my friends Pradnya, Antara, Neeraj, Pratik, Payal, Neha, Deepa Pooja, Meenu for keeping my spirits high and lending their helping hand.

I sincerely thank Dr. Praveen Bansal; Target Educare for giving me a platform to make this work possible. My special thanks to Mr S. K. Jain and Late Mr. B. R. Sharma from CBS Publishers and distributors for their valuable help and cooperation.

I will always fall short of words to express my feelings for my parents and brothers for their love, support and sacrifices that made it possible for me to pursue my academics. Words of gratitude are not enough for their support and well wishes.

Last, but not the least, thanks to ALMIGHTY for showering all his blessings.

Ambika Gupta

Contents

Developmental Disturbances

DEVELPOMENTAL DISTURBANCES OF JAWS

I) Micrognathia

Two Types

A. Congenital - Etiology is unknown.

        - May be associated with other congenital abnormalities like congenital heart disease and Pierre Robin syndrome.

B. Acquired - Usually results from a disturbance in the area of TMJ.

Pierre Robin syndrome

- Mandibular micrognathia
- Glossoptosis
- Cleft palate
- Absence of gag reflex
- Respiratory difficulties

II) Macrognathia

- *Pituitary gigantism* - There is increase in size of both jaws.
- *Paget's disease* - Overgrowth of the cranium and maxilla, occasionally in mandible occurs.
- *Acromegaly* - Enlargement of mandible.
- *Leontiasis ossea* - A form of fibrous dysplasia where there is enlargement of maxilla and facial bones.

Features of mandibular prognathism

A. Increased height of ramus.

B. Increased mandibular body length.

C. Increased gonial angle.

D. Anterior positioning of glenoid fossa.

    E. Decreased maxillary length.

    F. Posterior positioning of maxilla.

    G. Prominent chin button.

III) Facial hemihypertrophy

- Unilateral enlargement of one half of head.
- Localized or generalized enlargement of crown size on affected side
- Root of teeth may be proportionately enlarged, but may be short.
- Rapid eruption of permanent teeth and premature shedding of primary teeth.
- Tongue - Unilateral hypertrophy
  -     - Enlargement of lingual papillae
  -     - Soft pendulous folds on affected side
- Associated abnormalities
  - (a) Mental deficiency   - 28 %
  - (b) Skin abnormalities   - 47 %
    - - Nevi
    - - Telangiectasia
    - - Thicker hair
    - - Hemangioma
  - (c) Compensatory scoliosis - 17 %
  - (d) Varicose vein   - 7 %
  - (e) Umbilical hernia   - 5%
- Associated syndromes
  - – Beckwith Weidemann Syndrome
  - – Neurofibromatosis
  - – Klippel Trenaunay Weber Syndrome
  - – Proteus Syndrome
  - – Mc Cune Albright Syndrome
  - – Epidermal Nevus Syndrome
  - – Maffucci Syndrome
  - – Ollier Syndrome

IV) Facial hemiatrophy (Parry-Romberg syndrome)

- White line, furrow or mark on one side of face or brow near the midline.
- Hollowing of cheek.
- Eye may be depressed in orbit.
- Cartilage of nose, ear, larynx and palpebral tarsus may be involve.
- Contralateral Jacksonian epilepsy, trigeminal neuralgia and changes in eye and hair commonly occurs.

- Darkly pigmented skin.

Oral Manifestations

- Hemiatrophy of lips and tongue.
- Retarded eruption of teeth
- Stunted roots of teeth.

V) Segmental Odontomaxillary Dysplasia (Hemimaxillofacial Dysplasia)

- Unknown cause.
- Characterized by painless, unilateral enlargement of the maxillary bone, along with fibrous hyperplasia of the overlying gingiva.
- One or both maxillary premolars may be absent and primary teeth are usually hypoplastic.
- Thickened vertically oriented trabeculae with granular appearance.

DEVELOPMENTAL DISTURBANCES OF LIPS AND PALATE

I) Vander Woude's syndrome

- Pits of lower lip
- Cleft lip and/or palate

II) Double lip

- Congenital or acquired
- *"Cupid's bow"* when the upper lip is the double lip it resembles a cupid bow.

Ascher's Syndrome

- Acquired double lip
- Blepharochalasis
- Non toxic thyroid enlargement

III) Cheilitis glandularis

- Mostly lower lip is involved
- Lip becomes enlarged, firm & everted
- Three types :
  1. *Simple type*: Multiple, painless, pinhead-sized lesions with central depressions and dilated canals.
  2. *Superficial suppurative type*: (Baelz disease) : Painless swelling, induration, crusting and superficial & deep ulcerations.
  3. *The deep suppurative type*: Cheilitis glandularis apostematosa, myxadenitis labialis.

IV) Cheilitis granulomatosa (Miescher's syndrome)

- Diffuse swelling of lip

Melkerson Rosenthal syndrome
- Cheilitis granulomatosa
- Facial paralysis
- Scrotal tongue

V) Cleft lip & palate
- Incidence of cleft lip & cleft palate is 1 in 800 births.
- Mongoloid are mostly affected.
- Cleft lip alone - more common in males.
- Cleft palate alone - More common in females.
- Unilateral cleft lip - 80 %
- Left side clefts - 70 %
- Mode of inheritance is multifactorial.
- Maxillary cleft lip in due to failure of obliteration of the ectodermal grooves separating the maxillary process and mesial nasal process.
- Cleft palate is due to lack of forces, interference by the tongue or disparity in the size of palatal processes of maxilla and/or the globulomaxillary process.
- Mandibular cleft in very rare and is due to failure of copula to give rise to the mandibular arch or due to persistence of the central groove of the mandibular process.

Treatment of cleft lip
- *'Rule of 10'* is followed - Miller
  10 weeks of age.
  10 pounds weight.
  Hb not less than 10 gm %
  TLC - 10000/ cm^3

Treatment of cleft palate
- Treated at about 18 months of age.

Median cleft face syndrome
- Hypertelorism
- Median cleft of the premaxilla and palate.
- Cranium bifidum occultum.

VI) Peutz-Jeghers Syndrome (Hereditary Intestinal Polyposis Syndrome)
- Familial generalized intestinal polyposis.
- Pigmented spots on the face, oral cavity and sometimes the hands & feet, macules 1-5 mm in size.
- Usually present at birth.
- Facial pigmentation tends to fade later in life, mucosal pigmentation persists.
- Intestinal polyposis of colon may undergo malignant change.

VII) Ephelis
- Labial and oral melanotic macule.
- Solitary labial lentigo

DEVELOPMENTAL DISTURBANCES OF ORAL MUCOSA AND GINGIVA

I) Fordyce's Disease
- Heterotrophic inclusion of sebaceous glands in oral cavity in course of development of the maxillary and mandibular processes during embryonic life.
- Small yellow spots, either discretely separate or forming relatively large plaques.
- Usually innocuous, however very rarely adenomas may develop.

II) Heck's Disease (Focal epithelial hyperplasia)
- Multiple nodular lesions with sessile base usually on lower lip, 1-5 mm in size.
- Regress spontaneously after 4 – 6 months.
- Viral etiology has been postulated.

III) Fibromatosis Gingivae (Elephantiasis gingivae)
- Diffuse fibrous overgrowth of gingiva.
- Usually seen at the times of eruption of permanent incisors.
- May prevent the normal eruption of teeth.

IV) Retrocuspid papilla
- This is a small, elevated nodule located on the lingual mucosa.

DEVELOPMENTAL DISTURBANCES OF THE TONGUE

I) Microglossia

Hypoglossia- hypodactylia syndrome
- Microglossia
- Hypoplasia of mandible
- Hypodactylia
- Hypomelia
- Cleft palate, missing lower incisors
- Situs inversus

II) Macroglossia (Glossocele)

Congenital
- Vascular malformations like lymphangiohemangioma.

- Hemihyperplasia
- Cretinism
- Beckwith Weideman syndrome
- Down's syndrome
- Mucopolysaccharidosis
- Neurofibromatosis
- MEN 2B
- Lingual thyroid.

Acquired

1. Inflammatory
   - T.B
   - Actinomycosis
   - Dental infections
   - Syphilitic gumma
   - Ranula
2. Hypertrophic
   - Due to muscle hypertrophy
3. Neoplastic
   - Carcinomas
   - Sarcomas
   - Granular cell tumor
   - Neurofibroma
   - Leiomyoma
   - Lipoma
4. Traumatic
   - Dental irritation
   - Hematoma
   - Postoperative edema
5. Metabolic
   - Amyloidosis
   - Acromegaly
   - Lipoid proteinosis
   - Chronic steroid therapy
   - Myxoedema
6. Angioedema.

Beckwith – Wiedemann Syndrome

- Omphalocele
- Visceromegaly

- Neonatal hypoglycemia
- Macroglossia
- Postnatal somatic gigantism
- Increased risk of childhood tumors

III) Ankyloglossia

- Male : female = 4 : 1

Ankyloglossia superious syndrome

- Tongue attached to hard palate
- Limb malformation
- Jejunal and ileal atresias.

Fraser syndrome

- Ankyloglossia
- Cryptopthalmos
- Limb deformities

IV) Cleft tongue (Bifid tongue)

- Due to lack of fusion of lateral halves.
- Associated with oro-facial digital syndrome.

V) Fissured tongue (Scrotal tongue)

Classified as:

1. Foliaceous
2. Cerebriform
3. Transverse
   - Usually associated with geographic tongue.
   - May be associated with chronic trauma or vitamin deficiencies.
   - May be a component of Melkersson Rosenthal Syndrome.

VI) Median rhomboid glossitis (Central papillary atrophy of the tongue)

- Due to failure of tuberculum impar to retract or withdraw before fusion of the lateral halves of tongue.
- Localized chronic fungal infection specifically candida albicans has been found.
- There is absence of filliform papillae.
- Three times more frequent in men than in woman.
- Fungi are best visualized by PAS stain.

Familial dysautonomia

There is absence of circumvallate and fungiform papillae.

VII) Benign migratory glossitis (Geographic tongue / wandering rash of tongue / Glossitis areata exfoliativa /Erythema migrans)

Type 1 - Lesion confined to tongue with both active and remission phase.

Type 2 - Same as type 1 with similar lesion elsewhere in mouth.

Type 3 - Lesions on tongue that are not typical and may be accompanied by lesion elsewhere in mouth.

(a) Fixed form

(b) Abortive form

Type 4 - No tongue lesion but geographic areas elsewhere in oral cavity.

- Predilection for female.
- Microabcess or *Monro's abscess* may be formed near the surface.

VIII) Hairy tongue

- Hypertrophy of filliform papillae with lack of normal desquamation.
- May be related to microorganisms, systemic disturbances, and oral use of certain drugs, smoking, poor oral hygiene, use of mouthwashes and antacids, extensive X-ray irradiation.

IX) Lingual varices

- Red or purple shot like clusters of vessels on the ventral surface and lateral borders of the tongue and floor of month.
- Occurs due to loss of connective tissue tone supporting the vessel.

X) Caliber persistent artery

- A main arterial branch extends up into the superficial submucosal tissue, without a reduction in its diameter.
- Lesion presents as a linear, arcuate or papuler elevation, becomes conspicuous on stretching the lip.

XI) Lingual thyroid nodule

- Develops at site of foramen caecum
- Females: Males = 4 : 1
- Dysphagia, dysphonia, dyspnoea, haemorrhages with pain or feeling of tightness or fullness in the throat.
- Diagnosis is best established by thyroid scan using Technetium 99 m or Iodine isotopes.
- Biopsy is often avoided because of the risk of haemorrhage and because it may be the only thyroid tissue of the patient.

Developmental Anomalies of Teeth

I) Alterations in number

A. Anodontia - total lack of tooth development.

B. Hypodontia - lack of development of one or more teeth.

C. Oligodontia - lack of development of six or more teeth (a subdivision of hypodontia).

D. Hyperdontia - development of increased number of teeth.

Syndromes associated with hypodontia

1. Ankyloglossia superioris	2. Book syndrome
3. Cockayne syndrome	4. Coffin – lowry
5. Cranio – oculo – dental	6. Crouzon
7. Down	8. Ectodermal dysplasia
9. Cleft lip, palate	10. Ehler – Danlos
11. Ellis – van Crevald	12. Focal dermal hypoplasia
13. Freire – Maria	14. Frontometaphyseal dysplasia
15. Goldenhar	16. Gorlin
17. Gorlin – Chaudhary – Moss	18. Hallermann – Streiff
19. Hanhart	20. Hurler
21. Hypoglossia - hypodactylia	22. Incontinentia pigmenti
23. Johanson – Blizzard	24. Lipoid proteinosis
25. Marshall – White	26. Melanoleukoderma
27. Monilethrix – anodontia	28. Oro – facial - digital type 1
29. Otodental dysplasia	30. Palmoplantar keratosis
31. Progeria	32. Rieger
33. Robinson	34. Rothmund
35. Sturge – Weber	36. Tooth and nail
37. Turner	

Syndromes associated with hyperdontia

1. Apert	2. Angio-osteohypertrophy
3. Cleidocranial dysplasia	4. Craniometaphyseal dysplasia
5. Crouzon	6. Curtius
7. Down	8. Ehlers-Danlos
9. Fabry-Anderson	10. Fucosidosis
11. Gardner	12. Hollermann – Streiff
13. Klippel – Trenaunay – Weber	14. Laband
15. Nance – Horan	16. Oro – facial – digital, type I and III
17. Sturge - Weber	18. Tricho – rhino – phalangeal

- Hypodontia is uncommon in deciduous dentition. When present, it most frequently involves the mandibular incisors.
- Frequency of missing teeth in permanent dentition: 3rd molars > 2nd premolars > lateral incisors.
- Frequency of supernumerary teeth in permanent dentition: Mesiodens > maxillary 4th molar > mandibular 4th molar > premolars > canines > lateral incisors.
- Mesiodens – supernumerary teeth in maxillary incisor region.
- Supplemental tooth - Extra tooth with a normal morphology.
- Distomolar or distodens - an accessory 4th molar.
- Paramolar – posterior supernumerary tooth situated lingual or buccal to a molar tooth.
- Peridens- supernumerary tooth situated lingual or buccal to the normal arch.
- Natal teeth - teeth present in newborn.
- Neonatal teeth – those arising within 30 days of life.

II) Developmental alterations in size

1. Microdontia

   (a) True microdontia

     Peg lateral (maxillary lateral incisor) > 3rd molars

     • Congenital Heart Disease

     • Progeria

   (b) Relative microdontia / macrognathia

     • Down syndrome

     • Pituitary dwarfism

2. Macrodontia / megalodontia / megadontia

   • Pituitary gigantism

   • Pineal hyperplasia with hyperinsulinism

   • Hemifacial hyperplasia

   • Hemangioma

III) Developmental alterations in shape

1. Gemination (Twinning)

Single enlarged tooth or joined (i.e. double) tooth in which the tooth count is normal when the anomalous tooth in counted as one.

The pulp chamber is usually single and enlarged and may be partially divided.

2. Fusion (Syndontia)

Single enlarged tooth or joined (i.e. double) tooth in which the tooth count reveals a missing tooth when the anomalous tooth is counted as one.

3. Concrescence

Unions of two adjacent teeth by cementum alone without any confluence of dentin.

   • Fusion and gemination is most common in anterior and maxillary region.

- Concrescence is more frequent in posterior and maxillary regions.

4. *Cusp of carabelli*

- Present on mesiopalatal cusp of maxillary 1st molars.
- An analogous accessory cusp in seen occasionally on the mesiobuccal cusp of a mandibular permanent or deciduous molar – *protostylid*.

5. *Talon cusp*

- Frequency of occurrence: Maxillary lateral incisor > maxillary central incisor > mandibular incisors > maxillary canines.
- Associated syndromes:
  - Mohr Syndrome
  - Rubinstein – Taybi Syndrome
  - Sturge – Weber Syndrome

6. *Dens evaginatus / Central tubercle / Leong's premolar*

- Most common on mandibular premolars.
- May be seen in association with shovel – shaped incisors.
- Highest frequency in Asians and Native Americans.
- A fine pulp horn may extend into the tubercle, but this may not be visible radiographically.

7. *Dens invaginatus / Dens in dente / Dilated odontome/ Gestant odontome*

Type 1 - Confined to the crown.

Type 2 - Extends below the CEJ.

Type 3 - Extends through the root and perforates in the apical or lateral radicular area without any immediate communication with the pulp.

- Frequently occurs in permanent maxillary lateral incisor, followed by maxillary central Incisors, premolars and canines and less often in posterior teeth.
- Associated with risk of pulpal disease.

8. *Ectopic enamel / Enamel pearls/ Enameloma/ Enamel drop*

- Usually occur in furcation area below the crest of gingiva.
- Cervical enamel extension, also occurs along the surface of dental roots.
- Maxillary and mandibular molars are most commonly affected.
- Predisposes to development of buccal bifurcation cysts.

9. *Taurodontism / Bull – tooth*

- Normal   -   Cynodont
- Mild   -   Hypotaurodontism
- Moderate -   Mesotaurodontism
- Severe   -   Hypertaurodontism
- Peculiar radiographic feature is an extension of the rectangular pulp chamber into the elongated body of the tooth, short crown and shortened roots.

Syndromes associated with taurodontism

1. Amelogenesis imperfecta
2. Cranioectodermal
3. Ectodermal dysplasia
4. Hypophosphatasia
5. Hyperphosphatasia – oligophrenia – taurodontism
6. Klinefelter
7. Microdontia - taurodontia – dens invaginatus
8. Microcephalic dwarfism – taurodontism
9. Oculo–dento – digital dysplasia
10. Oro– facial – digital, type II
11. Rapp – Hodgkin
12. Scanty hair – Oligodontia – taurodontia
13. Sex chromosomal aberrations
14. Down
15. Tricho – dento osseous type I, II, III.
16. Tricho – Onycho – dental.

10. Hypercementosis

Usually associated with

- Acromegaly and pituitary gigantisms
- Paget's disease
- Arthritis
- Calcinosis
- Rheumatic fever
- Thyroid goiter
- Abnormal occlusal trauma
- Adjacent inflammation
- Unopposed teeth

11. Dilaceration

- Sharp bend or curve in the tooth.
- Maxillary incisors most frequently involved followed by maxillary premolars and mandibular incisors.
- Dilaceration in the apical end of an unaltered root appear as a rounded opaque area with a dark shadow in its central region cast by the apical foramen and root canal (bull's eye appearance on radiograph).

12. Supernumerary root

3rd molars > mandibular cuspids and premolars.

13. *Prostostylid*: An accessory cusp on the mesiobuccal cusp of a mandibular permanent or deciduous molar.

IV) Developmental alterations in structure

1. *Amelogenesis imperfecta*

- May be autosomal dominant, recessive or X-linked.
- Not related to any time or period of enamel development.
- Enamel may lack the normal prismatic structure. As a result, these teeth are more resistant to decay.
- Associated syndrome – Tricho-dento-osseous syndrome.
- HYPOPLASTIC TYPE:
  - Occurs as a result of some defect in ameloblasts.
  - Enamel of the affected teeth fails to develop to its normal thickness.
  - Yellowish brown color of the teeth.
  - Enamel may be pitted, rough, smooth and glossy.
  - Open contacts and anterior open bite may occur.
- HYPOMATURATION TYPE:
  - Enamel has a normal thickness but mottled appearance.
  - Softer than normal and may crack away from the crown.
  - Color may range from clear to cloudy white, yellow or brown (***Snow capped teeth***).
- HYPOCALCIFIED TYPE:
  - Enamel is poorly mineralized, so starts to fracture shortly after the tooth comes into function.
  - An explorer can penetrate into the enamel.
  - Enamel appears more radiolucent than dentin.

2. *Dentinogenesis Imperfecta*

- Autosomal dominant disturbance.
- Type I - Osteogenesis Imperfecta with opalescent teeth (Dentinogenesis Imperfecta). There is an inborn error in the synthesis of Type I collagen.
- Type II – (Hereditary opalescent teeth) Isolated opalescent teeth.
- Type III – (Brandywine isolate) Isolated opalescent teeth.
- Enamel may be thinner than normal, with amber like translucency and variety of colors from yellow to blue gray.
- Radiographs show bulbous crowns with a cervical constriction.
- Short slender roots.
- Obliterated pulp canals and chambers in Type I, II.
- ***Shell – teeth appearance*** in Type III.

3. *Dentin dysplasia*
   - Autosomal dominant disturbance
   - *Type I (Radicular dentin dysplasia / rootless teeth)*
     - Normal color or bluish brown translucency.
     - Crescent or chevron – shaped pulp chambers.
     - Shortened roots, no pulp canal. Roots of primary teeth may be thin spicules.
     - Periapical radiolucencies associated with non carious teeth is a characteristic feature.
     - *Lava- flowing around boulders* appearances.
     - A similar, but localized lesion occurs in fibrous dysplasia of dentin in which, teeth are normal clinically radiographically, teeth are normal in shape but demonstrates a radiodense product filling the pulp cavity.
   - *Type II (Coronal dentin dysplasia)*
     - Color and contour similar to Dentinogenesis Imperfecta.
     - Thistle tube or flame – shaped pulp anatomy of permanent teeth with pulp stones.
     - Deciduous teeth resemble Dentinogenesis Imperfecta
   - *Associated diseases:*
     1. Calcinosis universalis
     2. Rheumatoid arthritis
     3. Vitaminosis D
     4. Sclerotic bone and skeletal anomalies
     5. Tumoral calcinosis

4. *Regional Odontodysplasia (odontodysplasia / odontogenic imperfecta)*
   - Affects only a few teeth in a quadrant.
   - Teeth are small and mottled brown.
   - Susceptible to caries, are brittle, and are subject to fractures and pulpal infection.
   - May delay eruption.
   - Radiograph – **Ghost like appearance**.
   - Histopathology – Enameloid conglomerates.

V) Disturbances of growth (eruption of teeth)

1. *Premature eruption*
   - Common causes are hyperthyroidism and adrenogenital syndrome
   - Natal teeth – present at birth
   - Neonatal teeth - erupt within one month of life

2. *Delayed eruption*
   - Rickets
   - Cretinism
   - Cleidocranial dysplasia

- Local factors like fibromatosis gingiva.

3. *Multiple unerupted teeth*
- Cleidocranial dysplasia
- Gardner's syndrome

4. *Eruption sequestrum*
- Usually associated with erupting teeth
- Condition corrects itself
- No treatment required

5. *Embedded teeth*
- Unerupted due to lack of eruption forces.

6. *Impacted teeth*
- Have eruptive forces, but can't erupt due to physical barrier.
- 3rd molar > maxillary canine > premolar.

7. *Submerged teeth* (Ankylosed deciduous teeth)
- Usually mandibular second molars.

VI) Discoloration of teeth

- EXTRINSIC
  - Bacterial stains
  - Iron
  - Tobacco
  - Foods and beverages
  - Gingival hemorrarhage
  - Restorative material
  - Medication
- INTRINSIC
  - Amelogenesis Imperfecta
  - Dentinogenesis Imperfecta
  - Dental Fluorosis
  - Erythropoietic porphyria (Gunther disease)
  - Hyperbilirubinaemia
  - Trauma
  - Localized RBC breakdown
  - Medications

DEVELOPMENTAL DISTURBANCES OF LYMPHOID TISSUE

Kimura's Disease

- Angiolymphoid hyperplasia with eosinophils, eosinophilic granuloma, eosinophilic follicularis.
- Self limiting.

QUESTIONS

1. **Median rhomboid glossitis is due to:** [AIPGEE 2008]
   1. Trauma
   2. Nutritional deficiency
   3. Candidiasis
   4. None of the above

Ans. **3**

Median rhomboid glossitis occurs due to failure of tuberculum impar to retract or withdraw before fusion of the lateral halves of tongue. Localized chronic fungal infection specifically candida albicans has also been found.

2. **Benign migratory glossitis is also termed as:** [AIPGEE 2008]
   1. Erythema migrans
   2. Wandering rashes
   3. Geographic tongue
   4. All of the above

Ans. **4**

Other name is Glossitis areata exfoliativa.

3. **Ghost teeth are seen in:** [AIPGEE 2008]
   1. Dentin dysplasia
   2. Dentinogensis imperfecta
   3. Amelogenesis imperfecta
   4. Regional odontodysplasia

Ans. **4**

Amelogenesis imperfecta - Snow capped teeth
Dentinogenesis Imperfecta- Hereditary opalescent teeth, Shell – teeth
Dentin dysplasia - rootless teeth

4. **Shell teeth are associated with:** [AIPGEE 2008]
   1. Dentin dysplasia
   2. Dentinogensis imperfecta

3. Amelogenesis imperfecta

4. Regional odontodysplasia

Ans. **2**

5. **Taurodontism is usually seen in:**   [AIPGEE 2008]

1. Mandibular first molar

2. Mesiodens

3. Mandibular Incisor

4. Maxillary premolars

Ans. **1**

Also known as Bull – tooth. Peculiar radiographic feature is an extension of the rectangular pulp chamber into the elongated body of the tooth, short crown and shortened roots.

6. **Ectopic sebaceous glands present as:**   [AIPGEE 2008]

1. Melasma

2. Fordyce's granules

3. Melanosome

4. Papillary overgrowth

Ans. **2**

7. **Which of the following teeth is most likely to be congenitally missing?**   [AIPG 2005]

1. Maxillary central incisor.

2. Mandibular canine.

3. Mandibular second premolar.

4. Maxillary first premolar.

Ans. **3**

Most commonly missing teeth are third molars followed by maxillary lateral incisors and mandibular second premolars.

8. **The term refers to a type of fusion in which the formed teeth are joined only along the line of cementum.**   [AIPG 2005]

1. Gemination.

2. Fusion.

3. Concrescence.

4. Dilaceration.

Ans. **3**·

Gemination - attempt of tooth bud to divide into two.

Fusion - fusion of two buds.

Dilacerations - sharp bend in the root.

9. **In erythema migrans, which papilla of tongue is absent:**   [AIPG 2004]
   1. Fungiform
   2. Foliate
   3. Filliform
   4. Circumvallate

Ans. **3**

10. **Thistle-tube appearance of pulp chamber is a feature of:**   [AIPG 2004]
    1. Coronal dentin dysplasia
    2. Regional odontodysplasia
    3. Dentinogenesis imperfecta
    4. Amelogenesis imperfecta

Ans. **1**

   Regional odontodysplasia - Ghost teeth.

   Dentinogenesis imperfecta - Obliteration of pulp chamber and shell teeth.

11. **Which is degeneration disorder characterized by atrophic changes of the deeper structures (e.g. fat, muscle, cartilage and bone) involving one side of the face?**   [AIPG 2004]
    1. Scleroderma
    2. Parry Romberg syndrome
    3. Miescher's syndrome
    4. Peutz - Jeghers syndrome

Ans. **2**

   It is marked by hemifacial atrophy.

12. **The clinical picture of hairs in black hairy tongue is caused by hyperkeratinized hyperplastic:**   [AIPG 2004]
    1. Filliform papillae
    2. Fungiform papillae
    3. Vallate papillae
    4. Filliform and fungiform papillae

Ans. **1**

13. **A dens in dente is usually caused by:**   [AIPG 2003]
    1. An abnormal proliferation of pulp tissue.
    2. Dentin formation within the pulp tissue
    3. A deep invagination of the enamel organ during tooth formation.
    4. A supernumerary tooth bud enclaved within a normal tooth.

Ans. **3**

   It is a predisposing site for infection and caries.

Abnormal proliferation of pulp tissue is called a polyp.

Dentin formation within the pulp tissue is termed as reparative or secondary dentin.

14. Difference between accessory and supernumerary teeth is that a supernumerary tooth: [AIPG 2002]

1. Erupts in place of an absent tooth.
2. In addition to the normal number of teeth.
3. It shows no resemblance to any other tooth.
4. Normal feature of the oral cavity.

Ans. **2**

Accessory tooth shows no resemblance to any other tooth. Supplementary tooth is similar to the adjacent tooth in morphology.

15. Following are features of fissured tongue except: [AIPG 2002]
1. Malignant transformation
2. Accompanies GI disturbance
3. Associated with vitamin deficiency
4. May occur as a sequel to geographic tongue.

Ans. **1**

It is a benign condition.

16. A patient shows a smooth red circumscribed area devoid of papillae just anterior to the sulcus of the tongue. Histology reveals epithelial hyperplasia. It is most probably: [AIPG 2000]

1. Geographic tongue
2. Median rhomboid glossitis
3. Carcinoma in situ
4. Lingual thyroid.

Ans. **2**

It is a common developmental anomaly. Geographic tongue may occur anywhere on dorsum of tongue. Lingual thyroid is found on posterior third while carcinoma in situ usually occurs on lateral borders.

17. Generalized growth failure in the first year of life results in: [AIPG 2000]
1. Maxillary hypoplasia
2. Mandibular hypoplasia
3. Enamel hypoplasia
4. Dentinogenesis imperfecta.

Ans. **3**

Calcification of permanent teeth begins at birth. So any disturbance of growth leads to enamel hypoplasia.

18. Dentinogenesis imperfecta differs from amelogenesis imperfecta in that the former:

[AIPG 2000]

1. Is a hereditary disease.
2. Results in brown discoloration of enamel.
3. Results from increased fluoride intake.
4. Results in small pulp chambers and roots.

Ans. 4

Secondary dentin formation with obliteration of pulp chambers and canals is characteristic feature of dentinogenesis imperfecta.

19. Supernumerary teeth are present in all except:

[AIPG 2000]

1. Cleidocranial dysostosis
2. Ectodermal dysplasia
3. Cleft palate
4. Associated with megalodontia and double teeth.

Ans. 2

Ectodermal dysplasia is marked by oligodontia.

20. Midline cleft of the lip is due to the failure of merging of:

[AIPG 99]

1. Maxillary processes.
2. Maxillary process and lateral nasal process.
3. Maxillary and the medial nasal process.
4. Medial nasal process.

Ans. 4

Maxillary processes- leads to cleft palate.

Maxillary process and lateral nasal process- leads to oblique facial cleft.

Maxillary and the medial nasal process- lead to unilateral cleft lip and palate.

21. Mottled enamel is due to:

[AIPG 99]

1. Vitamin A deficiency
2. Excess of fluoride
3. Vitamin D deficiency
4. Teratogens

Ans. 2

Vitamin A and D deficiency can cause hypoplasia.

22. The commonest bone malignancy is:

[AIPG 99]

1. Metastatic tumor
2. Osteosarcoma
3. Osteoma
4. Ameloblastoma

Ans. 1

Ameloblastoma and osteoma are benign tumors. Metastasis to bones from primary carcinomas is more common than osteosarcoma. Mostly, metastasis occurs from lungs and breast tumors to mandible.

23. **Which of the following is incorrect of Peutz-Jehger's syndrome?** [AIPG 98]
    1. It is an autosomal recessive trait.
    2. Melanin pigmentation of oral mucosa is seen.
    3. Intestinal polyps are present.
    4. Pain in intestine due to intussusception.

Ans. 1

It is an autosomal dominant disorder.

24. **Midline swelling is seen in all except:** [AIPG 98]
    1. IInd brachial cyst
    2. Thyroglossal cyst
    3. Submental lymphadenopathy
    4. Substernal cyst

Ans. 1

Second branchial cyst appears as a lateral swelling in neck along the anterior border of sternocleidomastoid muscle.

25. **Torus mandibularis is a:** [AIPG 96]
    1. True exostosis
    2. Malignant growth
    3. Irritation fibroma
    4. None of the above

Ans. 1

26. **Oblique facial cleft results from nonfusion of:** [AIPG 96]
    1. Maxillary process and lateral nasal process.
    2. Maxillary process and medial nasal process.
    3. Maxillary and mandibular process.
    4. Midline of mandibular process.

Ans. 1

Maxillary process and medial nasal process - Cleft lip.

Maxillary and mandibular process - Macrostomia.

Midline of mandibular process - Median mandibular cleft.

27. **Amelogenesis imperfecta is associated with:** [AIPG 96]
    1. Enamel hypoplasia

2. Dentinal hypoplasia
3. Calcified pulp chamber
4. None of the above

Ans. **1**

Amelogenesis imperfecta is a hereditary condition associated with defective enamel formation. It can be hypoplastic, hypocalcified or hypomaturation type.

28. Oligodontia means: [AIPG 96]

1. Congenital absence of all teeth.
2. Congenital absence of a few teeth.
3. Presence of peg laterals.
4. Presence of supernumerary teeth.

Ans. **2**

Congenital absence of all teeth - Anodontia

Presence of peg laterals - Microdontia

29. Dentinogenesis imperfecta is: [AIPG 1995]

1. Autosomal dominant
2. Autosomal recessive
3. Sex linked recessive
4. Not a heritable trait

Ans. **1**

Dentinogenesis imperfecta is an autosomal dominant trait. The trait exhibits 100% penetrance but variable extremely both the dentition are affected.

Characteristics

- Blue to brown discoloration with distinctive translucence.
- Enamel frequently separated easily from underlying defective dents.

Radiographically

- Teeth have bulbous crowns, cervical constriction, thin roots, early obliteration of root canal and pulp chambers.

30. Hypoplastic defects in permanent central and lateral incisors are likely to result due to severe illness or other factors during: [AIPG 1995]

1. First nine months of life
2. First two years of life
3. First month of life
4. Two to three years of life

Ans. **1**

Hypoplastic defects in permanent central & lateral incisor are likely to result due to severe illness or other factors during-first year of life.

31. **Differentiation between amelogensis imperfecta and dentinogenesis imperfecta can be made on the basis that dentinogenesis imperfecta:** [AIPG 1995]

    1. Shows dentin dysplasia with rootless teeth
    2. Has short thin root canals with obliterated pulp chamber
    3. Shows delayed eruption
    4. May have complete absence of enamel

Ans. **2**

Features of dentinogenesis imperfecta-

- Enamel loss & dentin undergoes rapid attention.
- Constriction of cervical potion of tooth that imparts a bulbous appearance.
- Partial or complete obliteration of pulp chamber.
- Root canals may be absent or thread like or may be blunted.
- Periapical radiolucency without pulpal involvement & PDL space widening.

Features of amelogenesis imperfecta-

- *Hypoplastic type:* Localized portions of enamel do not reach normal thickness during development
- *Hypocalcified type:* The enamel is so soft that it can be removed by a prophylactic instrument. Enamel is so soft that it can be lost soon after eruption, leaving crown composed of only dentin. Enamel has a cheesy consistency.
- *Hypomaturation type:* The enamel can be pierced by an explorer point under firm pressure and can be lost by chipping away of indulging, normal appearing dentin.

32. **Patient with slanting eyes, protruding tongue, low level of IQ and enamel hypoplasia is probably suffering from:** [AIPG 1995]

    1. Craniofacial dysostosis
    2. Achondroplasia
    3. Down's syndrome
    4. Cleidocranial dysplasia

Ans. **3**

Down syndrome is caused by trisomy of 21st chromosome.

Systemic

- CVS- VSD, PDA, mitral valve prolapse.
- Hematological- increased risk of leukemia, impaired immunodeficiency.
- Musculoskeletal – atlantoaxial instability under developed midface, prognathism, open mouth, tongue-thrusting habit.
- Nervous- motor function is delayed, dementia, distorted phonation.
- Behaviour- gentleness, anxiety, stubbornness

Oral

- V-shaped palate, soft palate insufficiency

- Mouth breathing
- Drooling of saliva
- Macroglossia
- Hypoplasia and hypocalcification of teeth
- Delayed eruption
- Malocclusion
- Bruxism

33. A lesion on patient's tongue is diagnosed as geographic tongue what should be the treatment of choice? [AIPG 1995]

1. Excision of lesion under LA
2. Periodic observation
3. Enucleation of lesion and antibiotics
4. Radiotherapy

Ans. 2

Geographic tongue is associated with psoriasis, juvenile diabetes, pernicious anemia, rhinitis and intrinsic asthma.

Best treatment is periodic assessment of patient.

34. Delayed eruption of teeth occurs in: [AIPG 1995]

1. Craniofacial dyostosis
2. Hyperthyroidism
3. Cleidocranial dysostosis
4. Osteitis deformans

Ans. 3

Delayed eruption of teeth is seen in

- Rickets
- Cretinism
- Cleidocranial dysplasia
- Hypoparathyroidism
- Fibromatosis gingiva.

35. Patient reports with discolored teeth bearing brown stains. The teeth glow fluorescent in UV light. The most likely diagnosis is: [AIPG 1995]

1. Porphyria
2. Amelogenesis imperfecta
3. Hutchinson's teeth
4. Tetracycline staining of teeth

Ans. 4

Discoloration during formation period of tooth can be demonstrated as golden fluorescence in

UV light, which is more intense in dentin than enamel. Rods are more intense towards DEJ. The location of discoloration coincides with the part of tooth developing at the time of administration of tetracycline.

36. **Clinical evidence of dentinogenesis imperfecta is:** [AIPG 94]
    1. Defective enamel and dentine.
    2. Defective dentine and obliterated pulp chamber.
    3. Increased rate of caries.
    4. Oligodontia

Ans. 2

37. **Lingual tonsils arise:** [AIPG 94]
    1. As developmental anomalies.
    2. From carcinomatous transformation.
    3. As a result of hyperplasia.
    4. Due to repeated trauma in the area.

Ans. 1

Lingual tonsils are aggregates of lymphoid tissue present on the dorsum of the posterior part of tongue. It is a developmental anomaly and forms a part of Waldeyer's ring. Sometimes, hyperplasia of these structures may occur.

38. **Which of the following conditions is not hereditary?** [AIPG 92]
    1. Amelogenesis imperfecta
    2. Cleidocranial dysostosis
    3. Regional odontodysplasia
    4. Dentinogenesis imperfecta

Ans. 3

Etiology of regional odontodysplasia is unknown somatic mutation; local vascular defects and viral infection during odontogenesis have been postulated as the possible causes.

39. **Fordyce spots are:** [AIPG 92]
    1. Fat tissues embedded in buccal mucosa
    2. Red spots
    3. Present on cheek mucosa lateral to the angle of mouth
    4. All of the above

Ans. 3

Fordyces spots are embedded sebaceous glands in buccal mucosa, which appears as yellowish white dots.

40. **Dilaceration refers to:** [AIPG 91]
    1. Curvature of the root tip
    2. Cemental union of root

   3. Calcified root canals
   4. Dysplasia of dentin

Ans. 1

Cemental union of root - concrescence

Calcified root canals seen in dentinogenesis imperfecta

41. **A 4-years old child has a normal complement of primary teeth, but they are gray and exhibit extensive occlusal and incisal wear. Radiographic examination indicates some extensive deposits of secondary dentin in these teeth. This condition is:**   **[AIPG 1989]**
   1. Neonatal hypoplasia
   2. Amelogenesis imperfecta
   3. Cleidocranial dysostosis
   4. Dentinogenesis imperfecta

Ans. 4

Neonatal hypoplasia affects the teeth in their developmental stage. Usually a history of fever / antibiotic therapy / exanthematous fever. Localized hypoplasia of teeth is present.

Amelogenesis imperfecta- teeth are yellow brown in color; enamel is thin, contacts between teeth absent. Secondary deposits of dentin usually not seen.

Dentinogenesis imperfecta - obliteration of pulp chambers, root canals, amber like translucency (yellow to blue gray color of teeth) marked attrition.

2 Regressive Alteration of the Teeth

ATTRITION

- Physiological wearing away of the tooth material:
- Usually associated with aging.
- Polished facets on occlusal surfaces.
- Arch length decreases due to proximal attrition.
- Advanced attrition seen in Amelogenesis imperfecta and Dentinogenesis imperfecta.

ABRASION

- Pathological wearing of teeth.
- Usually occurs at exposed root surface of teeth.
- Appears as **V or wedge – shaped ditch** near cementoenamel junction with sharply defined margins.
- Abrasion is more on left side of right-handed persons.
- Associated with use of toothbrush, toothpicks, pipe stems, bobby pins, chewing tobacco biting thread and using dental floss.

EROSION

- Chemical loss of tooth substance without involving bacterial action.
- Shallow, broad, smooth, highly polished, scooped out depression on enamel adjacent to CEJ on labial and buccal surfaces.
- May result in *"ski slope like depression"*
- Caused by citrus juices, gastric acidity, carbonated drinks, anorexia nervosa and industrial workers dealing with acids.
- Erosion from dental exposure to gastric secretions is termed ***perimolysis***.

ABFRACTION

- Refers to loss of tooth structure from repeated tooth flexure caused by occlusal stresses.

DENTAL SCLEROSIS (TRANSPARENT DENTIN)

- Calcification of dentinal tubules due to caries, trauma or aging process.
- Most probable source of calcium salts is fluid in dentinal tubules.
- Leads to decreased conductivity of odontoblastic processes.
- Slows an advancing carious process.
- Sclerotic dentin is more highly calcified than normal dentin.

DEAD TRACTS

- Seen in ground section of teeth and are manifested as a black zone by transmitted light and as a white zone in reflected light.

SECONDARY DENTIN (Irregular or Adventitious Dentin)

- Occurs in response to normal aging process, trauma, caries, attrition etc. It develops when the irritant is mild.
- Tertiary dentin: - Forms with a more intense stimulus.
- Tubules are very irregular, tortuous reduced in number or absent.
- There is decrease in tooth sensitivity.
- Well demarcated from primary dentin by a deeply staining "resting line".

RETICULAR ATROPHY OF PULP

- With aging, there is reticular atrophy and vacuolization of the pulp tissue.
- Usually asymptomatic.

PULP CALCIFICATION

Discrete calcification (Pulp stones / Denticles / Nodules)

(i) *True Denticles*: - Resemble secondary dentin due to their tubular structure.
   - More common in pulp chambers.
(ii) *False Denticles*: - Localized masses of the calcified tissue, do not contain dentinal tubules
   - Made up of concentric layers or lamellae around a nidus.
   - More common is pulp chamber.
(iii) *Free Denticles:* - Lie within the pulp tissue, not attached to the dentinal walls.
(iv) *Attached Denticles*: -Continuous with dentinal walls.
   - More common than free denticles.
(v) *Interstitial Denticle*: - A false denticle eventually may become surrounded by secondary dentin; it is than referred to as Interstitial denticle.

Diffuse Calcification

- More common in root canals.

ROOT RESORPTION

A. **External Resorption** - due to
- Periapical inflammation
- Tumors and cyst
- Reimplantation
- Excessive mechanical or occlusal forces (eg. orthodontic treatment) especially in hypothyroidism
- Impacted teeth
- Idiopathic (maxillary premolars - maximum; mandibular incisors and molars - least)
- Trauma
- Hormonal imbalances

B. **Internal Resorption (pink tooth of mummery)** odontoclastoma / Internal Granuloma / chronic perforating hyperplasia of pulp)
- Idiopathic
- Due to inflammatory hyperplasia of pulp.

HYPERCEMENTOSIS (Cemental hyperplasia)

- Deposition of excessive amounts of secondary cementum on roots.
- Seen in -
    (a) Accelerated elongation of a tooth
    (b) Non functional teeth
    (c) Inflammation about a tooth
    (d) Tooth repair
    (e) Paget's disease or Osteitis deformans (In Paget's disease, there is generalized hypercementosis with loss of lamina dura.

CEMENTICLES

- Small foci of calcified tissue, not necessarily cementum, which lies in the PDL of lateral and apical root areas.
- Formed by calcification of epithelial rests or from focal calcification of connective tissue between Sharpey's bundles with no apparent central nidus or through calcification of thrombosed capillaries in PDL.

NOTES

3 Dental Caries

- Dental caries is a microbial disease of the calcified tissues of the teeth characterized by demineralization of the inorganic portion and dissolution of the organic substance of the teeth.
- Etiology is **multifactorial.**
- Most commonly accepted theories of etiology: -
    1. Acidogenic (Miller's chemico-parasitic theory)
    2. Proteolytic theory
    3. Proteolytic chelation theory – most accepted.

1. Acidogenic theory: W.D. Miller (1882)
- First decalcification of enamel and dentin occurs by lactic acid resulting in destruction of inorganic part. This stage appears as chalky lesion.
- Lysis of organic part by proteolytic enzymes occurs in second phase.
- Role of carbohydrate - carbohydrates, which are rapidly cleared from the oral cavity by saliva and swallowing, are least conducive to caries than those, which are slowly cleared.

$$\text{Sucrose} \longrightarrow \text{most cariogenic.}$$

Role of microorganisms
Streptococcus mutans is the most cariogenic microorganism
- Is aciduric
- Initiates smooth surface caries.

Lactobacillus
- Acidophilic
- Initiates pit and fissure caries
- Found in deep cavities

Actinomyces – Responsible for root surface caries.

Role of Dental plaque
- pH of plaque
  Normal – 7.3 to 7.6

In caries active person - 4.5 to 5.5

- Plaque has a greater buffering capacity than saliva due to proteins and HCO_3^- ions.
- Plaque is essential to hold lactic acid on the tooth surface and adherence of bacteria.
- An important component of dental plaque is acquired pellicle which forms from glycoproteins of saliva and serve as a nutrient for plaque microorganisms.
- Acid is produced in presence of cooked starch and sucrose. There is no acid production with meat, fat and only little with raw starches.
- Polysaccharides are less easily fermented by plaque bacteria than mono and disaccharides.
- Little acid is produced from sugar alcohols, mannitol and sorbitol.
- Filamentous microorganisms, which grow in long interlacing threads, have the property of adhering to smooth enamel surfaces, while smaller bacilli and cocci then become entrapped in this reticular meshwork.
- S. mutans have the ability to metabolize dietary sucrose and synthesize *glucan* by cell-surface and extra cellular glucosyl transferase. This glucose is an insoluble sticky and slimy gel, relatively inert and resistant to bacterial hydrolytic enzymes.
- Dextranase, an enzymes produced by penicillium funiculosum which hydrolyses *dextran (Glucan)* minimizes plaque formation and prevents smooth surface caries.

2. Proteolytic theory- By Gottlieb

- Believed that the organic material (lamellae) of enamel could serve as a pathway for microorganisms, and the acid produced by these bacteria destroys inorganic portion of enamel.
- Gottlieb suggested that yellow pigmentation was characteristic of caries and was due to pigment produced by proteolytic enzymes.
- There may be some softening of dentin even though the overlying enamel appears hard and intact.
- Nasmyth's membrane, mucoproteins yield sulfuric acid on hydrolysis. Also, Gram negative bacteria produce enzyme sulfatase. The liberated acid combines with calcium to form $CaSO_4$. This compound is found only in carious enamel and not in sound enamel.

3) Proteolytic chelation theory – Schwartz

- Chelation is independent of pH of medium, so that removal of calcium ions may occur from tooth even at neutral or alkaline pH.
- Various naturally occurring chelating agents in saliva are –
  - (a) Citrate
  - (b) Amino acids
  - (c) Hydroxy and keto esters
  - (d) Phosphorylated and non-phosphorylated compounds in HMP Pathway.
  - (e) Antibiotics
  - (f) Certain enzymes.
- This theory states that the bacterial attack on the enamel, initiated by keratinolytic microorganisms, consists in a breakdown of protein and other organic components of enamel, chiefly keratin.

This results in formation of substances that forms soluble chelates with inorganic components and thereby decalcifies enamel.

- Both organic and inorganic portions may be attacked simultaneously.
- Increased lactobacillus counts are the result of caries, rather than cause.
- Proteolysis may provide ammonia, which prevents the pH drop that would tend to inhibit growth of the lactobacilli.
- Release of Ca from hydroxyapatite by chelation might encourage the growth of lactobacilli.
- Incorporation of a chelating agent such as EDTA into cariogenic diet results in an increase in severity of dental caries.

CLINICAL ASPECTS OF DENTAL CARIES

1. **Pit and fissure caries**
   - Pit and fissures with high steep walls and narrow bases are most prone to develop caries.
   - Does not depend upon development of plaque.
   - Enamel appears brown or black and will feel slightly soft and "catch" a fine explorer point. Enamel directly bordering the pit or fissure may appear opaque bluish white as it becomes undermined.
   - There may be a large carious lesion with only a tiny point of opening, due to lateral spread of caries at DEJ. *(INTERNAL CARIES)*

2. **Smooth surface caries**
   - Generally proceeded by plaque formation.
   - Proximal caries usually begins just below the contact point and appears in early stage as "incipient lesion".
   - Spread is usually slow.
   - Cervical caries is crescent – shaped, is always an open cavity.

3. **Primary (virgin caries)**

4. **Secondary (recurrent caries)**

5. **Arrested caries** - occurs on smooth surfaces. It is an open cavity; the dentin gets burnished giving brown stained polished appearance and hard *(Eburnated Dentin)*. The progression of caries is stopped.

6. **Incipient caries**

7. **Chronic dental caries**
   - Slow progress, delayed pulp involvement
   - Usually painless
   - Mostly occurs in adults.
   - Undermining is absent
   - Large open cavity.
   - Secondary dentin may be there
   - Deep brown stained dentin

8. **Acute dental caries**
   - Rapid spread
   - Pain present
   - Mostly occurs in children and young adults.
   - Undermining of enamel
   - Pin point exposure
   - No secondary dentin formation
   - Dentin is stained light yellow.

Caries susceptibility

- Bilateral caries > unilateral
- Maxillary arch > mandibular
- Mandibular molars > maxillary molars.
- 1st molars > 2nd molars > maxillary 2nd bicuspid > upper 1st and lower 2nd bicuspid > upper central and lateral incisors > upper cuspids and lower Ist bicuspid > lower central and lateral incisors and lower cuspids.
- Occlusal surface > mesial > distal > buccal > lingual.

HISTOPATHOLOGY OF CARIES

1. **Caries in Enamel** - 4 zones from dentin outwards are

   Zone 1
   - Translucent zone
   - Slightly more porous than enamel
   - Pore volume is 1%
   - Advancing front of the lesion
   - 1 – 2 % demineralization
   - Radio opaque.

   Zone 2
   - Dark zone (Positive zone)
   - 5 – 6 % demineralization
   - Radiolucent
   - Actual demineralization.
   - 2 – 4 % pore volume

   Zone 3
   - Body of Lesion
   - 5 – 25 % pore volume
   - Greatest demineralization (20 – 25 %)
   - Radiolucent

   Zone 4
   - Surface zone
   - 1–10% demineralization
   - Pore volume 5%
   - More resistant to ingress of materials
   - Radio opaque
   - 1st step in smooth surface caries is dental plaque formation (absent in pit & fissure caries)
   - Loss of interprismatic or inter-rod substances of enamel

- Increased prominence of rods and roughening of rod ends
- Appearance of transverse striations of enamel rods, dark lines or bands perpendicular to enamel prisms.
- Accentuation of incremental stria of Retzius.
- Triangular lesion in enamel with base towards DEJ in pit and fissures caries and base towards surface in smooth surface caries.

2. **Caries is dentin**: - 5 zones from pulp outwards to dentin

   Zone 1 - Fatty degeneration of Tome's fibres.

   Zone 2 - Dentinal sclerosis (transparent dentin formation)

   Zone 3 - Decalcification of dentin.

   Zone 4 - Bacterial invasion, intact but decalcified dentin.

   Zone 5 - Decomposed dentin.

   - Sudan red stain is used to see fatty degeneration of Tome's layer.
   - Dentinal sclerosis – seals off dentinal tubules against further penetration.
   - Fatty degeneration also reduces permeability of dentin.
   - In the earliest stages of caries when only few tubules are involved, microorganisms may be found penetrating these tubules before there is any clinical evidence of carious process. (Pioneer bacteria).
   - Acidogenic bacteria predominate in early caries while proteolytic bacteria predominate in deep dental caries.
   - There is decalcification of walls of dentinal tubules leading to their confluence.
   - Increase in diameter of tubules occurs due to packing by bacteria and thickening of sheath of Neumann.
   - Tiny "liquefaction foci" are formed by focal coalescence and breakdown of dentinal tubules.
   - In areas of globular dentin decalcification and confluence of tubules occurs rapidly. So presence of considerable amount of globular dentin accounts for malacotic or soft teeth.
   - Softening of dentin occurs only after proteolysis of organic portion. Clefts are common in this softened dentin, formed at right angle to the dentinal tubules.

3. **Root caries** (Caries of cementum)
   - Filamentous, rather than coccal bacteria are involved.
   - Bacteria invade the cementum either along Sharpey's fibres or between bundles of fibres and spread laterally between the various layers.
   - Decalcification is followed by matrix degradation.
   - Rate of caries progression in root dentin is slower because of fewer tubules.

RADIOGRAPHIC FEATURES OF DENTAL CARIES

- Radiographs cannot reveal whether the lesion is active or arrested.
- Bitewing radiographs are needed for detection of proximal carious lesions.
- Proximal caries appears as a triangular lesion, notch, a dot, a band or a thin line.

- The fact that the lesion does not start below the gingival margin helps distinguishing a carious lesion from cervical burnout.
- Lesions confined to enamel may not be evident radiographically until approximately 30-40% demineralization has occurred.
- *Mach band phenomenon* - an optical illusion that occurs when there is a sharply defined density difference, such as enamel and dentin. In such cases a radiolucent lesion may appear immediately adjacent to the enamel.
- Bucccal or lingual lesions appear as a radiolucent lesion surrounded by a uniform radiopacity.
- Some radiolucent restorative materials like composite, plastic, silicate and calcium hydroxide may resemble a carious lesion.
- High contrast or short gray scale is needed in the radiograph for caries detection

ALTERNATIVE DIAGNOSTIC TOOLS FOR CARIES DETECTION

- Light Fluoroscence
- Digital subtraction radiography
- Diagnodent laser light
- Fiberoptic transillumination
- Electrical conductance measurements
- Ultrasound

CONTRIBUTING FACTORS IN DENTAL CARIES

- Surface enamel is more resistant to demineralization because it is highly mineralized.
- Malposed and hypoplastic teeth are more prone to caries.
- Ca and P contents of saliva are low in caries active person.
- Ammonia content of saliva is high in caries active state.
- Thick viscosity saliva in caries active state.
- Antibacterial factors in saliva reduce caries activity.
- Buffers in saliva neutralize the acid.
- Plaque acts as barrier to buffer ions.
- Ca and P metabolic disturbances, vitamin A, D deficiency and rickets – alter tooth structure, which predisposes to caries.
- Vitamin B deficiency – may have anticaries effect because vitamin – B is essential for growth and metabolisms of oral bacteria.
- Vitamin B_6 – anticaries action
- Vitamin C – No association with caries
- F, vanadium – Decrease caries
- Selenium – Increase caries.

METHODS OF CARIES CONTROL

1. **Chemical measures**

A. Substances, which alter the tooth surface or structure – F, chlorhexidine, alexidine, bisguanide, $AgNO_3$, $ZnCl_2$, Potassium ferrocyanide.

B. Substances, which interfere with carbohydrate metabolism
   - Vitamin k
   - Sarcosides like sodium N– lauryl sarcosinate, sodium dehydroacetate

C. Substances, which interfere with bacterial growth and metabolism – Urea, Ammonium compounds.

2. **Nutritional measures**
   - Restrict frequency of sugar intake
   - Avoid soft, sticky foods
   - Phosphated diet resists caries. (Sodium dihydrophosphate)

3. **Mechanical measures**
   - Brushing
   - Mouth rinsing
   - Fluoride mouthwashes
   - Flossing
   - Detergent foods
   - Pit and fissures sealants
   - Prophylactic odontomy.

QUESTIONS

1. **Cavity formation in a tooth, due to dental caries is due to -**   [AIPG 2005]
   1. Destructive potential of streptococcus mutans.
   2. Destructive potential of lactobacillus acidophilus.
   3. Lateral spread of caries along dentinoenamel junction and weakening of the overlying enamel.
   4. Masticatory force and unrelated to the extent of carious process.

Ans.   3

Caries progress from pit and fissure towards DEJ as a triangle with its apex towards the occlusal surface, following the direction of enamel rods. Once the caries reaches DEJ, due to decreased mineral content, there is lateral spread of caries, which undermines the enamel and cause cavitation.

2. **The extracellular polysaccharides synthesized by cariogenic streptococci in the presence of excess sucrose are best described as:**   [AIPG 2003]
   1. Amylase
   2. Amylopectin
   3. Mucopolysaccharide
   4. Dextran-like glucan

Ans.   4

3. **Oral foci of Miller's are seen in: [AIPG 94]**

   1. Dental caries
   2. Lichen planus
   3. Herpes simplex
   4. Syphilis

Ans. `1`

4. **If content of ammonia is increased in saliva it results in:** [AIPG 92]

   1. Increase in calculus formation
   2. Decrease in plaque formation
   3. Increase in plaque formation
   4. Increase in gingivitis

Ans. `2`

Increase in ammonia content of saliva leads to buffering action, which prevents plaque formation and dental caries.

5. **Caries activity is more in persons suffering with:** [AIPG 1990]

   1. Xerostomia
   2. Parkinsonism
   3. Downs syndrome
   4. All of the above

Ans. `4`

   1. Lack of protective effect of saliva
   2. Due to lack of manual dexterity
   3. Due to mental retardation and poor oral hygiene

6. **Caries activity can be expected to increase in the mouth of:** [AIPG 1990]

   1. Pregnant ladies
   2. Patient with xerostomia
   3. Lactating mothers
   4. None of the above

Ans. `2`

4 Diseases of Pulp and Periapical Tissues

Anatomic features, which alter the nature and course of inflammation in pulp, are –
- Pulp tissue lies enclosed in dental hard tissues, which preclude the excessive swelling.
- Fact that the blood vessels supplying the pulp enter through apical foramina, precludes the development of extensive collateral blood supply.

Etiological factors for pulpal pathosis
- (a) Bacterial invasion
    - Dental caries
    - Trauma
    - Anachoresis
- (b) Chemical irritation
- (c) Thermal injury
- (d) Mechanical injury
- Anachoretic pulpitis - pulpitis due to entry of bacteria at site of pulpal inflammation through blood stream.
- Aerodontalgia - Seen after decompression or ascent to high altitudes, in recently filled teeth.

CLASSIFICATION

I. (a) Acute pulpitis
   (b) Chronic pulpitis

II. (a) Partial pulpitis (focal)
    (b) Subtotal pulpitis
    (c) Total pulpitis (Generalized)

III. (a) Open pulpitis (pulpits aperta)
     (b) Closed pulpitis (pulpits clausa)

IV. (a) Reversible pulpitis
    (b) Irreversible pulpitis

FOCAL REVERSIBLE PULPITIS (PULP HYPEREMIA)

- Mild, transient pulpitis.
- Localized to pulpal ends of irritated dentinal tubules.
- Pain disappears on removal of irritant.
- Sensitive to thermal changes particularly cold.
- Responds to electric pulp tester at a lower level of current.
- "Self - strangulation" of pulp can occur due to increased arterial pressure, occluding the vein at apical foramen.

ACUTE PULPITIS

- Immediate sequela of focal reversible pulpitis or an acute exacerbation of chronic pulpits.
- Severe pain elicited by thermal changes and persists even after removal of stimulus.
- Pain is continuous throbbing type and increases on lying down.
- Intrapulpal abscess may be formed especially when opening of cavity is small.
- Pressure of pulp increases due to lack of escape of inflammatory exudates and leads to liquifaction necrosis of pulp. This is called acute suppurative pulpitis.
- Responds to electric pulp tester at lower threshold.

CHRONIC PULPITIS

- May develop directly or through quiescence of a previous acute pulpitis.
- No thermal sensitivity is seen.
- 2 forms – open and closed.
- Pain is often absent, even though the pulp may be exposed.
- Threshold for stimulation by electric pulp tester is increased.
- Histology shows chronic inflammatory cells and tissue reaction may resemble granulation tissue. When this occurs on the surface of pulp tissue in a wide – open exposure, it is called "Ulcerative pulpitis".

CHRONIC HYPERPLASTIC PULPITIS (PULP POLYP)

- An excessive, exuberant proliferation of chronically inflamed pulp.
- Seen almost exclusively in children and young adults.
- Pinkish - red globule of tissue protruding from pulp chamber, relative insensitive to manipulation because it contains fewer nerves.
- Teeth most commonly involved by this phenomenon are the deciduous molars and first permanent molars because they have an excellent blood supply and large root opening.

GANGRENOUS NECROSIS OF PULP (PULP GANGRENE)

- Refers to necrosis of pulp tissue due to ischaemia with superimposed bacterial infection.
- It is a most complete end result of pulpitis, in which there is total necrosis of tissue.

- A type of gangrene known as "Dry Gangrene" sometimes occurs when the pulp dies for some unexplained reason.

INTERRELATIONSHIPS OF PERIAPICAL INFECTIONS

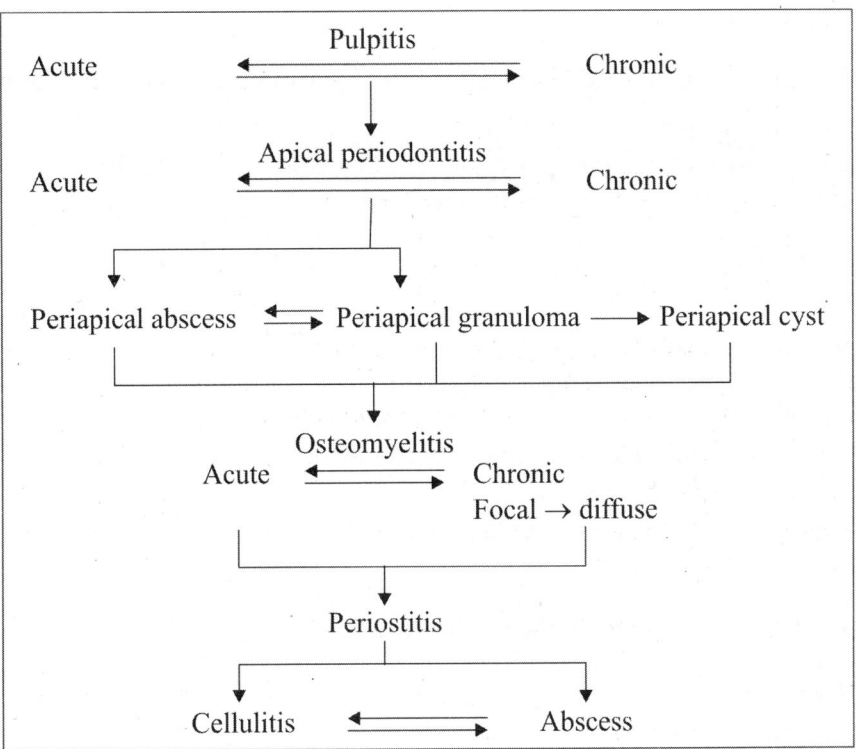

PERIAPICAL GRANULOMA

- 1st evidence is a noticeable sensitivity of the involved tooth to percussion or mild pain on chewing or biting.
- Tooth may feel slightly elongated in its socket.
- The earliest periapical change appears as thickening of PDL at root apex on radiograph. Later on, it appears as a well delineated lucency of size less than 1 cm.
- Histology shows predominantly macrophages, lymphocytes and plasma cells (*IMMUNE – TYPE GRANULOMA)*
- Many plasma cells contain **Russell bodies.**
- Bone and tooth resorption due to periapical granuloma may be related to T-Cell activity through the production of osteoclasts activating factor (OAF).
- In some granulomas, large number of phagocytes with ingested lipid (*FOAM CELLS*) is seen.
- Abundant mast cells.
- Cholesterol crystals (appear as clear needle like spaces or clefts.)

- Giant cell hyaline angiopathy – A condition consisting of inflammatory cell infiltration, foreign-body giant cells and ring-like structures composed of eosinophillic material resembling hyalinized collagen.
- *"Pulse- Granuloma"* term used when fragments of foreign material sometimes resembling legumes are seen.

APICAL PERIODONTAL CYST (Radicular cyst / Periapical cyst / Root end cyst)

- Common sequela of periapical granuloma.
- Epithelial lining is derived from rests of Malassez, respiratory epithelium of maxillary sinus, oral epithelium of fistulous tract or periodontal pocket.
- Mostly asymptomatic, only seldom sensitive to percussion.
- Radiographically, it is seen as well - delineated radiolucency usually > 1cm in size, exhibits a thin radiopaque border.
- Hyalin body (*Rushton body*) is found in histopathology of majority of cysts. These are tiny linear or arc–shaped bodies, amorphous, eosinophilic, and brittle. They are thought to arise from thrombus formation in capillaries (*Rouleau phenomenon*).
- Cholesterol slits with multinucleated giant cells are seen in wall of lesion.
- Lumen contains pale, eosinophilic fluid.
- **Residual cyst** – may develop if epithelial remnants remain after cyst enucleation or if a periapical granuloma is incompletely removed.

PERIAPICAL ABSCESS (Dento – alveolar abscess)

Acute abscess

- Tooth is extremely painful.
- Slightly extruded from socket.
- Regional lymphadenitis & fever may be associated.
- *No radiographic findings* except for slight thickening of PDL.

Chronic Abscess

- Asymptomatic
- May present as diffuse ill-defined periapical radiolucency.

OSTEOMYELITIS

- An inflammation of bone and bone marrow.
- 3 forms -Acute, Subacute, Chronic.

Acute suppurative osteomyelitis

- Causative organisms - Staphylococcus aureus, S.albus, various streptococci and sometime mixed organisms.
- Disease is usually fairly well localized in maxilla, while more diffuse and widespread in mandible.

- Severe pain, hyperthermia, lymphadenopathy, increased TLC.
- Little radiographic evidence initially. After 1-2 weeks, diffuse lytic changes may be visible **(Moth - eaten appearance).** There is an ill defined radiolucency, sequestra may be present.
- Histology shows mainly PMN'S, loss of viability of trabeculae and their resorption.

Chronic suppurative osteomyelitis

- Signs and symptoms are milder.
- Acute exacerbation of the chronic stage may occur periodically.
- Suppuration may perforate the bone and overlying skin or mucosa to form a fistula.
- Radiographically, the periphery of the lesion is better defined than in acute stage, dense radiopaque sequestra are usually present, surrounded by an involucrum.
- CT scan is the imaging modality of choice.
- Scintigraphy using bone scans, gallium or labeled WBC is not particularly helpful for differential diagnosis.
- Two phase nuclear medicine study composed of a technitium bone scan followed by a gallium citrate scan may help to confirm the diagnosis.

Chronic focal sclerosing osteomyelitis (condensing osteitis)

- Reaction of bone to infection seen in cases of low-grade infection and high tissue resistance.
- Almost exclusively in young persons (< 20 yrs).
- Most commonly involved tooth is mandibular first molar.
- On radiograph, it appears as a well- circumscribed radiopaque mass of sclerotic bone surrounding the root apex. The entire root outline is always visible (which is absent in cementoblastoma)
- "Bone scar"- Residual chronic focal sclerosing osteomyelitis after extraction of tooth.
- No surgical treatment is required for the radiopaque mass unless symptomatic.

Chronic diffuse sclerosing osteomyelitis (CDSO)

- More common in older age, especially edentulous mandibles.
- More in blacks.
- More common in females.
- Radiopaque diffuse sclerosis of bone is seen, sometime bilateral. May mimic *"cotton wool appearance"* of Paget's disease.
- Histological picture shows *"mosaic pattern"* indicative of repeated periods of resorption followed by repair. In some cases, the inflammatory component is completely "burned out" leaving only sclerotic bone fibrosis.
- Treatment is difficult. Usually conservative approach is taken.
- If a tooth is present in the sclerotic bone, it is surgically extracted, removing a liberal amount of bone and inducing fresh bleeding.

Sclerotic cemental masses (SCM)

- Usually in older black females.
- Similar to chronic diffuse sclerosing osteomyelitis except on histopathology, the tissue is cementum.

Florid osseous dysplasia (FOD)

- Closely related to CDSO and SCM.
- An additional feature is simultaneous occurence of simple bone *"cysts"*.

Chronic osteomyelitis with proliferative periostitis (Garre's osteomyelitis, chronic non-suppurative sclerosing osteitis, Periostitis ossificans)

- Focal gross thickening of periosteum with peripheral reactive bone formation, due to mild infection.
- Seen almost entirely in young persons (< 25 years).
- Predilection for long bones and mandible.
- Toothache, bony hard swelling on outer surface of jaw.
- Occlusal view shows a focal overgrowth of bone on the outer surface of the cortex, which may be described as a duplication of the cortical layer of bone.
- *Sequestrum* - separated fragment of dead bone seen in suppurative osteomyelitis, when the intensity of disease becomes attenuated. It is exfoliated spontaneously or may require surgical removal. It is more radiopaque than living bone.
- *Involucrum* – The new bone formed around sequestrum.
- Paraesthesia is often a feature of osteomyelitis in mandible.
- Pathological fracture can occur occasionally.

QUESTIONS

1. **Radiographically latent period of an acute periapical abscess is:** [AIPG 2004]
   1. 7-10 days
   2. 10-15 days
   3 2-5 days
   4. 3-7 days

Ans. **1**

There is no radiographic finding in the first 7 days. After this period apical PDL space widening can be seen. After 1-2 weeks, diffuse lytic changes may be visible.

2. **A patient feels that his molar is extruded from the socket and is tender to percussion. This can be due to:** [AIPG 2001]
   1. Periapical cyst
   2. Periapical granuloma

3. Periapical abscess

4. Furcation involvement

Ans. **3**

Tooth is extruded due to pressure exerted by the abscess in periapical region. In case of cyst and granuloma, the tooth may be tender to percussion, but it is not extruded. In case of periodontal involvement, tenderness on lateral percussion occurs.

3. **A non-vital asymptomatic tooth with a deep carious lesion shows radiopacity at the apex is possibly:** [AIPG 99]

1. Cementoma

2. Condensing osteitis

3. Periapical cyst

4. Periodontitis

Ans. **2**

Ill-defined radiopacity is usually seen at the apex of grossly carious teeth in young patients and when the infection is low grade. Mostly involves incisors and first molars. Cementoma occurs as a radiolucent, mixed or opaque lesion associated with vital teeth. Periapical cyst and periodontitis presents as radiolucent lesions.

4. **Diagnostic test commonly used to determine the status of vitality of pulp is:** [AIPG 1995]

1. Radiography

2. Thermal testing

3. Computerized axial tomography scanning

4. Percussion and palpation

Ans. **2**

Diagnostic tests commonly used to determine the status of vitality of pulp are-

• Electric pulp testing

• Thermal testing

• Heat testing

• Cold testing.

5. **On a radiograph internal resorption first appears as:** [AIPG 1995]

1. Dense radio-opaque shadow

2. Widening of periodontal space

3. Shortening of root at apical region

4. Increase in radiolucency of pulp chamber or canal

Ans. **4**

Internal resorption has the following radiographic features-

- Lesion is radiolucent, round, oval or elongated within the rods with widening of pulp chamber of canals.

- Margin of enlarged chamber are sharp and clearly defined.

6. Radiographic examination of permanent first molar with an early acute pulpal abscess in a 9-year-old child would reveal: [AIPG 91]

1. Involvement of the bifurcation
2. Little change from normal structure
3. A large area of periapical bone rarefaction
4. A disturbance in the integrity of the periodontal ligament

Ans. **2**

An early acute pulpal abscess usually has no radiographic manifestations. In some cases apical PDL space widening may be evident.

7. Periapical cyst is usually preceded by: [AIPG 1990]

1. Periapical granuloma
2. Periodontal abscess
3. Periapical abscess
4. All of the above

Ans. **1**

In response to inflammation in granuloma, epithelial proliferation begins which give rise to a cyst.

8. Reversible pulpitis changes to irreversible pulpitis primarily because of: [AIPG 1989]

1. Vascular strangulation
2. Reduced host resistance
3. Invasion of microorganisms
4. An increase in microbial virulence

Ans. **1**

Invasion of microorganisms reduced host resistance and increased microbial virulence increases the chances of periapical infection. But irreversible pulpitis is mainly due to strangulation of pulp.

Infections

BACTERIAL INFECTIONS

Disease (synonyms)	Etiology	Features
SCARLET FEVER	β - Hemolytic streptococci-erythrogenic toxin (scarlatina)	• Usually seen in children • Diffuse, bright scarlet skin rash in skin folds, due to toxic injury to vascular endothelium. • *"Stomatitis scarlatina"* mucosa is fiery red congested, particularly palate. • *"Strawberry Tongue"*- early stage, hyperemic papilla. • *"Raspberry tongue"* when coating in lost • Complication - peritonsillar abscess, rhinitis sinusitis, otitis media, mastoiditis, meningitis, rheumatic fever.
DIPHTHERIA	Corynebacterium diphtheriae (klebs loeffler bacillus) -gram-positive bacillus.	• Droplet infection • Usually in children • Involves upper respiratory tract. • *"Bull's neck"* • *"Diphtheritic membrane"* a pseudo-membrane, grayish thick, fibrinous exudate overlying necrotic, ulcerated areas of mucosa, tonsils, pharynx and larynx. It is adhesive and tends to leave a bleeding surface if stripped away. • Temporary paralysis of soft palate. • Nasal twang and nasal regurgitation. Complication – myocarditis, polyneuritis

Disease (synonyms)	Etiology	Features
TUBERCULOSIS	Acid-fast bacillus Mycobacterium tuberculosis Rarely, M. bovis.	• *Miliary T.B* microorganism may become disseminated by either blood stream or lymphatics to involve many organs like kidney, liver. • *Scrofula* - Tuberculous lymphadenitis of sub maxillary and cervical lymph nodes. • *Lupus vulgaris* – primary T.B. of skin. • Oral lesions are usually secondary to pulmonary infection. • Most common intra oral site is tongue followed by palate, lips, buccal mucosa, gingiva and frenulae. • Irregular, painful ulcer slowly increases in size. • Jaws affected by anachoretic effect or direct entry through open pulp chambers, cause periapical granuloma or tuberculoma. • Tuberculous osteomyelitis frequently occurs in late stages of disease and has unfavorable prognosis. • Histologic picture shows *caseous necrosis* surrounded by epitheloid cells, lymphocytes and multinucleated giant cells, AFB.
SARCOIDOSIS (Boeck's Sarcoid, Besnier-Boeck Schaumann disease)	-Etiology unknown -Multisystem granulomatous disease	• Depression of delayed type of hypersensitivity (CMI). • Oral lesions may resemble *"fever blisters"* or diffuse bone destruction. • Histology same as T.B except caseation necrosis and AFB are absent. • *Kveim – Siltzback Test* is diagnostic test for sarcoidosis.
UVEOPAROTID FEVER (Heerfordt's syndrome)	A form of sarcoidosis	• Firm painless, bilateral parotid enlargement and occasionally, sub maxillary and lacrimal glands are also involved. • Eye lesions • Unilateral / Bilateral 7th nerve paralysis.
LEPROSY (Hensen's disease)	Mycobacterium leprae (AFB)	• Tuberculoid and lepromatous types with 3 intermediate types. • Tuberculoid type – macular, erythematous lesions with dermal and peripheral nerve involvement.

Disease (synonyms)	Etiology	Features
		• Lepromatous – macules or papules leading to progressive thickening of skin and characteristic nodules may produce severe disfigurement • Facial paralysis may occur • Oral lesions consist of tumor like masses called lepromas on tongue, lips and palate. • Gingival hyperplasia with loosening of teeth. • Histologic picture – vacuolated macrophages called *"LEPRA CELLS"* containing bacilli
ACTINOMYCOSIS	A. israeli, A. naeslundi. Anaerobic gram positive, non-AFB. Chronic suppurative, granulomatous and fibrosing diseases.	• 3 form - (a) cervicofacial –most common. (b) Abdominal (c) Pulmonary • Formation of extra oral draining sinuses. Pus collected from sinus shows typical *"sulfur granu.es"* or tiny yellow grains which are colonies of organism. • Endogenous, opportunistic infection. • May cause osteomyelitis if bone of maxilla is invaded. • Periapical granulomas *"Ray – fungus"* Hematoxylin stained central colonies with eosinophilia of the peripheral club - shaped ends of filament.
BOTROMYCOSIS (Actinobacillosis, actinophytosis)	Staphylococcus, streptococcus, Escherichia and actinobacillus	• Granulomatous infection with multiple ulcers and sinuses, resembling actinomycosis. • *No "ray-fungus"* seen on histology.
TULAREMIA (rabbit fever)	Pasteurella tularensis (Gram negative bacilli)	• Several forms identified – cutaneous, ophthalmic pleuropulmonary, oral and abdominal. • Severe painful necrotic ulcers of oral mucosa and pharynx • Generalized stomatitis. • Lymphadenitis in sub maxillary and cervical lymph nodes.
TETANUS ('lock jaw')	Clostridium tetani (exotoxin)	• Disease of central nervous system characterized by intense activity of motor neurons and severe muscle spasm. • Incubation period- 14 days. • Pain and stiffness of jaws and neck muscles producing trismus and dysphagia. • *"Risus sardonicus"-* Rigidity of facial muscles.

Disease (synonyms)	Etiology	Features
		• *"Opisthotonus"*- whole body is involved.
		• *"Cephalic tetanus"*- either localized or generalized occurring in association with cranial nerve palsy (mainly 7th nerve)
SYPHILIS (Lues)	Treponema pallidum spirochaete	• Can be Acquired or congenital.
		• Congenital (prenatal) syphilis :-
		- Lesions similar to acquired secondary stage disease may be seen in neonates.
		- Frontal bossing of Parrot.
		- Olympian brow.
		- Sabre tibia, radius and ulna.
		- Cluttton's joints.
		- Hypoplastic maxilla and relative protuberance of mandible.
		- Saddle nose
		- High arched palate.
		- *Higoumenakis's sign* – irregular thickening of sterno clavicular portion of clavicle.
		- Rhagades - *Hutchinson triad* (hypoplasia of incisors and molars, eight nerve deafness and interstitial keratitis) screw -driver shaped incisors, mulberry molars / moon's / Fournier's molar.
		- Neurosyphilis may lead to convulsions, blindness and cranial nerve palsies.
	* Hexscheimer Reaction- After vigorous antibiotic use may cause palatal perforation	Acquired form
		(a) **Primary stage:** - Incubation period 3 weeks.
		• *Chancre*, which occurs mainly on genitalia.
		• May occur on oral mucosa and fresh extracts wound, as painful ulcers.
		• Highly infectious, positive serologic reaction.
		• Unilateral lymphadenopathy, non tender, rubbery nodes (buboes or shotty nodes).
		(b) **Secondary stage:** - (Metastatic stage)
		• Commences 6 weeks after 1° lesion
		• Oral lesions are *"mucous patches"*, occurs as multiple, painless, grayish – white plaque covered ulcers.
		• Generalized hematogenous spread of infection occurs.

Disease (synonyms)	Etiology	Features
		• **Coin like** circinate lesions on face.
		• Condyloma lata.
		• **Snail track** ulcers.
		• Pruritic syphilitic rash.
		• **"Split pea"** papules.
		• Laryngeal involvement.
		• Highly infectious, positive serological reactive.
		(c) **Tertiary stage** (late syphilis)
		• Non-infectious occurs several years later.
		• **"Gumma"**, mostly involving tongue and palate.
		• Palatal perforation may occur.
		• Stenosis of nasopharyngeal airway.
		• **Saddle nose** deformity.
		• Most common than primary and secondary lesions.
		• *Atrophic or interstitial glossitis or leutic glossitis* – may develop carcinomatous change.
		• Neurosyphilis is characterized by tabes dorsalis, *positive Romberg sign*, paraesthesias of extremities, Tabetic crisis, charcot's joint, *Argyll Robertson pupil*, personality changes.
GRANULOMA INGUINALE (Denovanosis Granuloma Venerum)	Denovania granulomatis or calymmatobacterium Granulomatis	• Primary lesions on external genitalia as granular lesions, pseudobulo (fluctuant swelling) and ulcers.
		• Oral lesions occurs secondary to genital lesions.
		• Presence of Denovan bodies in tissue from lesions.
		• 3 types of oral lesions
		- Ulcerative
		- Exuberant
		- Cicatricial Fibrous scars on cheek or lip may restrict oral opening.
RHINOSCLEROMA	Klebsiella spp.	• Proliferating nasal masses *"HEBRA NOSE"*.
		• Oral proliferating granulomas.
		• Anaesthesia of soft palate and enlargement of uvula.

Disease (synonyms)	Etiology	Features
MIDLINE LETHAL GRANULOMA (Malignant granuloma)	Unknown Etiology.	• Begins as superficial ulceration of palate or nasal septum, ultimately leading to progressive necrosis and sequestration of palatal, nasal and malar bones. • Hemorrhage occurs if blood vessels are eroded. • Diagnosis is mainly by exclusion of other conditions. • High dose radiotherapy is treatment of choice.
WEGENER'S GRANULOMATOSIS	Etiology unknown	• Involves vascular, renal and respiratory systems. • Intra orally, gingiva is the most common site. Oral lesions may be ulcerations, friable granular lesions or gingival enlargement. • Cyclophosphamide is treatment of choice. • *"Strawberry gingivitis"*
CHRONIC GRANULOMATOUS DISEASE	- Enteric bacilli and certain fungi - Defects of intracellular leukocyte enzyme functions, decreased oxidative metabolism, failure to destroy catalase positive micro organisms	• Oral lesions may be present as diffuse stomatitis or multiple ulcerations. • Histology shows small granulomas. • Diagnosis is established by neutrophil functions tests - the impairment of invitro microbicidal activity and failure of reduction of *nitro blue tetrazolium (NBT test).*
NOMA (Cancrum Oris, Gangrenous stomatitis)	Vincent's Organisms and complicated by other bacteria	• Usually begins as a small ulcer of gingival mucosa, which rapidly spreads and involves the surrounding tissue of jaws, lips and cheeks by gangrenous necrosis. • Predisposing factors include – malnutrition, infection other systemic diseases.
PYOGENIC GRANULOMA	- Non specific micro organism invading tissues - saprophytic organisms - Sulfahydryl radical is most essential stimulating agent.	• Overzealous proliferation of a vascular type of connective tissue. • Commonest site is gingiva. • Pus formation is not a characteristic finding inspite of the name. • Intravenous pyogenic granuloma - occurs on neck and upper extremities. • *"Pregnancy tumor"*- A Lesion histologically similar to pyogenic granuloma, occurs in pregnancy.

Disease (synonyms)	Etiology	Features
PYOSTOMATITIS VEGETANS		• Associated with Crohn's disease. • Oral lesions consists of large number of broad based papillary projections, tiny abscesses or vegetations. • *"Cobble stone"* appearance of oral mucosa • Refractory to antibiotic therapy.

VIRAL INFECTIONS

Condition	Etiology	Features
1. Herpes Simplex 2. Recurrent Herpes 3. Herpetic Whitlow 4. Recurrent Aphthae 5. Behcet's Disease 6. Herpengina 7. Acute Lymphonodular Pharyngitis 8. Hand Foot Mouth Disease 9. Chicken Pox 10. Herpes Zoster		*See Vesiculobullous And Ulcerative Lesions*
11. MEASLES (Rubeola, Morbilli)	Paramyxo virus	• Primarily affects children. • Occurs in epidemic form. • Incubation period 8 – 10 days. • Skin lesion begin on face, in hairline, behind the ears. • Blanch on pressure. • Oral lesions – *"Koplik's spots"* which usually occur on buccal mucosa. Bluish white specks surrounded by a bright red margin. • Palatal and pharyngeal petichae, ulceration, congestion. • Complications – pneumonia, encephalitis, otitis media. • Impaired CMI
12. RUBELLA (German measles)	Myxo virus	• "koplik spots" do not occurs. • Oral mucosa is not inflamed. • Infection during 1st trimester of pregnancy can lead to congenital defects such as

		blindness, deafness, cardio vascular abnormalities or miscarriage.
13. SMALL POX (Variola)	Pox virus	• Totally eliminated disease now. • Oral lesions reported are ulcers and vesicles.
14. MOLLUSCUM CONTAGIOSUM	Virus & pox group	• Nodules on eyelids, arms, legs, trunk and face. • Oral lesions are uncommon. • Histology shows large eosinophilic inclusion bodies – *Handerson – paterson inclusion or molluscum bodies.*
15. CONDYLOMA ACUMINATUM (Venereal wart)	– HPV group.Oral lesions by HPV – 6	• Small multiple nodules which coalesce and form papillomatous, bulbous masses scattered over tongue, buccal mucosa. palate, gingiva. • Intranuclear viral inclusions may be seen in the lesional epithelial cells. • Treatment – topical podophyllin.
16. CAT – SCRATCH DISEASE (Benign lymphoreticulosis)	Viral origin	• Lymphadenopathy. • *Oculoglandular syndrome of Parinaud* – localized granuloma of eye and preauricular lymphadenopathy • Self - limiting disease
17. CYTOMEGALIC INCLUSION DISEASE (Salivary gland virus Disease)	CMV	• Cause fetal encephalitis and CNS damage. • Transplacental infection may occur. • Most common cause of mental retardation. • Intranuclear and cytoplasmic inclusions in cells of salivary glands are constant features.
18. REITER'S SYNDROME	PPLO	• Typical *tetrad* of manifestations Urethritis Arthritis (usually bilaterally symmetrical polyarticular), Conjunctivitis and Muco cutaneous lesions

FUNGAL DISEASE

1. NORTH AMERICAN BLASTOMYCOSIS (Gilchrist's Disease)	Blastomyces dermatitidis	• Granulomatous Infection • Oral lesions may resemble Actinomycosis, although abscess formation is not usually prominent. • Resembles squamous cell CA.
2. SOUTH AMERICAN BLASTOMYCOSIS (lutz's disease paracoccidiomycosis)	B. Brasiliensis	• Organism may enter the body through periodontal tissues and subsequently reaches lymph nodes . • Can cause widespread oral ulcers.

		• Has been isolated from periodontal ligament and periapical granuloma.
		• Histopathology shows **"Pilots wheel"** or **"Micky mouse"** cells.
3. HISTOPLASMOSIS (darling's disease)	Histoplasma capsulations	• Specific predilection for the reticuloendothelial system.
		• Ulcerative, nodular and vegetative oral lesions.
		• Organism is usually seen intracellularly in phagocytes.
4. COCCIDIOIDO MYCOSIS (Valley fever, san Joaquin valley fever)	Coccidioides immitis	• 2 forms – Non disseminated and progressive disseminated.
		• Proliferative granulomatous and ulcerative lesions.
		• Lytic lesions of jaw are common.
		• Organisms are found in cytoplasm of giant cells.
5. CYPTOCOCCOSIS (Torulosis, European Blastomycosis)	C. bacillispora	• Opportunistic infection.
		• Skin, meninges and lungs are commonly involved.
		• Oral lesions occur as non specific ulcers.
		• Histology – *"Tissue microcyst"* - small organism with a large clear halo.
6. CANDIDIASIS (Candidosis, Moniliasis, thrush)	Candid alliance C tropicalis, C parapsiloes, C stellaloidea, C krusei.	• Most common opportunistic infection in world.
		• Occurs as mucocutaneous and systemic form. Pulmonary and gastrointestinal lesions may also occur.
		• *Acute pseudomembranous oral candidiasis* = thrush
		• *Acute atrophic candidiasis* = Antibiotic sore mouth
		• *Chronic atrophic candidiasis* = Denture sore mouth
		• *Chronic hyperplastic type* = "leukoplakia" type of Candidiasis
		• Histologically, sections are stained with PAS or methenamine silver.
		• *Id Reaction* of skin is often seen.
7. GEOTRICHOSIS	Geotrichum spp.	• Most commonly involves lungs and oral mucosa.
		• Oral lesions are identical to thrush.
8. PHYCOMYCOSIS	Phycomycetis rhizopus / mucor / absidia.	• Most frequently seen as a secondary occurrence in cancer patients.

		• Immunocompromised patients are more prone, especially diabetics. • 2 forms – Superficial, Visceral (Pulmonary Gastro intestinal Rhino cerebral). • Infections of head are characterized by the classical syndrome & uncontrolled diabetes, cellulitis, opthalmoplegia and meningioencephalitis. • Early clinical manifestation is reddish-black nasal turbinate and septum with nasal discharge. • Apparent predeliction for blood vessels.
9. SPOROTRICHOSIS	Sporotrichum schenckii	• Skin lesions *"Chancres"* at site of inoculation. • Non specific ulceration of oral, nasal and pharyngeal mucosa. • Histology shows chronic granulomatous lesion and pseudoepitheliomatous hyperplasia of overlying epithelium.
10. TINEA BARBAE (ringworm of the beard)	Trichophyton rubrum	• Inflammatory lesions involving beard, hair and skin of chin. • Rarely, vermilion border of lips may be involved.

QUESTIONS

1. **The best laboratory test to use in the diagnosis of Lupus vulgaris in the oral cavity is -** [AIPG 2005]

   1. Bacterial smear.
   2. Blood studies.
   3. Biopsy.
   4. Blood chemistry.

Ans. **3**

2. **In patients infected with HIV will have -** [AIPG 2005]
   1. Elevated blastogenesis.
   2. Depressed serum globulin levels.
   3. High T4-T8 ratio.
   4. Thrombocytopenia.

Ans. **4**

Due to decreased production of all blood cells.

3. **The time gap between appearance of Koplik's spot and cutaneous rash in measles is:**

   [AIPG 2004]

   1. 24 hrs
   2. 3-4 days
   3. 2 weeks
   4. 10 days

Ans. **2**

Usually Koplik's spots appear 2-3 days before cutaneous rashes. They are irregularly shaped flecks on buccal mucosa, which appear as bluish, white specks surrounded by a bright red margin.

4. **Which of the following medications shortens the recovery period of primary herpetic gingivostomatitis?** [AIPG 2004]

   1. Acyclovir
   2. Ziduvidine
   3. Kenalog in orabase
   4. All of the above

Ans. **1**

Acyclovir is drug of choice for herpes viral infection.

5. **In which of the following location there is collection of pus in the quinsy?** [AIPG 2004]

   1. Peritonsillar space
   2. Parapharyngeal space
   3. Retropharyngeal space
   4. Within the tonsil.

Ans. **1**

6. **Mulberry molars are characteristic features of:** [AIPG 2004]

   1. Severe fluorosis.
   2. Trauma at the time of birth.
   3. Congenital syphilis.
   4. Due to chronic suppurative abscess in over-lying gingival tissue

Ans. **3**

Congenital syphilis is marked by mulberry molar and screw shaped incisor.

7. **Which of the following features is not associated with acute osteomyelitis of mandible?** [AIPG 2004]

   1. Severe pain
   2. Purulent exudate
   3. Paraesthesia of lower lip
   4. Radiographic evidence of bone destruction

Ans. 4

That is seen with chronic osteomyelitis.

8. **Which of the following is true in case of AIDS patient?** [AIPG 2004]
   1. Acute pain
   2. Diffuse red lesion of the attached gingiva
   3. Gingiva covered with pseudomembrane
   4. Gingival itching

Ans. 2

9. **The organism that most commonly causes infective endocarditis is:** [AIPG 2003]
   1. Streptococcus mitis
   2. Staphylococcus aureus
   3. Streptococcus viridans
   4. Staphylococcus pyogenes

Ans. 3

10. **The most common complication of mumps is:** [AIPG 2003]
    1. Myocarditis
    2. Orchitis
    3. Uveitis
    4. Conjunctivitis

Ans. 2

Other complications include ovaries, pancreas, mammary gland, prostate, epididymis and heart. Meningoencephalitis, deafness and mastitis can also occur.

11. **Acute osteomyelitis is most frequently caused by which of the following microorganisms?** [AIPG 2003]
    1. Gonococcus
    2. Enterococcus
    3. Streptococcus
    4. Staphylococcus

Ans. 3

12. **The oral lesion of syphilis that is highly infective is a:** [AIPG 2003]
    1. Gumma
    2. Mucous path
    3. Koplik's spot
    4. Tabes dorsalis

Ans. 2

Secondary stage of syphilis most infectious.

13. **A high titer of serum heterophile antibodies is found in patients with -** [AIPG 2003]
    1. Herpangina
    2. Hepatitis A
    3. Actinomycosis
    4. Infectious mononucleosis

Ans. **4**

It can rise up to 1: 1049

14. **All the following are caused by EB virus except:** [AIPG 2002]
    1. Glandular fever
    2. Measles
    3. Burkitt's lymphoma
    4. Nasopharyngeal carcinoma

Ans. **2**

Measles is caused by paramyxovirus.

15. **A 23-year-old female complains of decreased mouth opening of 4 days duration. She is probably suffering from:** [AIPG 2002]

    1. Impacted lower third molar with pericoronitis
    2. Oral submucous fibrosis
    3. Oral candidiasis
    4. Bony ankylosis of the TMJ.

Ans. **1**

Pericoronitis in relation to impacted third molar is the most common cause of trismus in 18-25 years of age.

16. **All of the following are potential pathogens of oropharynx except:** [AIPG 2001]
    1. Streptococcus pneumoniae
    2. N. meningitidis
    3. E. coli
    4. Influenzae

Ans. **3**

E coli is a normal commensal of intestine.

17. **Incubation of period of mumps is:** [AIPG 2001]
    1. 1-5 days
    2. 7-10 days
    3. 14-21 days
    4. 3-6 weeks

Ans. 3

18. **Monospot test is used to diagnose:** [AIPG 2001]
    1. Pernicious anemia
    2. Sickle cell anemia
    3. Infectious mononucleosis
    4. Leukemia

Ans. 3

19. **Condensing osteitis is:** [AIPG 2000]
    1. Formed by proliferation of epithelial rests in the dental granuloma
    2. Area of hypercementosis within the intact lamina dura
    3. Osteosclerosis
    4. Circumscribed proliferation of peripheral bone due to mild irritation.

Ans. 4

It is usually seen in young individual with good immune defense and chronic low-grade infection

Choice 1 – Radicular cyst

Choice 2 – Cementablastoma

20. **Infection with which of the following has the greatest incidence of congenital malformations:** [AIPG 2000]
    1. Herpes zoster
    2. Herpes simplex
    3. Rubella
    4. Toxoplasma.

Ans. 3

Rubella usually affects the fetus during first trimester of pregnancy. The offspring has a high incidence of congenital defects.

21. **A patient with severe mycotic infection of the head and neck with a triad of uncontrolled diabetes, orbital infection and meningoencephalitis is suffering from:** [AIPG 2000]
    1. Candidiasis
    2. Mucormycosis
    3. Histoplasmosis
    4. Coccoidiomycosis.

Ans. 2

Mucormycosis or phycomycosis is the most common fungal infection in uncontrolled diabetes with rhinocerebral involvement.

22. **The commonest cause of a tender swelling in the submandibular triangle:** [AIPG 2000]
    1. Lipoma

2. Branchial cleft cyst
3. Lymphadenopathy
4. Obstruction of Stensen's duct.

Ans. **3**

Submandibular lymph nodes are commonly enlarged and become tender in odontogenic infections.

23. **Mycosis fungoides is a proliferation of:** [AIPG 99]
    1. Cutaneous T cells
    2. Cutaneous B cells
    3. Fungal hyphae
    4. All of the above

Ans. **1**

24. **Early manifestation of a patient infected with HIV virus is:** [AIPG 99]
    1. Elevation of p16
    2. Unexplained fever and weight loss
    3. Kaposi's sarcoma
    4. Hairy cell leukoplakia

Ans. **2**

Oral hairy leukoplakia is one of the indicator for conversion of HIV infection to AIDS.

25. **The most radiosensitive tumor is:** [AIPG 99]
    1. Ewing's sarcoma
    2. Osteosarcoma
    3. Lymphoma
    4. Seminoma

Ans. **3**

Sarcomas are radioresistant. Usually surgery is the treatment of choice. Lymphomas are most radiosensitive. They are usually treated by combination of radiotherapy and chemotherapy.

26. **A debilitated patient on oral penicillin has white lesions that can be stripped away from a tongue, leaving a raw surface. The patient probably has:** [AIPG 98]
    1. Candidiasis
    2. Lichen planus
    3. Histoplasmosis
    4. Mucosal dysplasia

Ans. **1**

Candidial infection is usually seen in immunocompromised patients, who are on prolonged antibiotic therapy. It appears as a curdy which scrapable white lesions, which leaves behind a raw bleeding surface.

27. Clinical diagnosis of candidiasis is confirmed by: [AIPG 98]
1. Characteristic odor
2. Response to injection of vitamin B_{12}
3. Response to administration of prednisolone
4. Demonstration of mycelia and spores in scrapings

Ans. 4

Cytological smears are made from the scrapings of oral lesions, which are fixed in KOH to demonstrate fungal hyphae and spores.

28. The usual incubation period for hepatitis B virus infection is: [AIPG 97]
1. 1-2 days
2. 1-2 weeks
3. 1-6 months
4. 1 year

Ans. 3

29. All of the following are features of tuberculosis of tongue except: [AIPG 96]
1. Giant cells are present
2. Presence of epitheloid cell
3. Presence of caseous necrosis
4. Presence of hyaline degeneration

Ans. 4

Tuberculosis of tongue shows granuloma formation, which consists of central area of caseation necrosis, surrounded by epitheloid cells and giant cells.

30. 'Risus sardonicus' is associated with: [AIPG 96]
1. Tetany
2. Lock jaw of tetanus
3. Grand mal epilepsy
4. Poliomyelitis

Ans. 2

Due to spasm of facial muscles, the patient acquires rigid facial expression, which is described as 'risus sardonicus'.

31. A child with a fever of 102°C and vesicles in the oral cavity is probably suffering from: [AIPG 96]
1. Herpes simplex type I
2. Juvenile periodontitis
3. Acute herpetic gingivostomatitis
4. Neutropenia

Ans. 3

32. **Cold abscess is related to:** [AIPG 96]
    1. Periapical pathology
    2. Mycobacterium tuberculae
    3. Streptococcus viridans
    4. None of the above

Ans. **2**

Cold abscesses are seen in tuberculous lymph nodes. It is so called because there are no signs of inflammation associated with it.

33. **Mumps is caused by:** [AIPG 96]
    1. Orthomyxo virus
    2. Paramyxo virus
    3. Rhino virus
    4. EB virus

Ans. **2**

34. **Drugs which cause ototoxicity and circumoral paraesthesia are:** [AIPG 96]
    1. Antileprotic drugs
    2. Antitubercular drugs
    3. Streptomycin
    4. Chloramphenicol

Ans. **3**

35. **The Epstein-Barr Virus (EBV) has been linked to:** [AIPG 1995]
    1. Breast cancer
    2. Prostate cancer
    3. Burkitt's lymphoma
    4. Leukemia

Ans. **3**

Epstein barr virus (EBV) is associated with
- Oral hairy leukoplakia (in AIDS patients)
- Infections mononucleosis/kissing's disease lymphomas like Africans Burkett's lymphoma
- Nasopharyngeal carcinomas
- Gastric carcinomas
- Some smooth muscle tumors.

36. **Other clinical signs and symptoms for AIDS related complex are:** [AIPG 1995]
    1. Diarrhoea
    2. Fatigue
    3. Night sweats
    4. All of the above

Ans. 4

Clinical course of HIV infection is divided into various groups:

1. Acute HIV infection – low-grade fever, lymphodenopathy malaise, headache, arthropathy, acute encephalopathy.
2. Asymptomatic or latent infection.
3. Persistent generalized lymphadenopathy.
4. AIDS related complex (ARC) – fatigue, unexplained fever persistent diarrhea, weight loss (more than 10% of body weight), opportunistic infections- oral candidiasis, herpes zoster, hairy cell leukoplakia, TB, salmonellosis.
5. AIDS- Dry cough, dyspnea, fever.

   Infections- P carinci, M tuberculosis, M. avinus intracellular, CMV, cryptococcus, histoplasma

   CNS- toxoplamosis, cryptococcosis.

   Malignances – Kaposi's sarcoma, NHL and HL.

37. **Laboratory studies in AIDS patient show all of the following except:** [AIPG 1995]
    1. Thrombocytopenia
    2. Increased serum globulin levels
    3. Increased hemoglobin levels
    4. Cutaneous allergy to skin tests

Ans. 3

Laboratory studies in AIDS patients show –

- Total leucocyte and lymphocyte count to demonstrate leukopenia & lymphocyte count below 2000 mm$^{3.}$
- T cell subset always- absolute CD4 + T cell count less than 200 mm^3 .
  T4:T8 ratio is reversed.
- Platelet count will show thrombocytopenia.
- Raised IgG & IgA level.
- Diminished CMI as indicated by skin tests.
- Lymph node biopsy showing profound abnormalities .

38. **Patient suffered from rubella during the first trimester of pregnancy. What are the likely effects on the child?** [AIPG 1995]
    1. Congenital heart disease or defects
    2. Encephalitis
    3. Saddle nose with frontal bossing
    4. Most likely the child may be normal

Ans. 1

Commonest malformations caused by rubella are cardiac defect, cataract of deafness which constitute the clinical congenital rubella syndrome. Several other features have been recognized in babies with congenital rubella. Hepatosplenomegaly, thromocytopenic purpura, myocarditis, bone lesions constituting the 'expanded rubella syndrome'.

39. **Oral prodromal symptoms are seen in:** [AIPG 1995]

    1. Rubella
    2. Rubeola
    3. Congenital syphilis
    4. Down's syndrome

Ans. 2

The oral lesions in measles are prodromal frequently occurring two to three days before cutaneous rash. These inter- oral lesions are called Koplik's spots. These characteristic spots, occurring on buccal mucosa are small irregularly shaped flecks, which appear as bluish, white specks surrounded by a bright red margin.

40. **Oral manifestations of infectious mononucleosis are most commonly:** [AIPG 1995]

    1. Bluish red spots opposite maxillary molar
    2. Pseudomembrane on gingiva
    3. Pinpoint petechiae on the palate
    4. Gingival hyperplasia

Ans. 3

Oral Manifestations of infections mononucleosis are:-
- Acute gingivitis & stomatitis
- Oral ulcers
- Palatal petechiae.

The disease is caused by EB virus (Epstein - Barr) and is characterized by fever, sore throat, headache, chills, cough, nausea, vomiting, lymphadenopathy, splenomegaly, hepatitis.

41. **Lupus vulgaris is associated with:** [AIPG 94]

    1. Tuberculosis of skin
    2. Ulcerations of oral mucosa
    3. White streaks on buccal mucosa
    4. Butterfly rash over bridge of nose

Ans. 1

White streaks are a feature of reticular lichen planus. Butterfly rash over the bridge of nose is seen in lupus erythematosus.

42. **Langerhan's giant cells are seen in:** [AIPG 94]

    1. Diabetes mellitus
    2. Diabetes insipidus
    3. Tuberculosis
    4. Candidiasis

Ans. 3

Langerhan's grant cells are multinucleated giant cells seen in tuberculous granuloma.

43. **A lesion in cervicofacial area has multiple abscesses and draining sinuses the lesion most likely is:** [AIPG 94]
    1. Parotitis
    2. Actinomycosis
    3. Gas gangrene
    4. Periodontal abscess

Ans. 2

The abscess collected from these sinuses shows yellowish granules due to presence of sulfur.

44. **Leutic glossitis is a condition associated with:** [AIPG 94]
    1. Pernicious anemia
    2. Treponema pallidum
    3. Tuberculosis
    4. Corynebacterium diphtheriae

Ans. 2

Leutic glossitis or interstitial glossitis is seen in tertiary stage of syphilis. It is more predisposed to development of cancer.

45. **Chancre is a:** [AIPG 93]
    1. Primary stage of syphilis
    2. Develops at site of inoculation
    3. Contains microorganisms
    4. All of the above

Ans. 4

46. **Recurrent herpes occurs due to:** [AIPG 93]
    1. Virus in oral mucosa
    2. Latent virus in skin supplying the area
    3. Latent virus in nerve ganglia
    4. None of the above

Ans. 3

Herpes virus remains latent in nerve ganglia and reactivated during immunosupression to cause recurrent infection.

47. **Spread of odontogenic infection into the lymphatic chain of the neck is detected by:** [AIPG 92]
    1. Angiography
    2. Laminography

3. Hematologic examination

4. Palpation of the cervical region

Ans. ■4

Angiography is used for detection of vascular lesions. Laminagraphy is a body section radiographic technique accomplished by moving the X-ray source and film in parallel planes and at predetermine angle to film surface. (Tomography)

48. Koplik's spots on the buccal mucosa are pathognomic for: [AIPG 92]

1. Rubella

2. Rubeola

3. Roseola

4. Varicella

Ans. 2

Koplik's spots are seen in measles or rubeola. They are yellowish white lesion with bluish halo seen during the prodromal phase, on bilateral buccal mucosa.

49. Oral lesions are found early in: [AIPG 92]

1. AIDS

2. Syphilis

3. Tuberculosis

4. Chronic alcoholism

Ans. 3

Oral lesions are found in early stages of tuberculosis in form of ulcer or osteomyelitis.

Initial symptoms in AIDS are related to gastrointestinal disturbances.

In syphilis, oral lesions are usually seen in secondary stage.

50. Oral tuberculosis lesions are most commonly found on the: [AIPG 92]

1. Soft palate

2. Hard palate

3. Gingiva

4. Tongue

Ans. ■4

Most common site for tuberculosis lesions in oral cavity is dorsum of tongue followed by gingiva and palate.

51. The coagulation time of blood is a diagnosis of: [AIPG 91]

1. Hemophilia

2. Leukemia

3. Pernicious anemia

4. Malignant neutropenia

Ans. 1

52. Which of the following antibiotics is effective in treating oral candidiasis? [AIPG 91]

1. Nystatin
2. Bacitracin
3. Penicillin
4. Tetracycline

Ans. **1**

Nystatin is the drug of choice for treatment of oral candidiasis. It is an antifungal agent. Others are antibacterial agents.

53. The reason why most patients suffering from recurrent herpes labialis rarely give a history of having acute form of the herpetic gingivostomatitis is because: [AIPG 91]

1. Aetiological agents differ.
2. The acute form occurs only in severely immunocompromised individuals.
3. The primary infection was subclinical.
4. The patient has received antibodies during intrauterine life and the antibodies have persisted.

Ans. **3**

54. The first clinical manifestations of herpes simplex virus infection are usually: [AIPG 1990]

1. Perleche
2. Gingivostomatitis
3. Keratoconjuctivitis
4. Involvement of the genital tract

Ans. **2**

Usually seen in 1-5 years of age.

55. Oral hairy leukoplakia may be classified as a: [AIPG 1990]

1. Viral infection
2. Bacterial infection
3. Fungal infection
4. Neoplasm

Ans. **1**

Seen in HIV positive patient on lateral border of tongue.

56. Which of the following lesions may create gingival deformities that require gingivoplasty to eliminate gingival defects? [AIPG 1990]

1. Erosive lichen planus
2. Desquamative gingivitis
3. Acute herpetic gingivostomatitis
4. Necrotizing ulcerative gingivitis

Ans. 4

Punched out lesions are formed in interdental papilla leaving hollowed out margins.

57. Sulfur granules are of diagnostic value in suspected cases of: [AIPG 1989]

1. Histoplasmosis
2. Actinomycosis
3. Lead sulfide tissue deposits
4. Scrofula

Ans. 2

Histoplasmosis - primary infection is mild, self-limiting, pulmonary disease that heals to leave fibrosis & calcification. Oral lesion occurs as a papule, nodule, ulcer or vegetation. The ulcer slowly enlarges. Cervical lymph nodes are enlarged & firm.

Biopsy shows small oval yeasts within macrophages.

Scrofula - tuberculosis infection of the lymph nodes.

58. A 30 years old patient presents with an asymptomatic, doughy, soft 2 cm swelling of the lateral neck, which has been present for months. The swelling recently enlarged as a result of an upper respiratory infection. The most likely diagnosis is: [AIPG 1989]

1. Scrofula
2. Hodgkin's disease
3. Cat scratch fever
4. Cervicofacial actinomycosis

Ans. 4

Cervicofacial actinomycosis - one of the characteristics of actinomycosis is lack of immediate tissue reaction after implantation of organ. It requires 6 weeks or longer for an actinomycotic swelling to break down. The adjacent tissues have a hard, doughy consistency.

Cat-scratch fever: - shows reactive lymphadenitis. H/O cat scratch- if the inflammation extends beyond the lymph nodes from cervical region to the eye it is known as Parinaud's syndrome.

59. The initial lesion of syphilis is a: [AIPG 1989]

1. Bubo
2. Gumma
3. Chancre
4. Pustule

Ans. 3

Chancre – Initial lesion in primary syphilis

Gumma-tertiary syphilis

Bubo- secondary syphilis

NOTES

6 Spread of Oral Infection

Spread of oral infection depends upon:

- Type of organism
- Physical state of the patient
- Anatomic features like thickness of cortex, muscle attachment, proximity to the tissue spaces.

CELLULITIS (Phlegmon)

- Acute diffuse inflammation of soft tissues that spreads along fascial planes and through tissue spaces.
- Cellulitis is usually seen with microorganisms that produce significant amounts of hyaluronidase (the spreading factor of Duran-Reynaulds) and fibrinolysins.
- Streptococci are common causative organisms.

SPREAD OF PERIAPICAL INFECTIONS

Tooth	Location of apex	Region of spread
1. Maxillary central Incisor	- Above orbicularis oris and dense subcutaneous tissue	- Oral vestibule
2. Maxillary lateral incisor	- Above orbicularis oris (labially located apex) - Above orbicularis oris (palatally located apex)	- Oral vestibule - Palate
3. Maxillary canine	- Above levator anguli oris - Below levator anguli oris	- Oral vestibule - Canine space
4. Maxillary premolar	- Above zygomaticus major and lavator labii superiors (Buccal root) - Palatal root	- Oral vestibule - Palate
5. Maxillary molars	- Buccal root apex above buccinator muscle - Buccal root apex below buccinator muscle - Palatal root	- Oral vestibule - Buccal space - Palate

Tooth	Location of apex	Region of spread
6. Mandibular central incisors and lateral Incisors	- Above mentalis muscle - Below mentalis muscle	- Oral vestibule - Submental space
7. Mandibular canine	- Below depressor labii inferioris, depressor anguli oris	- Oral vestibule
8. Mandibular premolars	- Below depressor labii inferioris, depressor anguli oris	- Oral vestibule
9. Mandibular 1st molars	- Below buccinator muscle (buccally) - Above buccinator muscle (buccally) - Lingually	- Oral vestibule - Buccal space - Sublingual space
10. Mandibular 2nd molar	- Below buccinator muscle (buccally) - Above buccinator muscle (buccally) - Below myelohyoid muscle (Lingually) - Above myelohyoid muscle (lingually)	- Oral vestibule - Buccal space - Sub mandibular space - Sub lingual space.
11. Mandibular 3rd molar	- Above myelohyoid	- Submandibular or pterygomandibular space.

LUDWIG'S ANGINA

- A severe cellulitis beginning usually in submaxillary space and secondarily involving sublingual and submental spaces as well.
- Manifests as board- like swelling of floor of mouth, elevation of tongue, edema of glottis may also occur.
- Cavernous sinus thrombosis and subsequent meningitis may be a sequela.

CAVERNOUS SINUS THROMBOSIS (Thrombophlebitis)

- Most common intracranial complication of dental infection.
- Infection from face and lip is carried by facial and angular veins, while dental infection from maxilla is carried by pterygoid plexus.
- Presents as exophthalmos with edema of lids and chemosis, paralysis of external ocular muscles, impaired vision, photophobia, and lacrimation.

FOCAL INFECTION

- Focus of Infection – refers to a circumscribed area of tissue which is infected with exogenous pathogenic microorganism and which is usually located near a mucous or cutaneous surface.
- Focal infection - refers to the metastasis from the focus of infection, of organism or their toxins that are capable of injuring tissue.

Disturbances in Metabolism

MINERAL METABOLISM

Mineral	Normal levels	Daily Requirements	Clinical features
Calcium	9 - 11 mg/dl • Phytic acid and oxalic acid interferes with calcium absorption • Vitamin D, citrates enhance absorption	• 300 mg in infants • 800 mg in children & adults • 1200 mg in pregnancy and Lactation	• Deficiency can cause hyperirritability, tetany, laryngospasm, convulsions, carpopedal spasm • >11 mg % - depressed nerve conductivity, muscle rigors. • Bone demineralization.
Phosphorus	2 – 4 mg / dl	• 240 mg in infants • 800 mg in adults	• Deficiency can occur due to long-term antacid use. It is characterized by weakness, malaise, anorexia and bone pain. • Bone demineralization.
Magnesium	1 – 3 mg / dl	• 50 mg in infants • 400 mg in adults	• Hypomagnesaemia due to magnesium containing antacids, results in CNS depression and severe voluntary muscle paralysis. • Deficiency causes neuromuscular and vascular disturbances, enamel hypoplasia. • Carpopedal spasm • Hypomagnesaemia and hypocalcaemia have identical effects on the parathyroid glands. • Magnesium – deficiency tetany - semi coma severe neuromuscular hyperirritability positive chvostek's sign, athetoid movements, marked susceptibility to auditory, visuals and mechanical stimuli.

Mineral	Normal levels	Daily Requirements	Clinical features
Sodium	160 mg %	0.5 gm	• Deficiency usually occurs in Addison's disease. • Characterized by weakness, fatigue, lassitude, apathy, anorexia, nausea, muscle cramps, peripheral vascular collapse.
Potassium	4 meq/ litre of plasma	2 – 4 gm	• Death in potassium deficiency may result from cardiac or respiratory failure or from paralytic ileus.
Chlorine	550– 650 mg %	6 – 9 gm	• Activates salivary amylase. • Deficiency can cause hyper excitability and convulsions.
Iodine		Traces	• Levels of Iodine are increased in hyperthyroidism and decreased in hypothyroidism.
Copper		Traces	• Deficiency leads to anaemia. • *Wilson's disease* (Hepato-lenticular degeneration). • *Menke's syndrome (steely or kinky hair syndrome).*
Iron		Traces	• *"One – way substance"* since little excretion occurs. • Deficiency leads to anaemia and *Plummer – Vinson syndrome.* • Iron overload - Hemochromatosis, Bantu's siderosis, Sideroblastic anaemia, Thalassemia.
Zinc		Traces	• Deficiency causes - Acrodermatitis enteropathica (diarrhea, mucocutaneous vesicles, eczema, alopecia, stomatitis, glossitis. • Taste disturbances • Keratogenesis • Disturbances in bone growth and wound healing.
Cobalt		Traces	• Constituents of vitamin B_{12}, used for treatment of pernicious anaemia.
Chromium		Traces	• Role in carbohydrate and lipid metabolism. • Potentiates action of insulin by forming Chromium Bridge.
Selenium		Traces	• Eliminates harmful peroxides and free radicals.

DISEASES OF VITAMIN METABOLISM

VITAMIN A

- Vitamin A has a role in vision, lysosomal stability and epithelial differentiation.

Deficiency

- Causes night blindness, xeropthalmia, keratomalacia.
- Hyperkeratosis of oral epithelium in adults.
- Disturbance in tooth formation (enamel and dentin).
- Retarded eruption rate.
- Alveolar bone is retarded.

Hyper vitaminosis A:

- Pronounced periosteal thickening.

VITAMIN D

- *Hypo vitaminosis D* - Causes 2° Hyperparathyroidism. Increased PTH level increase serum calcium at expense of bone, serum phosphorus decreases, and alkaline phosphatase increases.
- *Vitamin Deficient Rickets* - In children
  - Hypomineralized bone matrix
  - Craniotabes.
  - Swelling of wrists and ankles.
  - Failure of endochondral calcification
  - Increase in width of epiphyseal disk
  - Bowing of legs
  - Developmental abnormalities of enamel and dentin
  - Cortical structures of mandible may be thinned.
  - Delayed eruption
  - Malocclusion
- *Osteomalacia (Adult Rickets)*
  - Only flat bones and diaphyses of long bones are affected.
  - Most commonly seen in postmenopausal females.
  - Severe periodontitis (?)
  - Severe asymmetric deformities of all stress bearing bones.
  - Longitudinal hairline fractures are seen in the long bones.
  - Bone pain.
  - Peculiar waddling or penguin gait, tetany and greenstick fractures.
- *Vitamin D – Resistant Rickets*
  (Refractory Rickets; Familial hypophosphataemia)

- Hypophosphataemia
- Hyperphosphaturia
- Rickets or osteomalacia, which does not respond to the usual doses of vitamin D
- Normocalcaemia
- Short stature
- Normal vitamin D metabolism
- Absence of other related abnormalities
- Skull deformities
- "Sitting" deformity of legs
- Retarded eruption of teeth
- Elongated pulp horns
- Lamina dura is absent
- Abnormal cementum and alveolar bone.
- 10,000 to 25,000 I.U. per day of vitamin D along with oral phosphate is given.

• *Renal Rickets (Renal Osteodystrophy)*
- Negative calcium balance.
- Hyperphosphatemia.
- Secondary hyperparathyroidism.
- Superimposed osteitis fibrosis cystica.
- Softening and bowing of bones and frequent fractures.

• *Hypophosphatasia (Hypophosphatasemia)*
- Deficiency of alkaline phosphatase.
- Excretion of phospho-ethanol-amine in urine.
- Premature closure of skull sutures leading to gyral or convolutional markings, resembling hammered skull.
- Loosening and premature loss of deciduous teeth, chiefly incisors.
- Generalized radiolucency of maxilla and mandible.
- Rachitic rosary
- Three Forms: - 1. Infantile - lethal   2. Childhood   3. Adult
- Metaphyses of long bones show "spotty", "streaky" or "irregular ossification".
- Hypocalcified teeth, enlarged pulp chamber, loss of alveolar bone.
- Absence of cementum due to failure of cementogenesis.

VITAMIN E

• Deficiency causes decreased male fertility, impaired fetal – maternal vascular relationship, nutritional muscular dystrophy, encephalomalacia, and hemolysis.
• Degenerative changes in enamel organ.
• Anti oxidant effect on polyunsaturated fatty acids.

VITAMIN K

- Involved in both extrinsic and intrinsic systems of coagulation, particularly factor II synthesis.
- Secondary hypo vitaminosis K in adults is associated with impaired fat absorption, obstructive jaundice, sprue, and ulcerative colitis.
- Common oral findings are gingival bleeding. Spontaneous hemorrhages occur when prothrombin levels fall below 20 %.

VITAMIN C

- Vitamin C is necessary for hydrogen ion transfers, maintenance of intracellular oxidation-reduction potentials, as an antioxidant, facilitates Fe uptake and helps in formation of folinic acid.
- Needed for normal developments of intercellular ground substances in bone, dentin and other connective tissues.
- Deficiency causes **SCURVY.**
  - Swelling of marginal and inter dental gingiva.
  - Violaceous red color of gingiva.
  - Gingival enlargement may cover clinical crowns of the teeth.
  - Foul breath.
  - Fusospirochetal stomatitis
  - Hemorrhage and swelling of PDL.
  - Loss of bone, loosening of teeth.
  - Delayed healing due to failure of fibroblasts to form collagen.
- *Scorbutic lattice*: - Wide zone of calcified but non- ossified matrix in metaphysis due to failure of osteoblasts to form osteoid. These spicules are non resistant to weight – bearing and motion stresses and therefore liable to fracture.
- *Trummerfeld zone*: - As the "lattice" increases in size and fracture of spicules occur a region of complete disintegration is formed. This represents the classical picture of scurvy. Area beneath this zone is free of hematopoietic cells and made up of connective tissue cells, the so-called Geriistmark.
- There is atrophy and disorganization of odontoblasts, irregular dentin is formed and predentin becomes hyper calcified.

VITAMIN B – COMPLEX

(a) Thiamine Deficiency

  - **Beriberi-** this in characterized by multiple neuritis, often associated with congestive heart failure, generalized edema.
  - No oral lesions.

(b) Riboflavin (Vitamin B$_2$)

- It fluoresces green under UV illumination.

- Glossitis + dermatitis + ocular changes.
- Mild deficiency - glossitis, beginning at tip of tongue, atrophy of filliform papillae, fungiform papillae becomes mushroom shaped, giving a coarse, granular appearance, tongue has magenta color.
- Paleness of lips, especially at angles of mouth, followed by cheilosis.
- Scaly, greasy dermatitis of nasolabial folds and alae nasi.

(c) NIACIN

- Deficiency causes Pellagra.
- Mucous membrane lesions affect the tongue, oral cavity and vagina.
- Bilaterally symmetrical, sharply outlined dermal lesion.
- Mental symptoms and weight loss also occurs.
- Fiery red oral mucosa that is painful.
- Sialorrhea.
- Epithelium of entire tongue desquamates.
- ANUG may be a sequel.

(d) Pantothenic Acid

- Usually no evidence of deficiency is there in humans.

(e) Pyridoxine (vitamin B$_6$)

- Deficiency causes mental depression, mental confusion, albuminuria and leukopenia.
- Oral lesions are similar to pellagrous stomatitis.

(f) Choline

- No Oral lesions.

(g) Biotin

- Biotin deficiency causes scaly, greasy dermatitis and eventual alopecia.

(h) Folic acid Deficiency

- Macrocytic anaemia, sprue Addisonian (pernicious) anemia.
- Diarrhoea
- Glossitis - *fiery red* smooth tongue.
- Aminopterin therapy (for leukaemia) interferes with conversion of folic acid to folinic acid. So administration of folic acid in aminopterin toxicity reverses glossitis.

(i) Vitamine B$_{12}$ (cyanocobalamine)

- High doses are used for treatment of trigeminal neuralgia (> 1000 meq / day).
- Deficiency can cause pernicious anaemia and burning of mucosa.

DISEASES OF HORMONE METABOLISM

I. PITUITARY HORMONES

- Pituitary gland is made up of 2 lobes – anterior and posterior.
- Anterior lobe - epithelial origin, derived from Rathke's pouch.
- Posterior lobe – Nervous tissue, derived from floor of 3rd ventricle.
- Hormones of anterior pituitary
  - Somatotrophin
  - Thyrotrophin
  - Adrenocorticotrophin
  - Gonadotrophin
  - Lactogenin
  - In addition, it has ketogenic, anti-insulin, diabetogenic, parathyrogenic, pancreatotropic activity.
- Posterior lobe has vasoconstrictive, oxytocic and antidiuretic effects.
- **HYPOPITUITARISM-** Decreased levels of pituitary hormones (Mainly growth hormones and thyrotrophic hormone influences oral structures).
  - Retardation of tooth eruption and delayed exfoliation of teeth.
  - Thickening of dentinal walls at expense of pulp chambers.
  - Disturbances in amelogenesis.
  - Retarded dentino and cementogenesis.
  - *DWARFISM* in children but well proportioned body, fine, silky, sparse hair, and hypogonadism.
  - Small dental arches and malocclusion.
  - *SIMMOND'S DISEASE* in adults – no specific dental changes.
- **HYPERPITUITARISM**
  - *GIGANTISM* in infants, *ACROMEGALY* in adults.
  - Teeth in gigantism are proportional to the size of the jaws and the rest of the body. The roots may be longer than normal.
  - Hypercementosis and supraeruption of teeth.
  - Lips are thick and negroid.
  - Tongue is enlarged with crenations on lateral border.
  - Mandibular prognathism.
  - Ballooning of Sella turcica.
  - Enlargement of paranasal sinuses.
  - Diffuse thickening of outer table of skull.

II. THYROID HORMONES

- Thyroid hormone causes increased uptake of O_2 by body and controls many physiological functions.

- Calcitonin, secreted by "C" cells is responsive to hypercalcaemia and acts to lower the plasma calcium levels.

HYPOTHYROIDISM: *Cretinism* in infants and *myxoedema* in adults.

- *Cretinism*
  - Shortening of base of skull and numerous wormian bones.
  - Delayed closure of epiphyses.
  - Retraction of bridge of nose with flaring.
  - Overdeveloped maxilla and underdeveloped mandible.
  - Delayed eruption of teeth.
  - Over retained deciduous teeth.

- *Myxoedema*
  - Lips, nose, eyelids and suborbital tissue are edematous.
  - Enlarged tongue.
  - Periodontal disease and loss of teeth.
  - Spacing in jaws.
  - External root resorption.

HYPERTHYROIDISM

- Exopthalmic goiter and toxic adenoma .
- Alveolar atrophy.
- Premature exfoliation of primary teeth.
- Accelerated eruption of permanent teeth.
- Generalized decrease in bone density.
- Wide staring eyes.
- Sensitivity to epinephrine.

III. PARATHYROID HORMONE

- **PRIMARY HYPERPARATHYROIDISM**
  - Renal calculi, peptic ulcers, psychiatric problems or bone pains.
  - Pathological fracture may be the first symptom.
  - " *Giant cell tumor*" or " *cyst*" of jaws.
  - *"Osteitis fibrosa cystica / generalisata"*.
  - Generalized osteoporosis.
  - Malocclusion due to drifting of teeth.
  - *"Brown's tumor"*.
  - *"Ground Glass appearance"* of bone.
  - Loss of lamina dura.
  - Most reliable changes are subtle erosion of bone from subperiosteal surfaces of phalanges of hands.

- Pathological calcification of soft tissues.
- *"Pepper pot"* skull.
- Histology shows osteoclastic resorption of trabeculae of spongiosa.
- Serum Ca level is increased.
- **SECONDARY HYPERPARATHYROIDISM** (Von Recklinghausen's disease of bones)
    - Due to end – stage renal disease.
    - "Brown's tumor" is common finding .
    - Loss of lamina dura.
    - Serum alkaline phosphatase is increased.
- **HYPOPARATHYROIDISM**
    - Hypocalcaemia leading to tetany (carpopedal spasm).
    - Paraesthesia of hands, feet and around the mouth.
    - Neurological changes like anxiety, depression, chorea.
    - Calcification of brain.
    - Hypoplastic teeth, delayed eruption, external root resorption, root dilacerations.
    - Chronic candidosis refractory to anti fungal therapy. Chronic candidiasis may cause hypoparathyroidism by inducing an immune response.
    - Radiograph shows calcification of basal ganglia on PA skull view.
- **PSEUDOHYPOPARATHYROIDISM**
    - PTH extract has no effect in correcting the hypocalcaemia.

IV. ADRENAL HORMONES

Acute Insufficiency of Adrenal Cortex *(Waterhouse – Friderichsen syndrome)*

- Acute septicaemia, pronounced purpura and death within 48 - 72 hrs.

Chronic Insufficiency of Adrenal Cortex *(Addison's disease)*

- Bronzing of skin.
- Pigmentation of mucous membrane, spreading over buccal mucosa from angles of mouth, gingiva, tongue lips, may be the first evidence of the disease.
- Vomiting, diarrhoea, severe anaemia.
- Lesion shows acanthosis with silver positive granules in the cells of stratum germinativum.

Hyperfunction of Adrenal Gland

Adrenogenital syndrome – due to hyperplasia or tumor of adrenal cortex.

- Manifest as pseudo hermaphroditism.
- Premature eruption of teeth.
- Partial loss of lamina dura.
- Mottled appearance of teeth.

Cushing's syndrome.

- Mooning of face
- Buffalo hump
- Muscular weakness
- Vascular hypertension
- Glycosuria not controlled by insulin
- Albuminuria
- Osteoporosis
- Premature cessation of epiphyseal growth.

Stress and the "adaptation syndrome"

- Surgery is hazardous in hyperadrenocorticism because cortisone interferes with wound healing.

V. DIABETES MELLITUS

- Burning mouth
- Altered wound healing
- Increased incidence of infection
- Xerostomia
- Enlargement of parotid
- Increased incidence of oral candidiasis
- Gingivitis and periodontitis

VI. PROGERIA (HUTCHINSON – GILFORD SYNDROME)

- Alopecia, atrophic skin, pigmented areas on trunk, prominent veins and loss of subcutaneous fat.
- Beak – like nose, hypoplastic mandible.
- Accelerated formation of irregular secondary dentin.
- Delayed eruption of teeth.

QUESTIONS

1. **All can cause retardation of skeletal maturity except:**   [AIPG 2004]
    1. Chronic renal failure
    2. Hypothyroidism
    3. Protein energy malnutrition (PEM)
    4. Congenital adrenal hyperplasia

Ans. **4**

It usually causes hypertension, hirsuitism, cutaneous striae, weight gain, amenorrhoea.

2. **A 20-year-old male presented with chronic constipation, headache and palpitations. On examination he had marfanoid habitus, neuromas of tongue, medullated corneal nerve fibers**

and a nodule of 2x2 cm size in the left lobe of thyroid gland. This patient is a case of:

[AIPG 2004]

1. Sporadic medullary carcinoma of thyroid
2. Familial medullary carcinoma of thyroid
3. MEN II A
4. MEN II B

Ans. **4**

Thyroid adenomas are seen in MEN II (B) or MEN III

3. **A progressive increase in mandibular length and in mandibular interdental spacing in an adult patient is characteristic of:** [AIPG 2003]
   1. Periodontosis
   2. Hypothyroidism
   3. Hyperpituitarism
   4. Hypoadrenalism

Ans. **3**

This occurs due to excessive release of growth hormone from anterior pituitary.

4. **Abnormal pigment of skin and mucous membrane with generalized systemic symptoms of decreased blood pressure is seen in:** [AIPG 2002]
   1. Albright's syndrome
   2. Grinspan syndrome
   3. Addison's disease
   4. Von Recklinghausen's disease

Ans. **3**

Albright's syndrome is associated with polyostatic fibrous dysplasia, Grinspan syndrome with erosive lichen planus and Von Recklinghausen's disease with neurofibromatosis

5. **A child with low level of intelligence and delayed milestones is probably suffering from:**

[AIPG 1995]

   1. Hyperthyroidism
   2. Hypothyroidism
   3. Hyperpituitarism
   4. Hypoparathyroidism

Ans. **2**

Hypothyroidism is characterized by –

- Retracted mental & physical growth
- Delayed fusion of body epiphysis
- Delayed ossification of PNS

- Protuberant abdomen, umbilical hernia
- Hoarse cry
- Feeding problems in neonates.

6. **A female patient suffering from hypotension has perioral pigmentation. The most likely diagnosis will be:** [AIPG 1995]

    1. Cushing's disease
    2. Hypothyroidism
    3. Addisons's disease
    4. Menopause

Ans. **3**

Addison's disease is characterized by –

- Vomiting, diarrhea, severe anemia, feeble heart action, postural hypotension.
- Bronzing of skin, pigmentation of mucous membrane.
- Hypoglycemia
- Muscle weakness
- Infection, trauma.

7. **Which is/are common cause or causes of hyperparathyroidism?** [AIPG 94]

    1. Carcinoma of parathyroid glands
    2. Hyperplasia of parathyroid glands
    3. Adenoma of parathyroid glands
    4. All of the above

Ans. **4**

All the above are the causes of primary hyperparathyroidism.

8. **Endocrine disturbance is the primary cause of jaw deformity in patients with:** [AIPG 92]

    1. Acromegaly
    2. Achondroplasia
    3. Paget's disease
    4. Albright's syndrome

Ans. **1**

Due to overproduction of growth hormone in adults, there is unrestricted growth of mandible leading to class III malocclusion.

9. **Osteitis fibrosa cystica is caused due to:** [AIPG 91]

    1. Hyperparathyroidism
    2. Hypoparathyroidism
    3. Hypothyroidism
    4. None of the above

Ans. **1**

Osteitis fibrosa cystica and Brown's tumor are common manifestations of hyperparathyroidism. Also, there is loss of lamina dura.

10. **A 50 years old obese man complains of several recent abscesses in the gingiva with loosening of teeth. He also suffers from itching of skin and polyuria. The most probable aetiology is:**
    [AIPG 1989]
    1. Scurvy
    2. Myxoedema
    3. Diabetes mellitus
    4. Vitamin A deficiency

Ans. **3**

Diabetes mellitus
  - Dryness and burning sensation of oral mucosa
  - Severe periodontitis
  - Swollen gingiva
  - Loosened teeth
  - Polyuria, polydipsia, polyphagia.

Scurvy
  - Swollen bleeding gums.
  - Delayed wound healing early tooth loss.
  - Subcutaneous bruising & hematoma.

Vitamin A deficiency
  - Night blindness, xerosis, bitot spots, xeropthalmia, hyperkeratosis of oral mucosa

Myxoedema
  - Non pitting oedema- Hypothyroidism.

11. **All are manifestations of protein deficiency except:** [AIPG 2002]
    1. Degeneration of connective tissue of gingiva
    2. Osteoporosis
    3. Proliferation of epithelium
    4. Alveolar bone loss

Ans. **3**

12. **Moeller's glossitis is associated with:** [AIPG 97]
    1. Vitamin B_{12} deficiency
    2. Vitamin B_6 deficiency
    3. Niacin deficiency
    4. All of the above

Ans. **1**

Due to gradual atrophy of papillae, the tongue appears "bald" or smooth in vitamin B12 deficiency and is called Hunters or Moeller's glossitis. It is similar to "Bald tongue of Sandwith" seen in pellagra.

13. **The disease associated with copper metabolism is:** [AIPG 97]

   1. Carrhie's syndrome
   2. Wilson's syndrome
   3. Cruver's syndrome
   4. Globe's syndrome

Ans. **2**

Other disease caused due to copper deficiency is Menke's syndrome (Steely or kinky hair syndrome)

8 | Healing of Oral Wounds

HEALING OF BIOPSY WOUND

- Occurs by primary intention when the edges are in close apposition and secondary intention when the wound cannot be approximated.

HEALING OF EXTRACTION WOUNDS

1. *Immediate Reaction*
   - Coagulation of blood in socket, RBC's gets entrapped in fibrin meshwork and blood vessels in PDL are sealed off.
   - Mobilization of leukocytes.
2. *1st week* – Fibroblast proliferation
   - Osteoclastic activity in alveolar crest.
   - Endothelial proliferation.
   - Organization of blood clot.
   - Epithelial proliferation at edges of wound.
3. *2nd week*
   - Degeneration of remnants of PDL.
   - Organization of blood clot.
   - Walls of bony socket appear frayed.
   - Resorption of alveolar crest around socket.
4. *3rd week*
   - Completely organized clot.
   - Formation of osteoid matrix.
   - Rounding off of crest of alveolar bone.
   - Original cortical bone of alveolar socket undergoes remodeling.
5. *4th week*
   - Continuous deposition, remodeling and resorption of the bone filling the alveolar socket.
   - Due to resorption of crest, bone filling the socket does not extend beyond alveolar crest.

Radiographic changes
- Gradual loss of density of lamina dura.
- Bone develops at the base and sides of the socket.
- Consolidation of new bone.
- Cortical bone formation at the surface of alveolar process.

HEALING OF FRACTURES

1. Immediate effect
- Due to disruption of vessels along fracture line, there is a considerable extravasation of blood in that area.
- Osteocytes die due to tearing of vessels.
- Death of bone marrow.
- Formation of clot.

2. Callus formation
- Callus unites the fractured ends of bone and composed of varying amount of fibrous tissue, cartilage and bone.
- Periosteum is an important structure in callus formation and ultimate healing of fracture.
- Continuous proliferation of these osteogenic cells of periosteum forms a collar of callus around or over the surface of fracture.
- Differentiation of osteoblasts in callus.
- On the rapidly growing area of collar varying number cells of osteogenic layer differentiate into chondroblasts rather than osteoblasts and form cartilage.
- This cartilage fuses with bone and then begins to calcify by endochondral bone formation; calcified cartilage is gradually resorbed and replaced by bone.
- Internal callus forms from endosteum of haversian canals and undifferentiated cells of bone marrow.
- Both external and internal callus remodel to form indistinguishable bone.

Physical and Chemical Injuries

FRACTURES OF TEETH

Ellis classification.

Class

I - Enamel only

II - Enamel and dentin

III - Enamel, dentin and pulp.

IV - Tooth becomes non vital without loss of crown structure.

V - Avulsion

VI - Fracture of root with / without loss of crown structure.

VII - Displacement of tooth.

VIII - Fracture of crown en-masse.

IX - Trauma to deciduous teeth.

TRAUMATIC CYST / SOLITARY BONE CYST / HAEMORRHAGIC BONE CYST / SIMPLE BONE CYST

- Pseudo cyst, not lined by epithelium.
- Lies *above the mandibular canal* (as contrast to stafne's cyst which lies below the canal).
- Associated teeth are vital.
- Most common site is mandibular molar area.
- It contains only air, not blood.
- Treatment is surgical exploration to induce bleeding in the lesion.

IATROGENIC SOURCES OF PHYSICAL INJURY TO TEETH

(a) Speed of drill (>50,000 rpm with coolants is less injurious to pulp).

(b) Resins – Injurious agent is residual monomer that causes injury to pulp by marginal leakage and heat generation during setting. GIC and polycarboxylate cements are least irritating.

PHYSICAL INJURIES TO ORAL SOFT TISSUES

- *Riga-fede disease* – Traumatic ulcers on ventral surface of tongue due to natal and neonatal teeth.
- *Decubitus ulcers* – Traumatic ulcers.
- *Factitial injuries* – Accidentally self-induced injuries due to some habits.
- *Epulis fissuratum / inflammatory fibrous hyperplasia*: Hyperplasia along the margins of dentures due to chronic irritation by denture flanges.
- *Palatal papillomatosis* -Inflammatory papillary hyperplasia seen on palatal mucosa as red inflammatory papillary projections due to ill – fitted dentures.
- *Perleche / Angular cheilitis* – Candidal infection at angels of mouth due to over closure of jaws and saliva collection in folds at corners of mouth.
- *Mucocele* – Due to severance of the duct of minor salivary gland; can be retention or extravasation type. Most common site is lower lip.
- *Ranula* – Occurs on floor of mouth. Associated with injury to sublingual or submandibular glands.
- *Bednar ulcers* – Ulcers on palate of infants due to injudicious cleaning of palate with swab or cloth.

CHEMICAL INJURIES

- *Stomatitis Medicamentosa* – Drug allergy.
- *Stomatitis venenata* – Contact stomatitis.
- *Plumbism / Lead poisoning*
  - "Wrist-drop" or "foot-drop" phenomenon.
  - Peripheral neuritis.
  - Basophilic stippling of RBC's.
  - *Burtonian lines* – gray / blue line on marginal gingiva.
- *Bismuth line* – Blue-black line on marginal gingiva in areas of food stagnation due to bismuth sulfite precipitation.
- *Mercury poisoning*
  - Fine tremors of fingers, limbs, lips, tongue.
  - Ptylism
  - *Pink's disease / Swift's disease* occurs in infants, skin resemble "Raw beef," peeling of skin, severe pruritis, tearing of hair in patches is common.
  - BAL is treatment of choice.
  - Osteomyelitis may also occur.
- *Silver induced Argyria / Argyrosis:*
  Silver granules are prominently arranged in linear fashion along the collagen fibres and around blood vessels.
- *Arsenic* – necrosis of bone.

- *Chromium* – Necrosis of bone
                        – Oral ulcers.
- *Fluoride* – Osteosclerosis
- *Aniline* – Blue coloration of lips / gingiva.
- *Benzene* – Blue coloration of lips.
- *Acids* – Decalcification of teeth.
- *Cu, Fe, Ni, Cr etc* – staining of teeth.
- *Phenytoin* – Fibrous hyperplasia of gingiva.
  –"Test –tube" retepegs.
- *Tetracycline* – Yellowish or brown discoloration of teeth which increases after exposure to light, fluoresce under UV light as yellow / golden.
- *Quincke's edema / Angioneurotic edema*
  A biochemical abnormality due to absence of C_1 esterase enzyme in serum that causes increased consumption of C_2 and C_4 esterase. Kinin – like substances are formed leading to edema.

QUESTIONS

1. **Bronze discoloration of oral mucosa is seen in:** [AIPGEE 2008]
   1. Blue nevus
   2. Addison's disease
   3. Amalgam tattoo
   4. Hyperchromatosis

Ans. ◼ 2

Sprue – Brown

Aplastic anaemia – Olive brown.

Hyperparathyroidism.

Neurofibromatsis – Café –au-lait spots (Coast of California appearance)

Albright's syndrome - Café –au-lait spots (Coast of Maine appearance)

Amalgam tatto- bluish black

2. **Disturbance in calcification stage of tooth development results in:** [AIPGEE 2008]
   1. Transparent dentin
   2. Interglobular dentin
   3. Atypical dentin
   4. Osteodentin

Ans. ◼

3. **Calcitrions which do not fuse will result in the formation of:** [AIPGEE 2008]
   1. Transparent dentin

   2. Interglobular dentin

   3. Atypical dentin

   4. Osteodentin

Ans.

4. Which of the following is not responsible for the endogenous staining of teeth during development? [AIPGEE 2008]

   1. Tetracycline

   2. Rh incompatibility

   3. Neonatal liver disease

   4. Vitamin C deficiency

Ans. **4**

Tetracycline administration- Shows yellow to brown discoloration.

Neonatal Hepatitis – Yellowish brown color of primary teeth.

Erythroblastic fetalis – Green, bluish green to yellow brown or gray.

10 Discoloration of Teeth

- *Dentinogenesis Imperfecta* – Bluish grey or amber.
- *Dental fluorosis* – White flecks to yellow or brown discoloration.
- *Pink tooth of mummery* – Internal resorption.
- *Initial Enamel caries* – White chalky area.
- *Erythroblastic fetalis* – Green, bluish green to yellow brown or gray.
- *Neonatal Hepatitis* – Yellowish brown color of primary teeth.
- *Porphyria* – Red, brown or pinkish discoloration of primary & permanent teeth (Erythrodontia). Under UV light, the teeth always exhibit red fluorescence due to physical affinity to $Ca_3(PO_4)_2$.
- *Congenital defect in bile duct* – Green discoloration.
- *Tetracycline administration* - Minimum amount required to produce discoloration is 21 mg / kg body weight. Tetracycline reacts with calcium to form calcium orthophosphate complex.

  Seen in primary as well as permanent teeth.

  Demonstrated as golden fluorescence in UV light, which is more intense in dentin than enamel. Bands are more intense towards DEJ.

  Shows yellow to brown discoloration.

  Doxycycline causes no discoloration.
- *Congenital heart disease* – Milk color or bluish violet color.
- *Oxalosis* – Slate gray intrinsic stain.

Black stains
- Due to contact with certain metallic elements such as silver, iron and lead.

Green stains
- Usually seen in cervical 1/3rd of facial surface of maxillary incisions of children.
- Associated with poor oral hygiene, chromogenic bacteria or fungi action on remnants of enamel cuticle.

Orange stains
- Due to chromogenic bacteria.

• Associated with poor oral hygiene.

Brown stains

• Lingual surface of lower incisors and buccal surface of maxillary molars.

Formed due to altered salivary mucins which have undergone change through the action of bacterial enzymes.

NOTES

11 | Diseases of Bones

OSTEOGENESIS IMPERFECTA

("Brittle Bone" disease / Fragilitis Ossium / Osteopsathyrosis / Lobstein's Disease)

- Vrolik's type - congenital.
- Osteopsathyrosis or Tarda or Lobstein's type or Gravis or Levis - later in childhood
- There is an inborn error in the synthesis of type I collagen.
- Extreme fragility and porosity of the bones.
- Prone to fractures.
- Pale blue sclera.
- Deafness.
- Laxity of ligaments.
- May be associated with dentinogenesis imperfecta.
- Tendency for capillary bleeding.
- Class III malocclusion.
- Increased incidense of impaction of 1st and 2nd molars.

INFANITLE CORTICAL HYPEROSTOSIS

(Caffey Silverman syndrome / Caffey's disease)

- Development of tender, deeply placed soft tissue swellings and cortical thickenings of various bones.
- Arises in 1st three months of life.
- Mandibular swellings, usually in the angle and ramus, usually asymmetrical involvement.
- May be associated with fever, hyperirritability, pseudoparalysis, dysphagia, plurisy, anaemia, leukocytosis, monocytosis, elevated ESR.
- Increased alkaline phosphatase.

CHERUBISM

(Familial fibrous dysplasia of jaws / Disseminated juvenile fibrous dysplasia / familial multilocular

cystic disease of jaws / familial fibrous swelling of jaws / Hereditary fibrous dysplasia of jaws).

- Autosomal dominant inheritance with 100% male penetrance and 50-70% female penetrance.
- Manifests in early childhood (3-4 yrs), tend to regress with age.
- Progressive, painless, symmetric swelling of the jaws producing a chubby face.
- No associated systemic manifestation.
- Bilateral submandibular lymphadenopathy.
- Premature shedding of primary teeth.
- Defective permanent dentition.
- Serum calcium, phosphorus and alkaline phosphatase are within normal limits.
- Multilocular lesion, well defined, bilateral mandibular involvement.
- Causes anterior displacement of teeth.
- Narrow furrowed palate owing to bulging of alveolar processes.
- Multiple dentigerous cysts may be present.
- *Noonan's Syndrome*- Hypertelorism, webbed neck, mental retardation, cardiac defects, cryptorchidism, short stature, cherubism.
- *Ramon's Syndrome*- Cherubism, gingival fibromatosis, epilepsy, mental deficiency, insulin dependant diabetes mellitus.
- *Jaffe-Campanacci Syndrome*- Cherubism, Multiple non ossifying fibromas, café-au-lait spots, mental retardation, cryptorchidism, CVS and eye abnormalities.

CLEIDOCRANIAL DYSPLASIA

(Marie And Sainton's Disease, Scheuthauer Marie - Sainton's Syndrome, Mutational Dysostosis)

- Autosomal dominant malformation syndrome caused by mutation of RUNX2 gene on chromosome 6.
- Abnormalities of skull, shoulder girdle, teeth, jaws.
- Short stature.
- Delayed closure of fontanels, frontal, parietal and occipital bones are prominent.
- Brachycephalic (light bulb like shape), depressed nose with hypertelorism.
- Underdeveloped maxilla and paranasal sinuses.
- High, narrow arched palate.
- Cleft palate may be present.
- Prolonged retention of deciduous teeth.
- Delayed eruption of permanent teeth or impacted teeth, supernumerary teeth.
- Roots are thin and short due to absence of cellular cementum.

CRANIOFACIAL DYSOSTOSIS

[Crouzon Disease Or Syndrome, Apert syndrome (associated with syndactyly)]

- Early synostosis of sutures.

- Triangular frontal defect.
- Parrot beak nose.
- Hypoplastic maxilla.
- Mandibular prognathism.
- Hypertelorism, exopthalmos, strabismus.
  Radiograph - copper beaten appearance.

MANDIBULOFACIAL DYSOSTOSIS

(Treacher Collins syndrome / Franceschetti syndrome)

- Autosomal dominant disorder caused by mutation of TCOF1 gene on chromosome 5.
- Antimongoloid palpebral fissures with coloboma on eyelids.
- Hypoplasia of facial bones, especially the malar and mandible.
- Malformation of ear and absence of external auditory canal.
- Macrostomia.
- High palate.
- Underdeveloped paranasal sinuses.
- Angles class II anterior open bite malocclusion.
- Blind fistulas between the ears and angles of the mouth.
- Facial clefts.
- Bird like face.

PIERRE ROBIN SYNDROME (Robin Anomalad)

- Cleft palate + micrognathia (mandible) + glossoptosis
- Bird facies
- Respiratory difficulty.

MARFAN SYNDROME

(Marfan - Achards Syndrome / Arachnodactyly)

- Excessive length of tubular bones.
- Spidery fingers.
- Dolicocephalic.
- Hyper extensibility of joints and habitual dislocations.
- Cardiovascular complications.
- High, arched palate.
- Bifid uvula.
- Multiple odontogenic cysts of maxilla and mandible.
- TMJ dysarthrosis.

DOWN SYNDROME

(Trisomy 21 syndrome / Mongolism)

- Flat face.
- Large anterior fontanel, open suture.
- Class III malocclusion, high palate.
- Open mouth.
- Large tongue, enamel hypoplasia.
- Sexual underdevelopment.
- Cardiac abnormalities.
- Hyper mobility of joints.

OSTEOPETROSIS

(Marble bone disease / Albers Schonberg disease / Osteosclerosis fragilis Generalisata)

- Unknown etiology, defect in differentiation and function of osteoclasts, resulting in dense fragile bones susceptible to fracture and infections.
- 2 types   - Clinically benign dominant inherited
  - Malignant recessive
- Optic atrophy
- Hepatosplenomegaly.
- Poor growth
- Frontal bossing
- Pathological fractures
- Loss of hearing
- Facial palsy
- Genu valgum
- Osteomyelitis
- Medullary spaces of jaw are remarkably reduced.
- Enamel hypoplasia and increased caries incidence.
- Microscopic dentinal defects.
- Arrested root development.
- Delayed eruption, early tooth loss, missing teeth, malformed roots and crowns.
- Thickening of lamina dura.

Radiographs

- Diffuse homogenous symmetrically sclerotic appearance of all bones with clubbing and transverse striations of the long bones.
- Cortical thickening.
- Medullary cavities are replaced by bone.
- Internal structure and even roots of the teeth may not be apparent.

Lab findings
- Myelophthistic anaemia.
- Serum Ca, P- normal.
- Elevated serum acid phosphatase.

Histopathology
- Endosteal production of bone.

ACHONDROPLASIA (Chondrodystrophia Fetalis)

- Disturbance of endochondral bone formation.
- Dwarfism.
- Brachycephalic.
- Lumbar loridosis.
- Retruded maxilla.
- Relative mandibular prognathism.

Radiograph
- Clubbing at ends of long bones.
- Bones at base of skull fuse prematurely.
- Maxillary retrusion.

GENERALIZED CORTICAL HYPEROSTOSIS (Van - Buchem syndrome)

- Widening at angles of mandible and bridge of nose.
- Loss of visual acuity.
- Loss of facial sensation.
- Cranial nerve involvement.
- Overgrowth of alveolar process.

MASSIVE OSTEOLYSIS

(Vanishing Bone / Disappearing Bone / Phantom Bone / Progressive Osteolysis / Gorham Syndrome)
- Begins suddenly, advances rapidly unless a thin layer of fibrous tissue, surrounding a cavity, replaces the involved bone.
- Pathological fractures.

Histopathology
- Endothelial lined blood vessel proliferation in connective tissue.

PAGET'S DISEASE (Osteitis deformans)

- Etiology - Measles related virus has been suggested. It is a condition of abnormal apposition and resorption of osseous tissue in one or more bones.
- Disease of middle and old age (>40 years).
- Bone pain

- Severe headache
- Deafness
- Blindness
- Facial palsy
- Dizziness
- Weakness
- Mental disturbances
- Progressive enlargement of skull.
- Deformities of spine, femur and tibia.
- *"Simian appearance"* or Grotesque facial pattern.
- Increased vascularity of bones which become warm to touch
- Pathological fractures.
- Term Leontiasis Ossia was earlier used in case of facial bones involvement.
- Progressive enlargement of maxilla, widening of alveolar ridges with flattening of palate.
- Teeth become loose and migrate, leading to malocclusion.
- Maxilla to mandible involvement is 2.3:1.

Radiographs

- 3 radiographic stages- early radiolucent resorptive stage, a granular or ground glass appearing second stage and a denser, more radiopaque appositional late stage.
- *"Osteoporosis circumscripta"* - Isolated lesions on skull.
- *"Cotton wool"* appearance in skull and jaws.
- Hypercementosis.
- Loss of lamina dura.

Laboratory findings

- Serum Ca, P are normal
- Serum alkaline phosphatase in increased. Over 250 Bodansky units in osteoblastic phase.
- High levels of hydroxyproline in urine.

H/P

- *"Mosaic bone"* pattern
- *"Jigsaw - puzzle"* appearance

Treatment

- Calcitonin
- Diphosphonates like etidronate, pamidranone, tiludranone.
- Cytotoxic antibodies like mithramycin, plicamycin which inhibit osteoclastic activity.

Complication

- Osteosarcoma development
- Giant cell tumors

FIBROUS DYSPLASIA OF BONE

Polyostotic
- Jaffe's type
- Albright's syndrome

Jaffe's type
- FD involving a variable number of bones
- Pigmented lesions of skin called "cafe au - lait" spots

Albright's syndrome
- Polyostotic FD (more severe)
- Pigmented lesions of skin
- Endocrine disturbances
- Manifests early in life
- Deformity, bowing or thickening of long bones
- Often unilateral
- Recurrent bone pains
- Spontaneous fractures
- Commonly involved bones are clavicles, pelvic, scapulae, long bones and metacarpals and tarsal.
- Cafe - au - lait spots
- Precocious puberty in females.
- Endocrine disturbances related to pituitary, thyroid, parathyroid, and ovary.
- Multiple intramuscular myxomas.

Oral manifestations
- Mostly mandible is involved.
- Expansion and deformity of jaws.
- Eruption pattern of teeth disturbed .

Radiograph
- Medullary portions of bone are rarefied and present irregular trabeculation, often a multilocular cystic appearance.
- Cortical bone is usually thinned and often considerably expanded.

Lab findings
- Serum alkaline phosphatase is sometimes elevated.
- Serum Ca, P are normal

Histopathology
Fibrillar connective tissue within which is numerous trabeculae of coarse, woven fiber bone, irregular in shape but evenly spaced.

Treatment - surgical shaving

- Radiation induced sarcomas have been reported.

Prognosis

- May progress to Osteosarcoma.

Monostotic

- Term "leontiasis ossea" is applied to the cases of fibrous dysplasia which affect the maxilla or facial bones and give the patient a leonine appearance.
- Swelling of jaw usually involves the labial or buccal plate, seldom the lingual aspect.
- In mandible it sometimes causes protuberant excrescence of the inferior border.
- Malalignment, tipping or displacement of teeth can occur & tenderness may ultimately develop.

Radiograph

Extremely variable, 3 basic patterns seen:

- Unilocular radiolucency or somewhat larger multilocular lucency, both with ill circumscribed border containing a network of fine bony trabeculae.
- Similar pattern except for increased trabeculation renders the lesion more opaque and typically mottled appearance.
- Opaque with many delicate trabeculae (*'Ground glass' or orange peel appearance*)
- Roots of teeth may not be visible due to opaque bone.
- Swirling pattern of trabeculae resembling fingerprint pattern.
- Loss of lamina dura and narrowing of PDL space.
- Inferior alveolar canal is displaced superiorly.
- Expansion of sinus occurs from lateral wall.
- Fusiform expansion of mandible.

H/P

- Fibroblasts in a compact stroma of interlacing collagen fibres.
- Chinese character shaped or C- shaped arrangement of trabeculae.

QUESTIONS

1. **Ground glass appearance is seen in:**   [AIPGEE 2008]
    1. Hyperparathyroidism
    2. Fibrous dysplasia
    3. Osteopetrosis
    4. Condensing Osteitis

Ans. **1**

Ground glass appearance may also be seen in early stages of fibrous dysplasia; but it is a pathognomic radiographic feature in hyperparathyroidism. Osteopetrosis and condensing osteitis presents with ill-defined radiopacities.

2. **Blue sclera is characteristic feature seen with: (AIPGEE 2008)**
   1. Fluorosis
   2. Osteogenesis imperfecta
   3. Tetracycline hypoplasia
   4. Amelogenesis imperfecta.

Ans. **2**

Blue sclera is also seen in other conditions like
- Fetal rickets.
- Marfan syndrome
- Ehler Danlos syndrome
- Osteopetrosis
- Infants.

3. **Enamel hypoplasia is not a feature of:** [AIPG 2005]
   1. Osteopetrosis.
   2. Downs syndrome.
   3. Some types of epidermolysis bullosa.
   4. Cleidocranial dysplasia.

Ans. **4**

Cleidocranial dysplasia is marked by absence or paucity of cellular cementum on roots of permanent teeth, delayed eruption of permanent teeth, prolonged retention of deciduous teeth and sometimes partial anodontia.

4. **Café au lait spots are seen in:** [AIPG 2005]
   1. Paget's disease of bone.
   2. Cherubism.
   3. Von Recklinghausen disease.
   4. Von Willebrand disease.

Ans. **3**

Café au lait spots are highly characteristic of Von Recklinghausen disease. They vary in size from 1-2 mm to several cm. they are usually present at birth or may develop during first year of life. Other characteristics are neurofibromas, axillary freckling (crowe's sign), optic glioma, lisch nodules (iris hamartomas) and osseous lesions.

5. **The gold standard for the diagnosis of osteoporosis is:** [AIPG 2005]
   1. Dual energy X-ray absorptiometry.
   2. Single energy X-ray absorptiometry.
   3. Ultrasound.
   4. Quantitative computed tomography.

Ans. **1**

Other three methods are not reliable.

6. **All of the following can cause osteoporosis, except:** [AIPG 2005]
   1. Hyperparathyroidism.
   2. Steroid use.
   3. Fluorosis
   4. Thyrotoxicosis

Ans. 3

7. **In Treacher Collin's Syndrome there is:** [AIPG 2005]
   1. Upward sloping of the palpebral fissure.
   2. Poorly developed or absent malar bones.
   3. Progenia and Mandibular prognathism.
   4. No loss of hearing.

Ans. 2

Treacher Collin's syndrome or mandibulofacial dysostosis is characterized by antimongoloid palpebral fissures with a coloboma of outer portion of lower lid, hypoplasia of facial bones (especially malar and mandible), ear deformity and high palate.

8. **Pierre Robin Syndrome is associated with:** [AIPG 2005]
   1. Micrognathia.
   2. Cleft of the lip and palate.
   3. Tetrology of fallot.
   4. Syndactylly.

Ans. 1

Due to retrognathic mandible the tongue is unable to descend down which leads to cleft palate. Because of this mechanism, cleft lip is not formed.

9. **Hypercementosis of the entire dentition is a feature of:** [AIPG 2005]
   1. Alber Shonberge disease.
   2. Paget's disease.
   3. Lathyrism.
   4. Low grade periapical inflammation.

Ans. 2

Albers Shonberge disease usually shows enamel hypoplasia, dentinal defects and arrested root developments. Periapical infection of low grade shows condensing osteitis at apices.

10. **Which of the following is not a feature of torus mandibularis?** [AIPG 2004]
    1. Common in Mongoloids.
    2. Present on the lingual surface of mandible below the mylohyoid line.
    3. Usually bilateral.
    4. May or may not associated with torus palatinus.

Ans. **2**

Tori are located above the myelohyoid line.

11. **Bone marrow transplantation can be used as a treatment for all except:** [AIPG 2004]
    1. Osteopetrosis
    2. Adrenoleukodystrophy
    3. Hurler's syndrome
    4. Hemochromatosis

Ans. **4**

12. **Pseudoanodontia is seen is:** [AIPG 2002]
    1. Cleidocranial dysostosis
    2. Down's syndrome
    3. Fibrous dysplasia
    4. Cherubism

Ans. **1**

Because the permanent teeth are usually impacted, clinical picture is that of hypodontia.

13. **Which of the following is not true of cherubism?** [AIPG 2002]
    1. It is a strictly unilocular lesion.
    2. It is a hereditary disease.
    3. There is root resorption.
    4. Multiple displaced and unerupted teeth are present.

Ans. **1**

Cherubism is always bilateral.

14. **Which of the following is seen in hypervitaminosis D?** [AIPG 2002]
    1. Albuminuria
    2. Hypocalcemia
    3. Hypercalcemia
    4. Hyperphosphatemia

Ans. **3**

Due to excessive absorption of calcium.

15. **A 60-year old male complains of loss of hearing and visual acuity with gradual enlargement of the maxilla. The reason could be:** [AIPG 2000]
    1. Osteomalacia
    2. Osteoporosis
    3. Paget's disease
    4. Albright's syndrome.

Ans. **3**

Paget's disease is characterized by bone formation and lack of bone resorption. This leads to continuous enlargement of maxilla and facial bones. Other clinical features are due to compression of cranial nerves in their foramina at the exit from base of skull.

16. **Normal serum calcium, normal phosphorous and normal alkaline phosphatase is found in:**
    [AIPG 2000]

    1. Cherubism
    2. Hyperparathyroidism
    3. Paget's disease
    4. Hypoparathyroidism.

Ans. 1

In hyperparathyroidism calcium is increased, phosphorus decreased. Alkaline phosphatase is increased in Paget's disease.

17. **The dental finding in Paget's disease is:**
    [AIPG 2000]
    1. Widening of PDL
    2. Widening of pulp chamber
    3. Apical root resorption
    4. Internal resorption.

Ans. 3

Hypercementosis with apical root resorption is seen in Paget's disease.

18. **In which of the following does pathological fracture of maxilla and mandible not occur?**
    [AIPG 2000]

    1. Multiple myeloma.
    2. Primary and metastatic carcinoma.
    3. Myositis ossificans.
    4. Central giant cell tumour.

Ans. 3

Patient has rigid facial expressions and trismus.

19. **Florid osseous dysplasia is also called:**
    [AIPG 2000]
    1. Gigantiform cementoma
    2. Periapical osteofibrosis
    3. Cementoma stage II
    4. Cemental dystrophy.

Ans. 4

20. **Mosaic pattern and abnormal resorption is seen in:**
    [AIPG 98]
    1. Paget's disease
    2. Fibrous dysplasia
    3. Osteopetrosis

4. Cherubism

Ans. 1

Mosaic pattern seen in Paget's disease is due to partially resorbed and then repaired bone, which leaves deeply stained reversal lines. These lines form a "jig-saw-puzzle" pattern.

In fibrous dysplasia, C-shaped or Chinese- character shaped trabeculae are seen, cherubism is characterized by presence of large multinucleated giant cells.

21. Marble bone disease is: [AIPG 97]

1. Osteopetrosis
2. Osteoporosis
3. Osteogenesis imperfecta
4. Paget's disease

Ans. 1

There is normal appositional bone growth, but failure of physiologic bone resorption. This is seen radiographically as areas of diffuse, homogeneous, symmetrical sclerotic appearance. Increased serum alkaline phosphatase level is also seen.

22. Pebbled appearance is seen in radiographs of: [AIPG 97]

1. Periadenitis mucosa necrotica
2. Stomatoplasia
3. Hypercementosis
4. Cherubism

Ans. 4

It is marked by destruction of bone of one or both jaws with expansion and severe thinning of the cortical plates. Multilocular appearance on actual perforation of cortex may also occur.

23. Which of the following is associated with Paget's disease? [AIPG 96]

1. Fibroma
2. Osteolymphoma
3. Osteocarcinoma
4. Osteosarcoma

Ans. 4

Paget's disease, if left untreated may show malignant transformation into osteosarcoma.

24. Mandibulofacial dysostosis is also known as: [AIPG 96]

1. Marfan's syndrome
2. Treacher Collins syndrome
3. Pierre Robin syndrome
4. Paget's disease

Ans. 2

25. Which of the following is true about fibrous dysplasia?   [AIPG 96]

1. It is seen mostly in the maxilla.
2. Has a multilocular cystic appearance.
3. Level of serum calcium is increased.
4. Level of alkaline phosphatase is increased.

Ans. **1**

Radiographically, it usually appears as a radiolucent lesion initially, but later on appears as dense radiopacity. Serum calcium, phosphorous and alkaline phosphatase levels are within normal limits.

26. The histopathology of osteopetrosis shows: [AIPG 1995]

1. Endosteal bone formation and lack of normal bone resorption.
2. Periosteal bone formation and lack of normal bone resorption.
3. Presence of extra collagen fibres and less.
4. Presence of numerous osteoclasts and a few osteoblasts.

Ans. **1**

Osteopetrosis also called 'Marble bone disease' is a group of hereditary skeletal disorder characterized by marked increase in bone density resulting from a defect in remodeling cause by failure of normal osteoclast function.

Histopathology- Abnormal endosteal bone formation has been described. Numerous osteoclasts may be seen, which are nonfunctional because Howship's lacunae are not visible.

27. Bence Jones proteins are found in: [AIPG 94]

1. Multiple myeloma
2. Diabetes mellitus
3. Uremia
4. Anaemia

Ans. **1**

Bence jones proteins are found in 60-85% of myeloma patients. This is an unusual protein which coagulates when the urine is heated to 40-60^0 C and then disappears when the urine is boiled. It reappears as the urine is cooled. Besides multiple myeloma, they are also found in the urine of patients with leukaemia and polycythemia.

28. Albright syndrome is associated with: [AIPG 94]

1. Osteopetrosis
2. Polyostotic fibrous dysplasia
3. Paget's disease of bone
4. Hypofunction of adrenal cortex

Ans. **2**

It involves nearly all bones in the skeleton and accompanied by café-au-lait spots and endocrine disturbances of various types. Another variety of polyostotic fibrous dysplasia (Jaffe's disease) involves fever bones and café-au-lait spots with no endocrine disturbances.

29. **Radiographic picture of Paget's disease:** [AIPG 93]
    1. Ground glass appearance
    2. Sun-ray appearance
    3. Cotton wool appearance
    4. Honeycomb appearance

Ans. **3**

Cotton wool appearance is seen in Paget's disease and chronic diffuse sclerosing osteomyelitis.

30. **Gardner syndrome does not include:** [AIPG 93]
    1. Osteomas
    2. Epidermoid cysts
    3. Osteosarcoma
    4. Impacted permanent teeth

Ans. **3**

Gardner syndrome is characterized by multiple polyposis of large intestine, osteomas of the bones, multiple epidermoid or sebaceous cysts, desmoid tumors and impacted supernumerary and permanent teeth.

31. **Alkaline phosphatase increases in:** [AIPG 93]
    1. Paget's disease
    2. Osteopetrosis
    3. Cherubism
    4. All of the above

Ans. **1**

Alkaline phosphatase enzyme is increased in the diseases where bone formation is taking place. It is absent in hypophosphatemia, decreased in rickets, osteomalacia etc.

32. **Biochemical abnormality associated with osteogenesis imperfecta is an increase in:** [AIPG 92]
    1. Alkaline phosphatase
    2. Acid phosphatase
    3. Bicarbonate ion
    4. Phosphorylase enzyme

Ans. **4**

The basic defect appears to lie in the organic matrix with failure of fetal collagen to be transformed into mature collagen.

33. **Osteosarcoma's radiographic appearance is usually:** [AIPG 92]
    1. Leafless tree appearance
    2. Sun-ray appearance
    3. Cotton-wool appearance
    4. Soap-bubble appearance

Ans. 2

Leafless tree appearance is seen in sialogram of Sjogren's syndrome. Cotton wool appearance occurs in Paget's disease. Soap bubble appearance is seen in ameloblastoma, giant cell lesion and hemangioma.

34. Radiographically cleidocranial dysostosis is characterized by: [AIPG 91]
   1. Osteoporosis
   2. Multiple periapical radiolucencies
   3. Supernumerary teeth
   4. Hypercementosis

Ans. 3

Other features include abnormalities of skull, shoulder girdle, teeth, jaws, delayed closure of fontanelles, brachycephalic, underdeveloped maxilla, high narrow arched palate, cleft palate, prolonged retention of deciduous teeth, delayed eruption of permanent teeth, absence of cellular cementum.

35. Which of the following can undergo spontaneous malignant transformation? [AIPG 91]
   1. Osteomalacia
   2. Albright's syndrome
   3. Paget's disease of bone
   4. Osteogenesis imperfecta

Ans. 3

Paget's disease may spontaneously progress to osteosarcoma or giant cell tumors, if left untreated.

36. A common finding associated with Paget's disease is: [AIPG 1989]
   1. Hypercementosis
   2. Apical root resorption
   3. Internal resorption
   4. Widened periodontal ligament space

Ans. 1

Paget's disease: • Histology – "Jigsaw puzzle" appearance
                    • Alkaline phosphatase increased severely up to 700 BU

37. A patient with fibrous dysplasia can be treated by: [AIPG 1989]
   1. Surgical excision
   2. Removal of adjacent teeth
   3. Irradiation of the lesion
   4. Conservative surgery

Ans. 4

Conservative surgery – Fibrous dysplasia, surgical contouring.

Irradiation → malignant changes → osteosarcoma.

12 Salivary Gland Diseases

DEVELOPMENTAL DISTURBANCES OF THE SALIVARY GLANDS

APLASIA (AGENESIS)

- Congenital absence of major salivary glands is rare.
- Unknown etiology and not necessarily associated with other ectodermal dysplasias.
- Xerostomia is the chief complaint of such patients.
- Associated with several congenital conditions such as hemifacial microstomia, mandibulofacial dysostosis, cleft palate, lacrimoauriculodentodigital syndrome, Treacher Collins syndrome and anopthalmia.

CHEILITIS GLANDULARIS

- Involves minor salivary glands of lower lip, occasionally upper lip, and palate.
- Etiology is unknown. Various factors suggested are – actinic damage, tobacco, syphilis, poor oral hygiene and heridity.
- Due to hypertrophy and inflammation of the glands, lower lip becomes swollen and everted.
- 3 types:
  - Simple
  - Superficial suppurative (*Baelz's disease*)
  - Deep suppurative (*cheilitis glandularis apostematosa*)
- A significant percentage (18 –35 %) cases have been associated with the development of squamous cell carcinoma of overlying epithelium of lip.

XEROSTOMIA (DRY MOUTH)

Xerostomia is a clinical manifestation of salivary gland dysfunction and doesn't in itself represent a disease entity.

Causes

a. Developmental
   - Salivary gland aplasia

b. Water / metabolite loss
   - Impaired fluid intake
   - Hemorrhage
   - Vomiting / diarrhoea

c. Iatrogenic
   - Medications like antihistaminics, decongestants, antidepressants, antipsychotics, antihypertensives, and anticholinergics.
   - Radiation therapy to head and neck.

d. Systemic diseases: -
   - Sjogren's syndrome
   - Diabetes mellitus
   - Diabetes insipidus
   - Sarcoidosis
   - HIV infection
   - Graft Vs host disease
   - Psychogenic disorders.

e. Local factors:
   - Decreased mastication
   - Smoking
   - Mouth breathing

Clinical features

- Foamy or thick and "ropey" saliva.
- Dry mucosa.
- Positive *"Lipstick sign"and "tongue blade sign"*.
- Unstimulated salivary flow rate of <0.1 ml/min and stimulated whole saliva flow rate of <1.0 ml/min are considered abnormally low.
- Tongue – fissuring and atrophy of filliform papillae.
- Difficulty in mastication, swallowing, speaking.
- Increased prevalence of oral candidiasis.
- Dental decay, especially cervical and root carries.

Treatment

- Symptomatic treatment.
- Use of oral hygiene products that contain lactoperoxidase, lysozyme, lactoferrin (Biotene tooth paste mouthrinse, oral balance gel, WET MOUTH, Bio Xtra)
- Systemic pilocarpine 5- 10 mg TDS or QID

- Cevimeline hydrochloride
- Frequent fluoride applications.

HYPERPLASIA OF PALATAL GLANDS

- May represent a benign adenoma
- Etiology unknown may be due to-
  - Endocrine disorders
  - Gout
  - Diabetes
  - Menopause
  - Hepatic disease
  - Starvation
  - Alcoholism
  - Inflammation
  - Benign lymphoepithelial lesion.
  - Sjogren's syndrome
  - Adiposity, hyperthermia, oligomenorrhea, parotid swelling syndrome.
  - Aglossia – adactylia syndrome
  - Waldenstrom's Macroglobulinemia
  - Uveoparotid fever
  - Felty's syndrome
  - Certain drugs
  - Aging process
- Usually presents, as a small to localized swelling, measuring several mm to 1 cm is size, firm, sessile on the hard palate or at junction of hard and soft palate.

ATRESIA

- Congenital occlusion or absence of one or more of salivary gland ducts.
- May cause xerostomia or form retention cysts.

ABERRANCY

- Salivary glands are found farther than normal from their usual location like body of mandible.
- No clinical significance except for the site of retention cyst or neoplasm.

DEVELOPMENTAL LINGUAL MANDIBULAR SALIVARY GLAND DEPRESSION

(Static Bone Cyst / Static Bone Defect of Mandible / Static Bone Cavity / Lingual Mandibular Bone Cavity / Stafne Cyst or Defect)

- Occurs due to inclusion of glandular tissue within or more commonly adjacent to the lingual surface of the body of mandible.

- More common in men
- Usually asymptomatic
- Occasionally bilateral
- Radiographically it appears as an ovoid radiolucency, generally situated between the mandibular canal and the inferior border of mandible, commonly in second or third molar area or just anterior to the angle.
- Sialography can be used as an aid in diagnosis.

ANTERIOR LINGUAL DEPRESSION

- Represents a cavity or depression or the lingual surface of mandible caused by sublingual glands or an anatomic variation relates to digastric or sublingual fossa.
- Radiographically, appears as an ovoid radiolucency in anterior segment of mandible.

TUMORS OF SALIVARY GLANDS

- Most common site for salivary gland tumors is the parotid gland, accounting for 64 – 80 % of all cases out of these parotid tumors, 2/3 to ¾ are benign.
- 8-11 % salivary gland tumors occur in submandibular gland out of which 37-45% is malignant.
- Tumors of sublingual glands are rare (1%). But 70 – 90% of sublingual tumors are malignant.
- Minor salivary glands accounts for 9-23 % of all tumors (2nd common site) out of which 50 % are malignant.
- Most frequent site for minor salivary gland tumors is palate (42 – 54 %) followed by lip (21-22%), buccal mucosa (11-15%).
- Labial tumors are more common on upper lip (77 – 89%) while mucocoeles are more common on lower lip.

PLEOMORPHIC ADENOMA (Benign mixed tumor)

- Earlier known as enclavoma, Branchioma, endothelioma, enchondroma.
- Most common salivary gland neoplasm. It accounts for 53 – 77% of parotid tumors, 44 – 68 % of submandibular and 38 – 43 % of minor gland tumors.
- Derived from a mixture of ductal and myoepithelial elements. But rarely the individual cells are actually pleomorphic. Likewise, although the tumor often has a prominent mesenchyme appearing "stromal" component, it is not truly a mixed neoplasm that is derived from more than one germ layer. Its morphogenic complexity is the result of differentiation of tumor cells and the fibrous, hyalinized, myxoid, chondroid and even osseous areas as a result of metaplasia or is actually products of tumor cells.
- Usually appears as small, painless quiescent nodule with slow or intermittent growth pattern.
- Not fixed to deeper tissue or overlying skin.
- Seldom ulcerates.
- These tumors are radio resistant. Surgical excision is the treatment of choice.

- May undergo malignant transformation into adenocarcinomas or cylinderoma.

MONOMORPHIC ADENOMA

- W.H.O. sub divides monomorphic adenoma into 3 groups –
    - Adenolymphoma (Warthin's tumor)
    - Oxyphilic adenoma
    - Others
- *Histological classification*
  Basal cell adenoma
  Canalicular adenoma

A) Basal Cell Adenoma

- Primarily involves major glands, mainly parotid.
- Intercalated duct or reserve cell is the histogenetic source of basal cell adenoma.
- Tumor cells are arranged in solid nests with palisaded arrangement of peripheral cells, in ribbons or cords. Scanty stroma is found between cell nests.

B) Canalicular Adenoma

- Mainly involves accessory salivary glands, usually in upper lip.
- Histologically, it is composed of long strands or cords of epithelial cells, almost invariably arranged in a double row and usually showing a "party wall". Supporting stroma is loose and fibrillar with delicate vascularity.

WARTHIN'S TUMOR

(Adenolymphoma / Papillary Cystadenoma Lymphomatosum)

- Occurs almost exclusively in parotid glands.
- Numerous theories have been advance to account for the peculiar nature of this tumor. It is believed to arise from-
    1. Salivary gland tissue entrapped within paraparotid or intraparotid lymph nodes during embryogenesis.
    2. A delayed hypersensitivity disease.
    3. Exaggerated secretory immune response.
- Exhibits a definite predilection for men.
- Generally superficial, lying just beneath the parotid capsule.
- Made up of 2 histologic components- epithelial and lymphoid tissue.
- The lesion is essentially an adenoma exhibiting cyst formation, with papillary projections into the cystic spaces and a lymphoid matrix showing geminal centers. An eosinophillic coagulum in seen in cystic spaces. Oncocytes are seen under electron microscope.
- Surgical excision is the treatment of choice.
- Malignant transformation is rare.

OXYPHILIC ADENOMA (Oncocytoma / Acidophilic Adenoma)

- Rare benign tumor, which usually occurs in parotid gland.
- More common in women.
- Tumor cells resemble oncocytes, which have an eosinophillic cytoplasm and distinct cell membrane and choked with mitochondria.
- Oncocytes are normal cells found in a great number of other locations, including salivary glands, respiratory tract, breast, thyroid, pancreas, parathyroid, pituitary, liver, stomach etc.

MYOEPITHELIOMA

- Constitutes < 1% of all salivary tumors.
- Parotid and palate are common sites.
- Tumor is composed of spindle shaped or plasmacytoid cells. Definitive diagnosis lies in the ultra structure identification of myoepithelial cells.

DUCTAL PAPILLOMAS

- Arise from excretory ducts of major and especially minor salivary glands.
- 3 forms: -
    (a) Simple ductal papilloma
    (b) Inverted ductal papilloma
    (c) Sialadenoma papilliferum

MIKULICZ'S DISEASE (Benign Lymphoepithelial Lesion)

- Exhibits both inflammatory and neoplastic characteristics.
- Autoimmune etiology.
- Manifests as a unilateral or bilateral diffuse enlargement of the parotid and/or submaxillary glands.
- May be associated with mild local discomfort, occasional pain and xerostomia.
- Sometimes lacrimal glands are also enlarged.
- Far more frequent in women, particularly those in middle or later life.
- There is sometimes a history of an alternating increase and decrease in size of mass from time to time.
- Histological picture shows an orderly lymphocytic infiltration of salivary gland tissue, destroying or replacing the acini. *"Epimyoepithelial islands"* are present.
- Treatment is by surgery and radiation. However, there are chances of radiation-induced malignancy.
- Individuals with Miculicz's disease have an increased risk of lymphoma – either in the affected gland or in an extra salivary site.

Mikulicz's Syndrome

Used to describe the condition of salivary gland enlargement usually accompanied by node enlargement due to some generalized specific diseases such as lymphomas or T.B. or sarcoidosis.

Sjogren Syndrome

- Chronic systemic autoimmune disorder with genetic influence.
- *Sicca syndrome* = Xerostomia + Xeropthalmia.
- *Primary Sjogren's syndrome* -Sicca syndrome alone with no other autoimmune disorder.
- *Secondary Sjogren's syndrome* -Sicca syndrome in addition to another autoimmune disease like rheumatoid arthritis, SLE etc.
- *San Diego criteria for Sjogren's syndrome*

   1. Primary Sjogren's syndrome

   Symptoms and signs of ocular dryness

   (a) Schirmer's test less than 8 mm wetting per 5 minutes.

   (b) Positive Rose Bengal staining of cornea or conjunctiva.

   Symptoms and signs of dry mouth

   (a) Decreased parotid flow rate using lashley cups or other methods.

   (b) Abnormal findings from biopsy of minor salivary glands (focus score of [3] 2 based on average of 4 evaluable lobules).

   Serological evidence of a systemic autoimmunity

   (a) Elevated Rheumatoid factor > 1:320.

   OR

   (b) Elevated Antinuclear Antibody (ANA) > 1:320

   OR

   (c) Presence of anti SS-A (Ro) or anti SS- B (La) antibodies.

   2. Secondary sjogren syndrome

   - Characteristic signs and symptoms of Sjogren's syndrome PLUS.
   - Clinical features sufficient to allow a diagnosis of rheumatoid arthritis, SLE, polymyositis, scleroderma, Billiary cirrhosis.

   Treatment is symptomatic-

   - Artificial tears.
   - Artificial saliva.
   - Sugarless candy or gum.
   - Sialogogues such as pilocarpine and cevimeline.
   - Patients with Sjogren's syndrome have an increased risk for lymphoma (44 times high).

Sialography

Helpful in diagnosis and staging of the disease.

- Early stage – punctate appearance (<1mm).
- This is followed by globular appearance (1-2mm).
- Late stages – cavitary sialectases (>2mm).

MALIGNANT TUMORS OF SALIVARY GLANDS

MALIGNANT PLEOMORPHIC ADENOMA (Malignant "Mixed" Tumor / Carcinoma ex pleomorphic adenoma)

- Specific criteria for recognizing a malignant "Mixed" tumor are not completely established. They show nuclear changes held as indicative of malignancy invasion of blood vessels, lymphatics or nerves, focal necrosis and obvious peripheral infiltration and destruction of normal tissue.
- Malignant cell pattern of transformation appears to be resembling epidermoid carcinoma or adenocarcinoma or both.

ADENOID CYSTIC CARCINOMA (Cylinderoma, adenocystic Basal cell carcinoma / Basaloid mixed tumor)

- Palatal mucosa in the most common site. Parotid, submaxillary and accessory glands are most commonly involved.
- Clinical manifestations include:
  - Early local pain.
  - Facial nerve paralysis
  - Fixation to deeper structures
  - Local invasion
  - Surface ulceration
- Histologic features
  - Typical cribriform "Honey – comb" or " Swiss – cheese" patterns.
  - Stromal connective tissue becomes hyalinized and surrounds tumor cells, forming a structural pattern of cylinder.
  - Perineural spread is a common feature.
  - Mitotic figures are extremely rare.
- Treatment - surgery + Radiation.

ACTINIC CELL CARCINOMA (Acinar cell or serous cell adenoma and Adeno carcinoma)

- Occurs chiefly in parotid. Most common intra oral site is lips and buccal mucosa.
- 4 Histological patterns
  Solid
  Papillary cystic
  Follicular
  Micro cystic
- Lymphoid elements common.

MUCOEPIDERMOID CARCINOMA

- Majority of cases involve parotid gland and intra oral accessory gland.
- Most common malignant salivary gland tumor of children.
- Because of their tendency to develop cystic areas, these intra oral lesions may resemble mucocele, especially those in retro molar area.
- Histologically, it is a pleomorphic tumor composed of mucus secreting cells, epidermoid - type cells and intermediate cells.
- Treatment - surgery for mild grade. Radiotherapy for intermediate and high grade.
- Central mucoepidermoid carcinoma of the jaw usually occurs in mandible in premolar - molar region and less in maxilla. It usually resemble dentigerous cyst, clinically and radiographically.

CLEAR CELL CARCINOMA (DONATH – SEIFERT TUMOR)

- Originates from intercalated duct and myoepithelial cells.
- Must be differentiated from a metastatic renal malignancy.

EPIDERMOID OR SQUAMOUS CELL CARCINOMA

- SCC in salivary glands has a grave prognosis since it exhibits infiltrative properties, metastasizes early and recurs readily.
- Treatment is by combined use surgery and radiotherapy.

OTHER SALIVARY GLAND DISEASE

NECTROTIZING SIALOMETAPLASIA

- It is a benign, inflammatory reaction of salivary gland tissue, which mimics malignancy.
- Most common cause is coagulation necrosis due to local ischaemia.
- More common in men.
- Palate in the most common site.
- Predisposing factors include -
  Trauma
  Dental injections
  Ill– fitted prosthesis
  Upper respiratory infections.
  Previous surgery
  Adjacent tumors
  Tobacco and alcohol.
- Self – limiting disease.

MUCOCELE (Mucus – extravasations phenomenon / mucus escape reaction)

- It is not a true cyst because it lacks an epithelial lining.

- Forms due to trauma and rupture of a salivary gland duct and spillage of mucin in surrounding tissue.
- Lower lip is the most common site.

RANULA

- Refers to mucocele that occurs in the floor of the mouth. ·
- Source of mucin spillage is usually the sublingual gland.
- *Plunging or cervical ranula* – A clinical variant where the spilled mucin dissects through the mylohyoid muscle and produces swelling within the neck.
- Treatment consists of marsupialization or removal of the feeding sublingual gland.

SALIVARY DUCT CYST (Mucus Retention cyst or sialocyst)

- It is true cysts, which arise, in salivary ducts.
- Cysts of major glands are more common in parotid. Intra oral cysts occur most frequently in the floor of mouth, buccal mucosa and lips.

SIALOLITHIASIS (Salivary Calculi / Stones)

- Most often develop within submandibular gland ducts due to long, tortuous upward path of duct, high calcium and phosphorus levels, mucoid secretions and dependent position of submandibular glands.
- May or mayn't be visible on standard radiographs due to varying degree of calcification.
- Sialography is helpful to diagnose radiolucent calculi (appears as ductal filling defect) and to differentiate sialolith from phlebolith or lymph node calcification.

SIALADENITIS (Inflammation of salivary glands)

- Occurs due to -
  - A. Infectious causes
    1. Viral - Mumps
       - Coxsackie A
       - ECHO
       - Choriomeningitis
       - Parainfluenza
       - CMV
    2. Bacterial - staphylococcus aureus
       - Streptococci
  - B. Non- infections causes (sialadenosis)
    - Sjogren's syndrome
    - Sarcoidosis
    - Radiation therapy
    - Various allergens.

- Sialography is contraindicated in acute infections.
- Chronic infections may give sac like acinar areas (sialectasia) on sialogram.
- Abscess cavities appear on CT as walled off areas of lower attenuation within an enlarged gland.
- USG may differentiate between diffuse inflammation (echo-free light image) and suppuration (less echo-free dark image).
- MRI shows inflamed glands as enlarged with a lower tissue signal on T1 weighed images.

KUTTNER TUMOR

Persistent enlargement of submandibular gland secondary to ducal obstructions.

SIALODOCHITIS

- Inflammation of ductal system of salivary glands.
- Apparent in sialograms as *"sausage string"* appearance, if interstitial fibrosis develops.

SIALORRHEA (Ptylism, Excessive salivation)

- Usually seen with gastroesophageal reflux disease, rabies, and heavy metal poisoning, certain medications such as lithium and cholinergic agonists.
- Treatment – Anticholinergics

  Transdermal scopolamine

  Ductal relocation in mentally retarded or cerebral palsy patients.

  Bilateral tympanic neurectomy.

QUESTIONS

1. **Etiology of mucocele is related to:**   [AIPG 2004]
   1. Mechanical trauma to the minor salivary gland excretory duct.
   2. Salivary calculi in the excretory duct of major salivary gland.
   3 Acute infections.
   4. Smoking tobacco.

Ans. **1**

2. **A 98 year old woman has sudden swelling in right floor of her mouth, the swelling is fluctuant, bluish pink and painless. The most likely diagnosis is:**   [AIPG 2003]
   1. Irritation fibrosis
   2. Schwannoma
   3. Hematoma
   4. Ranula

Ans. **4**

3. **Which of the following is the commonest benign tumor of the parotid in the child?**

[AIPG 2000]

1. Lymphangioma
2. Pleomorphic adenoma
3. Warthin's tumor
4. Adenocarcinoma

Ans. **3**

4. **Which of the following parotid mucous shows perineural spread?** [AIPG 99]
   1. Pleomorphic adenoma
   2. Adenoid cystic carcinoma
   3. Warthin's tumor
   4. Ductal papilloma

Ans. **2**

Perineural spread is seen in adenoid cystic carcinoma.

5. **Mucocele is a/an:** [AIPG 97]
   1. Retention cyst
   2. Extraction cyst
   3. Inclusion cyst
   4. None of the above

Ans. **1**

Mucocele can either be a retention cyst or can be due to extravasation of saliva from minor salivary glands.

6. **Sialography is used to detect anomaly of:** [AIPG 97]
   1. Salivary duct only
   2. Salivary gland
   3. Salivary gland and duct
   4. Salivary gland tumours

Ans. **3**

With help of sialography any calcification in duct or gland, strictures, inflamed duct, acinar enlargement etc. can be assessed.

7. **Which of the following is of salivary gland origin?** [AIPG 96]
   1. Acinic cell carcinoma
   2. Granular cell myoblastoma
   3. Chondrosarcoma
   4. All of the above

Ans. **1**

Granular cell myoblastoma arise from neural tissue and chondrosarcoma from cartilage.

8. Which of the following is not true for ranula? [AIPG 96]

1. It forms insidiously in floor of the mouth
2. It is painless
3. Involves partial blockage of sublingual sali-vary gland duct
4. None of the above

Ans. **4**

9. The aetiology of Mikulicz's disease is: [AIPG 94]

1. Bacterial
2. Viral
3. Autoimmune
4. Genetic

Ans. **3**

This benign lymphoepithelial lesion exhibits both inflammatory and neoplastic feature. There is bilateral enlargement of parotid and submandibular glands.

10. The most common neoplasm of the parotid gland is: [AIPG 93]

1. Warthin's tumour
2. Benign mixed tumour
3. Monomorphic adenoma
4. Adenoid cystic carcinoma

Ans. **2**

Benign mixed tumor or pleomorphic adenoma is the most common tumor of parotid gland. Warthin's tumor occurs exclusively in parotid, but the frequency is less. Palatal accessory glands are most common site for adenoid cystic carcinoma.

11. Common cause of dry mouth in the adults is: [AIPG 93]

1. Tranquilizers
2. Radiation
3. Salivary gland atrophy
4. Sialolithiasis

Ans. **1**

Tranquilizers are the most common cause of xerostomia in adults.

12. Which tumour does not occur in minor salivary gland? [AIPG 93]

1. Pleomorphic adenoma
2. Adenocarcinoma
3. Mucoepidermoid carcinoma
4. Warthin's tumour

Ans. **4**

Warthin's tumor almost exclusively occurs in parotid, rarely in submandibular glands.

13. **Which of the following salivary gland neoplasm is least likely to occur in minor glands?**
[AIPG 92]

1. Warthin's tumor
2. Adenocarcinoma
3. Pleomorphic adenoma
4. Acinic cell carcinoma

Ans. **1**

Warthin's tumor chiefly involves the parotid glands. Adenocarcinoma most commonly involves minor salivary glands. Pleomorphic adenoma involves parotid followed by minor salivary glands of palate and lips.

14. **A painful crater like 1.5 cm ulcer develops with in one week on the hard palate mucosa of a 50 year old female. The most likely diagnosis:**
[AIPG 92]

1. Actinomycosis
2. Squamous cell carcinoma
3. Pleomorphic adenoma
4. Necrotizing sialometaplasia

Ans. **4**

Nectrotizing sialometaplasia occurs as a painful ulcer on hard palate due to local ischaemia. It may also be seen on buccal mucosa, lip and retromolar area. It is marked by acinar necrosis and squamous metaplasia of salivary duct.

15. **A mixed tumor of intraoral accessory glands most frequently occurs on the:**
[AIPG 91]

1. Tongue
2. Palate
3. Lower lip
4. Buccal mucosa

Ans. **2**

Mixed tumor accounts for 38-43% of minor gland tumor, of which plate is the most common site, followed by lips and buccal mucosa. 53% - 77% of parotid tumors are benign mixed tumors.

16. **A cyst occurs under the tongue, caused by obstruction of a salivary gland. Such a cyst is called:**
[AIPG 91]

1. Mucocele
2. Ranula
3. Dermoid cyst
4. Dentigerous cyst

Ans. **2**

It is an extravasation or intravasation type of salivary cyst, which contains saliva. Appears as a bluish dome shaped swelling on floor of mouth.

17. **Sialoliths are most commonly found during radiographic examination of the: [AIPG 1990]**

    1. Parotid gland
    2. Maxillary Sinus
    3. Submandibular duct
    4. Sublingual gland duct

Ans. 3

Submandibular duct – 80-90%

Parotid- 5-15%

Sublingual 2-5%

This is because; Wharton's duct is longer, more tortuous course.

NOTES

13 Diseases of Skin

HERIDITARY ECTODERMAL DYSPLASIA

- Syndrome characterized by a congenital dysplasia of one or more ectodermal structures:
    - Hypohidrosis (or Anhidrosis)
    - Hypotrichosis
    - Hypodontia
- X- linked recessive character. Males more commonly affected.
- Soft, smooth, thin, dry skin.
- Lack or absence of sweat glands leading to hyperpyrexia.
- Bridge of nose is depressed, frontal bossing and protuberant lips.
- Growth of jaws is not impaired.
- Sometimes, salivary glands are hypoplastic leading to xerostomia.

CHONDRO – ECTODERMAL DYSPLASIA (Ellis–Van Creveld Syndrome)

- Ectodermal tissues are affected.
- Sweat mechanism is normal.
- Involvement of nails (koilonychia), Bilateral polydactyly, chondrodysplasia, congenital heart disease.
- Fusion of middle portion of upper lip to the maxillary gingival margin eliminating the normal mucolabial sulcus.
- Natal teeth, prematurely erupted deciduous teeth, delayed eruption of permanent teeth, malformed teeth, and enamel hypoplasia.

PSORIASIS

- Small, sharply delineated dry papules, each covered by a delicate silvery scale, which resembles a thin layer of mica.
- *AUSPITZ'S SIGN:* If the deep scales are removed, one or more tiny bleeding points are disclosed.

- Papules enlarge at the periphery; tend to become infiltrating and elevated.
- Roughly symmetrical lesions, involve extensor surfaces of extremities, more severe in winters.
- Uncommon in children.
- Etiology is unknown. Polygenic inheritance pattern is seen linked to HLA antigen.
- Increase in serum IgG, IgA, salivary IgA, and IgE.
- Oral involvement is rare.
- May be associated with angular cheilosis, fissured tongue, geographic tongue, and Reiter's syndrome.
- Histologic features - Parakeratosis.
  Absence of stratum granulosum.
  Elongation and clubbing of retepegs.
  Monro's abscesses (Intra epithelial micro abscesses).
  Perivascular and periadenal lymphocytic and histiocytic infiltration.
  Very rapid turnover rate of skin epithelial cells (3-4 days).

PITYRIASIS ROSEA

- Acute skin eruption of unknown etiology.
- Primary lesion or *herald spot* (bright red) occurs 7-10 days prior to generalized outbreak.
- Individual exanthematous lesions are ovoid with long axis parallel to natural lines of cleavage of skin, covered by silvery scale.
- Asymptomatic oral lesions can occur which heals spontaneously.

MUCOCUTANEOUS LYMPH -NODE SYNDROME (Kawasaki Disease)

- Believed to be viral or "collagen-vascular" disease.
- Occurs mainly in children.
- Fever, bilateral conjuctival congestion, edema of extremities; dryness, redness and fissuring of lips; acute, non-purulent cervical lymphadenopathy.

KERATOSIS FOLLICULARIS (Darier's Disease / Darier – White's Disease)

- Genodermatosis, autosomal dominant inheritance.
- Related to vitamin A metabolism.
- Palmer, plantar keratosis, nails changes, firm papules over head, scalp, neck, shoulders.
- Oral mucosa shows *cobblestone appearance* with rough, verrucous plaques.
- Histological picture – typical cells called *corps, ronds and grains*.
- Suprabasilar cleavage.
- Hyperplasia of epithelial rests of Malassez in PDL.
- *"Leafing out"* pattern of parabasal cells.
- There is a defect in the desmosome tonofilament complex.
- Sevenfold decrease in turnover time of epithelium.

INCONTINENTIA PIGMENTI (Bloch-Sulzberger syndrome)

- Heavy melanin pigmentation of epithelium is the hallmark of the syndrome.
- Lethal in males.
- Onset shortly after birth, vesiculo bullous lesions are accompanied with marked eosinophilia.
- Delayed eruption of teeth, congenitally missing or malformed teeth (cone- shaped).

POROKERATOSIS OF MIBELLI

- Faulty keratinization of skin followed by atrophy.
- Epidermoid carcinoma may develop from atrophic skin.
- "Cornoid lamella" on histologic section.

DYSKERATOSIS CONGENITA

- X - Linked recessive inheritance. Occurs in males only.
- Predispose to high incidence of oral cancer.
- Associated with *fanconi's anaemia*.
- 3 typical signs –
  - Oral leukoplakia
  - Dystrophy of nails
  - Pigmentation of skin

ACANTHOSIS NIGRICANS

- 3 main types-
  (a) Benign
  (b) Malignant
  (c) Pseudoacanthosis nigricans
- 4th type called syndromal acanthosis nigricans is associated with other diseases like:
  - Insulin resistant diabetes.
  - Congenital lipodystrophy
  - Lupoid hepatitis
  - Hepatolenticular degeneration.
  - Hepatic cirrhosis
  - Bloom's syndrome
  - Corticosteroids and nicotinic acid therapy.
- Verrucous, pigmented skin lesions.
- Papillomatous growths on lips.
- Hypertrophy of filliform papillae.
- Gingival enlargements.

EPIDERMOLYSIS BULLOSA

- Classified as: -
    - (i) Epidermolysis bullosa simplex
        - a. Generalized form
        - b. Localized from (Weber- Cockayne syndrome)
    - (ii) Epidermolysis bullosa dystrophic- dominant.
    - (iii) Epidermolysis bullosa dystrophic- recessive
    - (iv) Junctional epidermolysis bullosa (Herlitz's disease).
    - (v) Epidermolysis bullosa acquisita.
- There is destruction of basal and suprabasal cells, PAS - positive basement membrane remains on the dermal side of separation.
- Nikolsky's sign positive in recessive form.
- Bullae are painful, heals by scarring, which may obliterate the sulci and cause restriction of tongue, dysphagia and esophageal strictures.
- Dental defects like rudimentary teeth, congenitally absent teeth and hypoplastic teeth.
- 3 criteria for diagnosis of junctional form -
    - (i) Onset at birth.
    - (ii) Absence of scarring, milia or pigmentation.
    - (iii) Death within 3 months of age.

DERMATITIS HERPETIFORMIS (Duhring – Brocq disease)

- Associated with malabsorption enteropathy.
- Unrelated to herpes virus.
- Accumulation of neutrophils and eosinophils in dermal papillae produce micro abscesses.
- Presence of eosinophils is a typical finding.
- DIF staining positive at epidermal dermal junction in a granular pattern.
- Sulfapyridine is the treatment of choice.

ACRODERMATITIS ENTEROPATHICA

- Related to malabsorption of zinc.
- Lesions occur in crops.
- Zinc supplements should be given.

LUPUS ERYTHRMATOSUS

- Two basic forms
    - (a) Systemic LE (SLE)
    - (b) Discoid LE (DLE)
- Etiology includes genetic, immunological abnormality, viral infection, and autoimmunity.
- Female: male ratio is 8 : 1

SLE

- Butterfly shaped erythematous patches over cheek and nose.
- *"Wire loops"* pattern of fibrinoid thickened glomerular capillaries in kidneys.
- Cardiac involvement.
- Considered a "collagen disease".

DLE

- Slightly elevated red or purple macules, often covered with scales, forceful removal of scales reveals *"Carpet – tack"* extensions which had dipped into enlarged pilosebaceous canal.
- Exhibits scarring.

Laboratory findings

- L.E cells inclusion phenomenon -In SLE. Rosette of neutrophils surrounding a pale nuclear mass derived from lymphocytes.
- γ - Globulin in serum is elevated.
- Positive Coombs test.
- Anaemia, leukopenia, thrombocytopenia, elevated ESR, antinuclear antibodies.
- Immuno fluorescence - Detect IgG, IgM and IgA at epidermal – dermal junction or basement membrane zone in a *"particulate" (or "speckled") pattern* also known as *"shaggy", "granular – band"* pattern or *positive lupus band test.*

SYSTEMIC SCLEROSIS (Scleroderma, Dermatosclerosis, Hidebound disease)

- 2 forms
    - (a) Diffuse systemic
    - (b) Localized or morphea type
        - Circumscribed
        - Linear
- Progressive fibrosis of skin and multiple organs by vascular insufficiency in diffuse form.
- Raynaud's phenomenon is nearly always present.
- Acrosclerosis = Raynaud's phenomenon + sclerodactyly + sclerosis of neck and face.
- Females: males = 2: 1
- **CREST SYNDROME** – A variant of systemic sclerosis
    - C - Calcinosis cutis
    - R - Raynaud's phenomenon
    - E - Esophageal dysfunction
    - S - Sclerodactyly
    - T - Telangiectasia
- Morphea or circumscribed form is manifested by appearance of well defined slightly elevated or depressed, cutaneous patches, white with violaceous halo.

- Linear form occurs as linear bands, made up of a furrow with an elevated ridge on one side (*coup de sabre appearance*).
- Tongue, soft palate and larynx are commonly involved which manifest as dysphagia, dysphonia, microstomia reduced oral opening.
- Salivary glands show changes similar to Sjogren's syndrome.
- Generalized PDL widening.
- Sometimes, resorption at angle of mandible and condyle or coronoid process may also occur.

EHLERS -DANLOS SYNDROME

- 8 forms of disease are recognized out of which EDS I, II, III are common.
- Characterized by hyperelasticity of skin, hyper extensibility of joints, Excessive bruising due to fragility of blood vessels, Defective wound healing.
- Circus *"Rubber man"* where hyperelasticity of skin is pronounced.
- Ecchymotic type - EDS IV.
- Scars tend to spread rather than contract in time.
- Oral mucosa becomes fragile and bruised easily.
- Recurrent dislocations of jaw due to hyper mobility of TMJ.
- Lack of normal scalloping of DEJ.
- Increased tendency to form pulp stones.
- Enamel hypoplasia
- Extensive periodontal destruction.
- Positive capillary fragility test.

FOCAL DERMAL HYPOPLASIA SYNDROME (GOLTZ - GORLIN SYNDROME)

- Meso ectodermal dysplasia.
- Characterized by focal absence of dermis, skin atrophy, streaky pigmentation, telangiectasia, and multiple papilloma of mucosa.
- Papillomas of oral mucosa are common.
- Microdontia, enamel hypoplasia.

SOLAR ELASTOSIS (Senile Elastosis / Actinic Elastosis)

- A degenerative condition of skin.
- Such skin is termed sailor's skin or farmer's skin
- Connective tissue shows basophilic degeneration.

QUESTIONS

1. Ectodermal dysplasia is -   [AIPG 2005]

   1. Autosomal recessive.

2. Autosomal dominant.

3. X-linked dominant.

4. X-linked recessive.

Ans. 4

Ectodermal dysplasia is a triad marked with partial or complete anodontia, decreased sweating and thinning of hair. Manifested in males more frequently than females. However, it may also be transmitted as autosomal dominant or recessive trait in some cases.

2. All are findings in ectodermal dysplasia except: [AIPG 2002]

1. Hereditary disorder

2. Depressed nasal bridge

3. Lip withdrawn inside

4. Defective mental development.

Ans. 4

These is no mental deficit

3. Scleroderma involves: [AIPG 94]

1. Tighting of oral mucosa and periodontal involvement

2. Multiple palmar keratosis

3. Raynaud's phenomenon

4 All of the above

Ans. 4

Other features are diffuse systemic sclerosis of many internal organs like GIT, lungs, cardiovascular, renal, musculoskeletal and central nervous systems, CREST syndrome.

4. Darier's disease is associated with: [AIPG 94]

1. Pernicious anemia.

2. Rickets with involvement of teeth and bones.

3. Vitamin A deficiency and involvement of oral epithelium and skin.

4. Diffuse tender ulceration on the palate predo-minantly.

Ans. 3

Darier's disease or keratosis follicularies is a genodermatosis, which is transmitted as an autosomal dominant characteristic. It gives a cobblestone appearance to oral mucosa and thought to be related to vitamin A deficiency. Corps, ronds and grains are important histological findings.

5. Premature exfoliation of teeth is seen in: [AIPG 94]

1. Papillon-Lefevre syndrome

2. Hypophosphatasia

3. Juvenile diabetes

4. All of the above

Ans. 4

6. **A 3-year old child presents with only deciduous canine and molars. The child has light fine hair, light complexion and over all appearance of an older person. The findings suggest:**

[AIPG 1989, 1992]

1. Cleidocranial dysostosis
2. Osteogenesis imperfecta
3. Crouzon's disease
4. Hereditary ectodermal dysplasia

Ans. 4

Hereditary ectodermal dysplasia is marked by hypodontia, hypohidrosis and hypotrichosis.

14 Diseases of Blood

DISEASE OF RED BLOOD CELLS

PERNICIOUS ANAEMIA / ADDISON'S ANAEMIA / BIEMER'S ANAEMIA

- Due to atrophy of gastric mucosa, resulting in failure to secrete the "intrinsic factor".
- Generalized weakness.
- *"Beefy-red"* tongue with glossitis, glossodynia and glossopyrosis.
- Gradual atrophy of papillae of tongue which leads to "bald" tongue also known as *"HUNTER"S / MOELLER'S GLOSSITIS"*.
- Numbness or tingling of extremities.
- RBC'S - macrocytic, polychromatophilic cells, stippled cells, nucleated cells.
- *Howell- Jolly bodies* and *Cabot's rings.*
- Achlorhydria or lack of gastric HCl secretion with reduction of parietal cells.
- Hypersegmented neutrophils and enlarged platelets.
- Schilling test is positive.

APLASTIC ANAEMIA

- Pancytopenia due to depression of bone marrow.
- *Fanconi's syndrome* – congenital and sometimes familial aplastic anaemia associated with a variety of other congenital defects like bone abnormalities, microcephaly, hypogenitalism and a generalized olive brown pigmentation of skin.
- Secondary aplastic anaemia may occur due to radiation, allergy, drugs.
- Presents as petechiae, purpura, frank hematomas, spontaneous gingival hemorrhage, ulcerative lesions, lack of resistance to infection.
- RBC count decreases
  - CT normal
  - Clot retraction poor
  - BT Increases
  - Tourniquet test positive.

THALASSEMIA / COOLEY'S ANAEMIA / MEDITERRANEAN DISEASE / ERYTHRO BLASTIC ANAEMIA

- Heterogeneous group characterized by diminished synthesis of α or β globin chain of Hb-A.
- 2 types –
  - (a) Heterozygotes or Thalassemia minor or Thalassemia trait.
  - (b) Homozygous β thalassemias or thalassemias major.
- 2 forms of α - Thalassemia –
  - (a) Hb-H disease (mild).
  - (b) Hb Bart's disease with hydrops fetalis.
- Mongoloid features, flaring of maxillary anteriors depressed bridge of nose, unusual prominence of premaxilla, poor spacing of teeth, a marked open bite, prominent malar bone.
- Ashen gray skin due to combination of pallor, jaundice and haemosiderosis.

Laboratory findings

- Hypochromic microcytes anaemis.
- WBC count elevated.
- Presence of *"safety-pin"* cells and *"Target-cells"*.
- *Heinz bodies* are formed by the precipitation of alpha chains.
- Increased serum bilirubin.
- Cellular hyperplasia of bone marrow.

Radiographic features

- Extreme thickening of diploe producing *"crew-cut"* or *"Hair-on-end"* appearance of surface of skull.
- Osteoporosis of skull and long bones.
- Intraoral radiographs show *"salt and pepper appearance"*.

SICKLE CELL ANAEMIA

- Normal adult Hb A is genetically altered to produce sickle Hb (HbS) by the substitution of valine for glutamine at the sixth position of the β - globin chain.
- Patient is weak dysphonic, pain in joints, limbs and abdomen.
- Systolic murmur and cardiomegaly also occur.
- Jaundice and pallor of oral mucosa.
- Delayed eruption and hypoplasia of teeth.
- Predispose the bone to osteomyelitis.

Radiographic features

"Hair-on-end" pattern on skull radiograph.

Step ladder or chicken mesh appearance on dental radiographs.

Areas of sclerosis or radiopacity.

Osteoporosis.

ERYTHROBLASTOSIS FETALIS

- Congenital hemolytic anaemia due to Rh incompatibility. Transplacental leakage of RBC'S from fetus to the mother results in immunization of the mother and formation of antibodies which, when transferred back to the fetus by the same route produces fetal hemolysis.
- Rh negative mothers are given anti-D gamma globulin to prevent immunization since it binds to antigenic receptor sites on fetal red cells, making them non immunogenic.
- Present as anaemia, jaundice, compensatory erytheropoesis, and fetal hydrops.
- Green, brown or blue hue to the teeth (intrinsic stains).
- *"Rh hump"* – ring like defect due to enamel hypoplasia, seen at the incisal edges of the anterior teeth and the middle portion of deciduous cuspid and first molar crown.

IRON DEFICIENCY ANAEMIA / PLUMMER VINSON SYNDROME / HYSTERICAL DYSPHAGIA / PATTERSON KELLY SYNDROME

- Predisposes to CA of upper GIT.
- Angular chelitis, glossodynia, dyphagia due to esophageal stricture or web, dry mouth and koilonychias.

POLYCYTHEMIA VERA / VAQUEZ'S DISEASE / OSLER'S DISEASE

- Absolute increase in RBC count and total blood volume.
- Hb concentration increases to 18-24 gm%, leading to increased blood viscosity and thrombosis.
- Hyperuricemia and hyperuricosuria are seen in 40% cases.
- Leukocyte alkaline phosphatase is increased.
- Headache, dizziness, tinnitus, visual disturbances, mental confusion, slurring of speech, spleenomegaly.
- Purplish red oral mucosa, ruddy cyanosis of face and extremities.
- Crystal violet tongue.
- Gingiva is swollen, engorged and often bleeding.
- Secondary polycythemia is seen in hypoxic conditions such as at high altitudes, chronic pulmonary disease, congenital heart disease and renal disease.
- Apparent polycythemia occurs in diabetic ketoacidosis, postsurgical dehydration, vomiting and diarrhoea.

DISEASES INVOLVING WHITE BLOOD CELLS

AGRANULOCYTOSIS

- More common in adults, particularly women, health professions.
- High fever, chills, sore throat, regional lymphadenitis.
- Necrotizing ulcerations of oral mucosa, tonsils and pharynx, particularly involving gingiva and palate.

- Ragged necrotic ulcers covered by a gray or even black membrane with little or no inflammatory cell infiltrate.
- WBC count is often less than 2000 per cubic millimeter with an almost complete absence of granulocytes.

CYCLIC NEUTROPENIA / PERIODIC NEUTROPENIA

- Unusual form of agranulocytosis characterized by a periodic or cyclic diminution in circulating polymorphonuclear neutrophils.
- Mostly seen in infants or young children.
- Unlike other types of primary agranulocytosis rampant bacterial infection is not a significant feature, presumably because the neutrophil count is low for such a short time.
- Severe gingivitis and ulceration correspond to period of neutropenias.
- In children, repeated gingivitis lead to considerable loss of supporting bone (prepubertal periodontitis).
- The cycle commonly occurs often every three weeks.

CHEDIAK- HIGASHI SYNDROME

- Genetic disease, an autosomal recessive trait.
- Oculocutaneous albinism, photophobia, nystagmus, recurrent infections.
- Hair will have gray streaks.
- Neuropathy and ataxia are prominent features in some patients.
- Oral ulceration, severe gingivitis, glossitis, periodontal break down.
- Giant abnormal granules in circulating leukocytes are the hallmark of the syndrome.

INFECTIOUS MONONUCLEOSIS / GLANDULAR FEVER / KISSING DISEASE

- Caused by EBV.
- Chiefly occurs in children and young adults.
- Oral lesion include stomatitis, acute gingivitis, appearance of a white or gray membrane in various areas, palatal petechiae and occasional ulcers, oronasopharyngeal bleeding.
- Laboratory findings.
  - Atypical lymphocytes in the circulating blood.
  - Antibodies to EBV.
  - Increased neutrophil antibody title (1:4096) i.e. Positive Paul-Bunnell test.
  - Increase in WBC.
  - Thrombocytopenia.
- Bed rest, adequate diet and short-term steroid therapy is the usual form of therapy.

LEUKAEMIA

- 3 types –
- (a) Myeloid (Myelogenous, Myelocytic)

(b) Lymphoid (Lymphogenous, Lymphocytic, Lymphatic)

(c) Monocytic.

- Etiology is unknown EBV, radiation, chemicals may be the cause.
- Chromosomal abnormalities commonly occur in leukaemic patients. *Philadelphia chromosome* occur in CML. It is a translocation of chromosomal material from chromosome 22 to 9.
- Acute leukemia is common in children and young adults, while chronic form is seen in middle or older age.
- Males are more commonly affected.

Acute Leukaemia	Chronic Leukemia
(a) Sudden onset, fever, headache, generalized swelling of LN, petechial and ecchymotic hemorrhages.	(a) Chronic disease patient may appear in excellent health or may exhibit pallor.
(b) LN enlargement is usually 1st manifestation.	(b) LN enlargement is common in CLL, but uncommon in CML.
(c) Spleen, liver and kidney may enlarge due to leukaemic infiltration.	(c) Spleenomegaly, hepatomegaly, salivary gland enlargement usually seen.
	(d) Skin is usually involved – petichiae or ecchymosis, papules, pustules, bullae, areas of pigmentation, herpes zoster, itching and burning.
	(e) Destructive lesions of bone may occur which results in pathologic fracture or osteomyelitis.

- *"Sub leukemia" or "Aleukaemia"* – WBC count of the peripheral blood is normal or even subnormal in which abnormal or immature leukocytes may or may not be present.
- *Acute leukemia* – Both BT and CT are prolonged.
- Tourniquet test is positive.
- WBC count may be sub normal in early stage, but it usually rise in terminal stage to 100,000/cmm.
- *"Stem cell leukemia"* – when it is not possible to distinguish the exact type of leukemic cells.
- Oral manifestations are more common in acute stage and in AML. These include cervical lymphadenopathy, oral bleeding, gingival infiltrates, oral infections and oral ulcers.
- Gingival hyperplasia is most constant features except in edentulous patients, usually generalized, boggy, edematous and deep red which easily bleeds.
- Spontaneous bleeding occurs when platelet count fall below 20,000/cmm.
- Chloromas- Localized tumors consisting of leukaemic cells. The surface of these tumors turns green when exposed to light because of the presence of myeloperoxidase.
- AML – worst prognosis.
- ALL – CNS involvement is common.
  - Least likely to produce oral lesions.

DISEASES INVOLVING PLATELETS

NON-THROMBOCYTOPENIC PURPURA

- There is increased permeability of capillaries.
- Etiology includes autoimmune disorders, viral and bacterial infections, structural malformation (eg. Connective Tissue disorders).

THROMBOCYTOPENIC PURPURA

- Abnormal reduction in no. of circulating blood platelets.

PRIMARY THROMBOCYTOPENIA /WERLHOF'S DISEASE / PURPURA HEMORRHAGICA AND IDIOPATHIC PURPURA)

- Acute form is seen in children while chronic form occurs in adults.
- Oral lesions – profuse gingival hemorrhage, petichae on palate.
- Laboratory findings
  - Platelet count < 60,000 /cmm
  - BT is prolonged.
  - CT is normal.
  - Capillary fragility increased.
  - Torniquet test is positive.
- Secondary thrombocytopenia is usually associated with radiation, drugs and chemicals, fanconi's anaemia, idiopathic, infections etc.

THROMBOTIC THROMBOCYTOPENIC PURPURA

- Immunologically mediated.
- Characterized by thrombocytopenia, hemolytic anaemia, fever, neurologic dysfunction and renal failure.
- Major finding is microthrombi in blood vessels.

ALDRICH SYNDROME (WISKOTT – ALDRICH SYNDROME)

- X linked recessive trait, occurs in males.
- Characterized by thrombocytopenic purpura, eczema, increased susceptibility to infection due to inability to form antibody against polysaccharide containing organisms such as pneumococci, H. influenza, and coliform bacilli.
- Malignant lymphoma often occurs.
- Lab. Findings –
  - Both qualitative and quantitative defects of platelets.
  - Platelet count 18,000 to 80,000 per cmm.
  - Anisocytosis.
  - Deficiency of ADP nucleotide storage pool.

THROMBAESTENIA / GLANZMANN DISEASE

- Qualitative defect in platelets.
- Mostly familial.
- BT prolonged
- Clot retraction is impaired.
- Platelet count is normal.
- There is a reduced amount of certain membrane glycoproteins on surface of platelet.

THROMBOCYTOPATHIC PURPURA / THROMBOCYTOPATHIA

- Platelet count is normal.
- Severe bleeding tendency, although petichae are rare.
- BT prolonged or normal.
- Generally due to defective platelet aggression.
- *"Storage pool Disease"* - in this form there is deficiency of the non metabolic storage pool of platelet adenine nucleotides.
- *"Portsmouth syndrome"* – there is normal ADP-induced platelet aggregation but abnormal collagen induced aggregation.
- *Bernard Soulier syndrome* – normal platelet aggregation to collagen and ADP but an abnormal response to fibrinogen.

THROMBOCYTHEMIA / THROMBOCYTHOSIS

- Increase in number of circulating blood platelets. High concentration interferes with formation of thromboplastin.
- Abnormal platelet aggregation.
- CT, PT, Clot retraction and tourniquet test are all normal, BT prolonged.
- Most common treatment is administration of radioactive phosphorus.

DISEASE INVOLVING SPECIFIC BLOOD FACTORS

HEMOPHILIA / BLEEDER'S DISEASE / DISEASE OF HAPSBURG / DISEASE OF KINGS

- X-linked recessive disorder.
- Hemophilia A - Factor VIII Deficiency.
    B - Factor IX Deficiency (Christmas disease)
    C - Factor XI Deficiency
    Parahaemophilia- Factor V Deficiency.
- Oral manifestations include gingival hemorrhage, severe prolonged hemorrhage during tooth eruption and exfoliation.
- *"Pseudo tumor"* of hemophilia – There is subperiosteal bleeding, with reactive new bone formation causing tumor like expansion of the bone.

- *"Rubber band"* extraction is usually indicated which causes exfoliation of tooth through pressure necrosis of PDL.
- CT is prolonged, BT, PT normal.

VON-WILLEBRAND'S DISEASE / PSEUDOHEMOPHILIA / VASCULAR HEMOPHILIA

- Normal platelet count, CT, serum fibrinogen, PT.
- BT prolonged to an extremely high range.
- Tourniquet test is positive.
- Whereas classic hemophilia is caused by a deficiency of only one of the three components of factor VIII; classic Von- Willebrand's disease is caused by decreases in all three functional components of factor VIII.

PARAHEMOPHILIA

- Due to deficiency of factor V (proaccelerin).
- CT, PT are prolonged, BT normal.

AFIBRINOGENEMIA AND HYPOFIBRINOGENEMIA

- In congenital forms, there is usually complete absence of fibrin while in acquired form; there is deficiency of fibrin.
- Clinically indistinguishable from hemophilia, but hemarthrosis is not prominent.
- CT and PT are infinite.
- Tourniquet test is normal.
- ESR is zero.
- The peripheral blood fails to clot even after the addition of thrombin.

DYSFIBRINOGENEMIA

- There is impairment of the rate at which thrombin cleaves fibrinopeptides from fibrinogen.
- There may be replacement of one amino acid residue by another in the $-NH_2$ terminal part of the Aα chain of fibrinogen.

MACROGLOBULINEMIA / MACROGLOBULINEMIA OF WALDENSTROM

- It is related to
  - (a) A variant of multiple myeloma.
  - (b) *Bing –Neel syndrome* (hyperglobulinemia with CNS involvement).
  - (c) Variant of plasmacytoma.
  - (d) Altered immunologic reaction.
  - (e) Plasma cell dyscrasia so that there is excessive proliferation of B- lymphocytes.
- Associated with bleeding tendencies.
- Xerostomia.
- Severe anaemia (Hb-4-6gm/dl)

- Gelling of serum upon cooling at room temperature or lower temperature.
- Bone marrow smear shows increase in mononuclear cells.
- Bence Jones proteinuria may be present in few patients.
- Chlorambutol is treatment of choice along with plasmapheresis.

CRYOGLOBULINEMIA

- Presence of cryoglobulins in blood, which precipitates on exposure to cold.
- Mild cryoglobulinemia may be present in rheumatoid arthritis, periarteritis nodosa, SLE, Lymphoma, cirrhosis polycythemia, heart disease.
- May be associated with spontaneous bleeding from nose and mouth, decubitus ulcers and gangrene of lower extremities.

RESULTS OF HEMOSTATIC SCREENING TESTS FOR SELECTED BLEEDING DISORDERS

BLEEDING DISORDER	SCREENING LABORATORY TEST			
	PLATELET COUNT	PT/INR	aPTT	BT
Thrombocytopenia, Leukaemia	↓	N	N	↑
F VIII, IX, XI deficiency, heparin anticoagulant	N	N	↑	N
F II, V, X deficiency, Vitamin K deficiency, intestinal malabsorption	N	↑	↑	N
F VII deficiency, Coumarin anticoagulant, Liver disease	N	↑	N	N
Von Willebrand's disease	↓		↑	↑
DIC, Severe liver disease	↓	↑	↑	↑
F XIII deficiency	N	N	N	N
Vascular wall defect	N	N	N	↑

N= NORMAL, ↓ = DECREASED, ↑ = INCREASED

LABORATORY TESTS FOR ASSESSING HEMOSTASIS	
TEST	NORMAL RANGE
Platelet Count	1.50,000-4,50,000/cmm
Bleeding time	<7 min (by Simplate), 1-6 min(modified Ivy's test)
Prothrombin time/International normalized ratio	Control+/- 1 sec (PT=11-13 sec, INR=1 sec)
Activated partial thromboplastin time	Comparable to control (15-35 sec)
Thrombin time	Control+/- 3 sec (9-13 sec)
Coagulation factor assays	60-100% F VIII activity

PRINCIPAL PRODUCTS FOR MANAGEMENT OF PATIENTS WITH BLEEDING DISORDERS

- Platelets 1 unit raises the count by 10-12,000/cmm
- Fresh frozen plasma
- Cryoprecipitate
- F VIII concentrate
- F IX concentrate
- DDAVP
- ε-Aminocaproic acid
- Tranexamic acid.

15 Diseases of Muscles

MILD RESTRICTED MUSCULAR DYSTROPHY

- Primarily involves muscles of face and shoulders.
- *"Myopathic facies"* - weakness of facial muscles. Patient is unable to smile, whistle.
- *"Tapir – lips"*- lips develop a characteristic looseness and protrusion.

DYSTROPHIC MYOTONIA

- There is ptosis of eyelids and atrophy of masseter and sternocleidomastoid muscles.
- Characteristic *"myopathic - facies"*.
- *"Swan-neck"* appearance.
- Occasional myotonia of tongue muscles and recurrent dislocations of TMJ.

CONGENITAL MYTONIA (Thomsen's disease)

- *"Percussion contraction"* occurs with electrical or physical stimulation of muscles.
- There is delay in relaxation of contracted muscles.
- *"Herculean- Appearance"* due to muscular hypertrophy.
- Blinking with strong closure of eyes can produce prolonged contraction of lids.

ACQUIRED MYOTONIA

- Facial muscles are often involved in cases of:
  - Epilepsy
  - Tetany
  - Infectious myositis
  - Diseases of Central Nervous system.
  - Pericoronal infection
  - Hysteria

PARAMYOTONIA

- Non progressive myotonia.
- Cramping attacks are precipitated by exposure to cold.
- The eyelids are closed and face assumes "mask-like appearance".

HYPOTONIA

- Complete absence or reduction of tonus of muscles.
- *"Floppy infant syndrome"*- There in generalized weakness so that the body of infant hangs limply with inability to sit, stand or walk.

MYASTHENIA GRAVIS

- Progressive weakness of skeletal muscles, particularly those innervated by cranial nerves.
- There is a defect in neuromuscular transmission; fault in Acetyl choline mechanism.
- Occurs chiefly in middle aged females.
- Muscles of mastication and facial expression are involved.
- *"Sorrowful appearance"* of face.
- Thymic hyperplasia or tumors may be associated with this disease.
- Physostigmine administered intramusculary for diagnosis as well as to improve the strength of muscles.

DERMATOMYOSITIS (Polymyositis / neuromyositis)

- *"Calcinosis cutis"* or *"calcinosis universalis"* are often associated with acute form.
- Chronic form may not show dermal involvement.
- Oral lesions presents as diffuse stomatitis, pharyngitis, telangiectasia, dysphonia, dysphagia.
- Creatinuria, elevated serum aldolase and transaminase is a constant finding.

GENERALIZED MYOSITIS OSSIFICANS (Progressive / Interstitial myositis ossificans)

- *"Petrified man"* appearance due to bony transformation of muscles.
- Masseter muscle is often involved leading to fixation of jaw.
- Death occurs due to respiratory embarrassment (involvement of inter costal muscles).

TRAUMATIC MYOSITIS OSSIFICANS (Myositis ossificans circumscripta/Ossifying Hematoma)

- Ossification in muscle following either a single acute traumatic episode or a series of minor traumatic injuries to muscle.
- May occur as an occupational disease e.g. *"Rider's bone"* in thigh of horseback riders and jockeys, *"Drill or exercise bone"* in infantrymen in deltoid muscles.
- *"Fascitis ossificans"* - when ossifying lesions occurs in superficial tissue away from muscle.
- *"Feathery type"* calcification in muscle is seen on radiographs.

CONGENITAL FACIAL DIPLEGIA (Mobius syndrome)

- Facial diplegia with bilateral paralysis of ocular muscles, particularly abducens.
- Everted lips, failure to close eyes during sleep, partial or complete facial paralysis, and mouth may remain open.

16 Diseases of Nerves

TRIGEMINAL NEURALGIA (TIC DOULOUREUX, FOTHERGILL'S DISEASE)

- Possibly retated to circulatory insufficiency of gassarian ganglion.
- Frequently found in multiple sclerosis.
- Common in older adults.
- Usually involves right side of face.
- Searing, stabbing or lancinating type of pain.
- *"Tic douloureux"*- when patient suffers from spasmotic contraction of facial muscle.
- *"Pre trigeminal Neuralgia"*- Early pain; resembling toothache.
- *"Trigger zones"* are often elicited. It is usually the key for diagnosis.
- *"Trigeminal neuritis or trigeminal neuropathy"* - differs from TN by nature of pain. It is burning, boring, pulling, drawing or pressure sensation, continuing for hours to weeks.
- Carbamazepine is most commonly used drug for management. Other drugs include gabapentin, phenytoin, lamotrigine, pimozide.
- Other modalities include peripheral neurectomy, alcohol injections, injection of boiling water in gasserian ganglion, surgical sectioning of sensory root, microsurgical decompression of the trigeminal root.
- *Anaesthesia dolorosa* may occur as a surgical complication i.e. numbness combined with severe intractable pain.

PARATRIGEMINAL SYNDROME (Raeder's syndrome)

- Severe headache in area of trigeminal distribution with signs of ocular sympathetic paralysis, without vasomotor or trophic disturbances.

SPHENOPALATINE NEURALGIA (Lower – Half Headache, Sluder's Headache, Vidian Nerve Neuralgia, Horton's Syndrome, Atypical Facial Neuralgia, Cluster Headache, Histamine Cephalgia)

- A symptom complex referable to the nasal ganglion or vidian nerve

- May be caused by vasodilatation of internal maxillary artery.
- *"Alarm clock headache"-* pain occurs at exactly the same time of day.
- No trigger zones are elicited.
- Usually associated with epiphora, sneezing, swelling of nasal mucosa.

AURICULOTEMPORAL SYNDROME (Frey's syndrome, Gustatory sweating)

- Occurs due to damage to auriculotemporal nerve and subsequent innervation of sweat glands by parasympathetic salivary fibres.
- Flushing and sweating from temporal area during eating.

BELL'S PALSY (Facial paralysis)

- Caused by ischemia of the nerve near the stylomastoid foramen, resulting in edema and compression of nerve.
- Women are more commonly affected.
- Middle aged is most susceptible.
- *Bell's phenomenon* – Rolling of eyeball upwards when the patient closes eye.
- Drooping of corners of mouth, epiphora drooling of saliva, inability to close eye or wink, loss of wrinkling of forehead, *"mask like expressionless face"*.
- *Melkersson – Rosenthal syndrome* - Recurrent attacks of facial plasy + multiple episodes of non-pitting, non- inflammatory painless edema of face, cheilitis granulomatosa and fissured tongue.
- *Ramsay Hunt syndrome* – facial palsy + herpes zoster of Geniculate ganglion.
- *Bogorad syndrome*- (Crocodile tears) generally follows Bell's palsy, result of herpes zoster or head injury, leading to a salivary lacrimal reflex arc. Manifested as lacrimation on eating.

GLOSSOPHARYNGEAL NEURALGIA

- Sharp shooting pain in ear, pharynx, nasopharynx, tonsil and posterior portion of tongue.
- Trigger zone located in posterior oropharynx or tonsillar fossa.
- May be associated with vagal symptoms such as syncope and arrhythmias.

MULTIPLE SCLEROSIS (Disseminated sclerosis)

- Demyelinating disease.
- *Charcot's triad* - Triad characteristic of multiple sclerosis but not invariably present. Consists of intention tremor, nystagmus, and dysarthria.
- Bell's palsy and trigeminal neuralgia may be present.

OROFACIAL DYSKINESIA

May occur as a result of disruption of dental proprioception.

TEMPORAL ARTERITIS (Giant Cell Arteritis)

- A focal granulomatous inflammation of temporal arteries.
- Temporal arteritis is particularly prone to develop.
- May lead to loss of vision.
- Abnormal C reactive protein is an early finding; elevated ESR, biopsy from the temporal artery is diagnostic.

CAUSALGIA

- Severe pain that arises after injury due to sectioning of a peripheral sensory nerve.
- It usually follows extraction of multirooted tooth.

ATYPICAL FACIAL PAIN (Facial causalgia)

- Vague deep pain in the regions supplied by 5th and 9th cranial nerves and 2nd and 3rd cervical nerves.
- *Eagle's syndrome* - Consists of either elongation of styloid process or ossification of stylohyoid ligament causing dysphagia, sore throat, otalgia, glossodynia, headache, vague orofacial pain.

CAROTID ARTERY SYNDROME

Pressure exerted by either a deviant styloid process or an ossified ligament, on carotid arteries.

HORNOR'S SYNDROME

- Miosis + ptosis + Anhidrosis + vasodilatation.
- Involvement of carotid sympathetic plexus by lesions of the gasserian ganglion.
- May produce atypical facial sweating defect and facial pain.

JAW-WINKING SYNDROME (Marcus-gunn Phenomenon/ Pterygoid – Levator Synkinesis)

- Congenital unilateral ptosis, with rapid elevation of the ptotic eyelid occurring on movement of the mandible to the contralateral side.
- *Marin – Amat syndrome or Inverted Marcus – Gunn phenomenon-* Eye closes automatically when the patient opens his mouth and tears may flow.

TROTTER'S SYNDROME

- Caused by nasopharyngeal tumors.
- There is asymmetry and defective mobility of the soft palate on affected side.
- Trismus may occur.
- Neuralgic pain due to involvement of the mandibular nerve in the foramen ovale.

POST HERPATIC NEURALGIA

- Pain usually involves the ophthalmic division of the 5th cranial nerve.

- Particularly seen in elderly and immuno compromised people.
- Pain persists for longer than 1 month after shingles, manifest as persistent pain, paraesthesia, hyperaesthesia and allodynia.
- Topical capsaicin is helpful in treatment.

QUESTIONS

1. Eagle's syndrome is characterized by: [AIPGEE 2008]
   1. Dysphagia & elongation of the Styloid process
   2. Paralysis of tongue
   3. Multiple sclerosis
   4. Ptosis

Ans. **1**

Consists of either elongation of styloid process or ossification of stylohyoid   ligament causing dysphagia, sore throat, otalgia, glossodynia, headache, vague orofacial pain.

2. Which of the following statements best represents Bell's paralysis? [AIPG 2004]
   1. Hemiparesis and contralateral facial nerve paralysis
   2. Combined paralysis is of the facial, trigeminal and abducens nerves
   3. Idiopathic ipsilateral paralysis of the facial nerve
   4. Facial nerve paralysis with dry eyes

Ans. **3**

3. What is not characteristic of Eagle's syndrome? [AIPG 2004]
   1. Excessive lacrimation
   2. Pain during mandibular movement
   3. Stabbing type pain originate in the tonsillar region
   4. When the jaws are closed the pain subsided

Ans. **1**

Excessive lacrimation is a feature of Bogorad syndrome.

4. A 40-year-old female patient experiences severe throbbing headache of left craniofacial region. She also has nausea with paresthesia of right upper and lower lip. She may be suffering from: [AIPG 2001]
   1. Trigeminal neuralgia
   2. Glossopharyngeal nerve neuralgia
   3. VII cranial nerve neuralgia
   4. Migraine

Ans. **4**

In (1) and (2), trigger zones are elicited, (3) is marked by facial palsy.

5. **Damage to the facial nerve of the right side can cause:** [AIPG 2000]
   1. Paralysis of the masticatory muscles
   2. Paralysis of muscles of facial expression
   3. No loss of taste sensation in the anterior 2/3 of tongue
   4. Loss of secretion of the glands.

Ans. 2

Facial paralysis cause weakness of muscles of facial expression which leads to loss of wrinkling, inability to whistle, blow, accumulation of food in buccal vestibule, drooping of corner of mouth with dribbling of saliva.

6. **Thickening of styloid process causing difficulty in swallowing is seen in case of:** [AIPG 97]
   1. Diabetes
   2. Eagles syndrome
   3. Ramsay Hunt syndrome
   4. Trigeminal neuralgia

Ans. 2

Due to elongation of styloid process or ossification of the stylohyoid ligament, there is dysphagia, sore throat, otalgia, glossodynia, headache and pharyngeal pain.

7. **Eagle's syndrome is caused by:** [AIPG 1995]
   1. Ossification of stylohyoid ligament
   2. Sensitisation of trigger zones in oropharynx region
   3. Fracture of styloid process
   4. Nasopharyngeal tumour

Ans. 1

Eagles syndrome is characterized by elongation of styloid process or ossification of stylohyoid ligament.

Features- dysphagia, sore throat, otalgia, glossodynia, headache, vague oro-facial pain.

8. **Paresthesia of the lower lip most often results from:** [AIPG 93]
   1. Fracture of the condyle
   2. A traumatic mandibular bone cyst
   3. A benign lesion of the mandible
   4. Removal of a mandibular third molar

Ans. 4

Paresthesia of lower lip occurs as a result of injury to inferior alveolar nerve during surgical extraction of mandibular third molars.

9. **A neuralgia with trigger zones in the oropharynx and pain in the ear, pharynx, nasopharynx, tonsils and posterior tongue is most likely:** [AIPG 91]
   1. Trigeminal neuralgia

2. Bell's palsy

3. Glossopharyngeal neuralgia

4. Sphenopalatine neuralgia

Ans. **3**

In trigeminal neuralgia, trigger zones are elicited usually near ala of nose, cheek, lips, chin and gingiva. There are no trigger zones or neuralgia in Bell's palsy. Sphenopalatine neuralgia (Horton's syndrome) shows no trigger zones.

10. **During removal of a parotid tumour, the auriculotemporal nerve is injured. This could result in:** **[AIPG 91]**

    1. Facial paralysis

    2. Trigeminal neuralgia

    3. Gustatory sweating

    4. Orolingual paraesthesia

Ans. **3**

Due to damage to auriculotemporal nerve and subsequent innervation of sweat glands by parasympathetic salivary fibres. There is flushing and sweating from temporal area during eating.

11. **Which of the following drugs is often used successfully to treat trigeminal neuralgia?** **[AIPG 1990]**

    1. Clonazepam

    2. Carbamazepine

    3. Acetazolamide

    4. Carbamylcholine (carbachol)

Ans. **2**

Carbamazepine is the drug of choice followed by gabapentin and clonazepam.

17 Temporomandibular Disorders

JAW JERK REFLEX

It is a stretch reflex whereby stretching the jaw-closing muscles (by applying a downward tap on the chin) produces a reflex contraction of these muscles. This reflex is thought to relate to the fine control of jaw movements to take into account different consistencies of food.

JAW-OPENING REFLEX

Stimulating mechanoreceptors within the mouth or nociceptors from the mouth or face triggers the jaw-opening reflex. The reflex results in an inhibition of the activity of the jaw-closing muscles. This reflex is thought to help prevent injury when biting or chewing objects that may cause damage.

Disk Displacements

The steep and more vertical form of the fossa has been associated with articular disk displacements. Chronic recurring condyle subluxation or dislocation has also been related to the form and steepness of the fossa and articular eminence. Demonstration of the lateral pterygoid's attachment to the anterior articular disk has led to the theory that at least some anterior disk displacements may be related to lateral pterygoid-muscle dysfunction.

PREDISPOSING FACTORS FOR MPDS

1. Parafunctional habits (e.g, nocturnal bruxing, tooth clenching, lip or cheek biting).
2. Emotional distress.
3. Acute trauma from blows or impacts.
4. Trauma from hyperextension (e.g, dental procedures, oral intubation for general anesthesia, yawning, hyperextension associated with cervical trauma).
5. Instability of maxillomandibular relationships.
6. Laxity of the joint.
7. Comorbidity of other rheumatic or musculoskeletal disorders.
8. Poor general health and an unhealthy lifestyle.

Trigger Point Therapy

Trigger point therapy has used two modalities: the cooling of skin over the involved muscle and stretching and the direct injection of local anesthetic into the muscle. Spray and stretch therapy is performed by cooling the skin with fluoromethane (a refrigerant spray) and then gently stretching the involved muscle. Intramuscular trigger point injections have been performed by injecting local anesthetic, saline, or sterile water or by dry needling without depositing a drug or solution.

ANTERIOR DISK DISPLACEMENT WITH REDUCTION

- Complain of pain during mandibular movement, the pain is most noticeable at the time of the click.
- Palpation and auscultation of the TMJ will reveal a clicking or popping sound during both opening and closing mandibular movements (the so-called reciprocal click).
- The clicking or popping sound due to anterior disk displacement with reduction is characterized by a click that occurs at a different point during opening and closing.
- Tenderness will be present when ADD is accompanied by capsulitis or synovitis.
- TMJ effusion may be noted on a T2 weighted MRI scans.

ANTERIOR DISK DISPLACEMENT WITHOUT REDUCTION (CLOSED LOCK)

- It is detected more frequently in patients with clicking joints that progress to intermittent brief locking and then permanent locking.
- A patient with an acute closed lock will often have a history of a long-standing TMJ click that suddenly disappears with a sudden restriction in mandibular opening.
- Other findings include pain directly over the joint during mandibular opening (especially at maximum opening) and limited lateral movement to the side away from the ADD since disks are most frequently displaced medially as well as anteriorly.
- During maximum mandibular opening, the mandible will deviate towards the side of the displacement. Palpation of the joints will reveal decreased translation of the condyle on the side of the disk displacement.

POSTERIOR DISK DISPLACEMENT

- The disk is folded in the dorsal part of the joint space, preventing full mouth closure.
- The clinical features are:
  1. A sudden inability to bring the upper and lower teeth together in maximal occlusion.
  2. Pain in the affected joint when trying to bring the teeth firmly together.
  3. Displacement forward of the mandible on the affected side.
  4. Restricted lateral movement to the affected side.
  5. No restriction of mouth opening.

DEGENERATIVE JOINT DISEASE (OSTEOARTHRITIS)

- Degenerative joint disease (DJD), also referred to as osteoarthrosis, osteoarthritis, and degenerative arthritis, is primarily a disorder of articular cartilage and subchondral bone, with secondary inflammation of the synovial membrane.

- It is a localized joint disease without systemic manifestations.
- The process begins in loaded articular cartilage, which thins and clefts (fibrillation) and then breaks away during joint activity. This leads to sclerosis of underlying bone, subcondylar cysts, and osteophyte formation.
- Some degenerative changes may be underdiagnosed by conventional radiography because the defects are confined to the articular soft tissue. These soft-tissues changes are better visualized with MRI. Radiographic findings in degenerative joint disease may include narrowing of the joint space, irregular joint space, flattening of the articular surfaces, osteophytic formation, anterior lipping of the condyle, and the presence of *Ely's cysts*. These changes may be seen best on tomograms or CT scans. The presence of joint effusion is most accurately detected in T2 weighted MRI images.

SYNOVIAL CHONDROMATOSIS

- Synovial chondromatosis (SC) is an uncommon benign disorder characterized by the presence of multiple cartilagenous nodules of the synovial membrane that break off resulting in clusters of free-floating loose calcified bodies in the joint.
- Extension of SC from the TMJ joint to surrounding tissues (including the parotid gland, middle ear, or middle cranial fossa) may occur.
- Slow progressive swelling in the pretragus region, pain, and limitation of mandibular movement is the most common presenting clinical picture.
- TMJ clicking, locking, crepitus, and occlusal changes may also be present. The extension of the lesion from the joint capsule and involvement of surrounding tissues may make diagnosis difficult, causing SC to be confused with parotid, middle ear, or intracranial tumors.

RHEUMATOID ARTHRITIS

- The disease process starts as a vasculitis of the synovial membrane. It progresses to chronic inflammation marked by an intense round cell infiltrate and subsequent formation of granulation tissue. The cellular infiltrate spreads from the articular surfaces eventually to cause an erosion of the underlying bone.
- The TMJs are usually bilaterally involved in RA.
- The most common symptoms include limitation of mandibular opening and joint pain.. Other symptoms often noted include morning stiffness, joint sounds, and tenderness and swelling over the joint area.
- The most consistent clinical findings include pain on palpation of the joints and limitation of opening. Crepitus also may be evident.
- Micrognathia and an anterior open bite are commonly seen in patients with juvenile RA.
- Radiographic changes in the TMJ associated with RA may include a narrow joint space, destructive lesions of the condyle, and limited condylar movement. There is little evidence of marginal proliferation or other reparative activity in RA in contrast to the radiographic changes often observed in degenerative joint disease. High-resolution CT of RA patients – TMJs will show erosions of the condyle and glenoid fossae that cannot be seen by conventional radiography.

PSORIATIC ARTHRITIS

Psoriatic arthritis (PA) is an erosive polyarthritis occurring in patients with a negative rheumatoid factor who have psoriatic skin lesions. The skin lesions precede the joint involvement by several years. PA affects 5 to 7% of patients with psoriasis.

SEPTIC ARTHRITIS

- Septic arthritis of the TMJ most commonly occurs in patients with previously existing joint disease such as rheumatoid arthritis, or underlying medical disorders (particularly diabetes).
- Patients receiving immunosuppressive drugs or long-term corticosteroids also have an increased incidence of septic arthritis. The infection of the TMJ may result from blood-borne bacterial infection or by extension of infection from adjacent sites such as the middle ear, maxillary molars, and parotid gland.
- Gonococci are the primary bloodborne agents causing septic arthritis in a previously normal TMJ while Staphylococcus aureus is the most common organism involved in previously arthritic joints.

GOUT AND PSEUDOGOUT

- Gouty arthritis is caused by long-term elevation of serum urate levels, which results in the deposition of crystals in a joint, triggering an acute inflammatory response.
- Acute pain in a single joint (monoarticular arthritis) is the characteristic clinical manifestation of gouty arthritis.
- An attack of gouty arthritis is most accurately diagnosed by examination of aspirated synovial fluid from the involved joint by polarized light microscopy. The detection of monosodium urate crystals confirms the diagnosis of gout.
- The deposition of other crystals, such as calcium pyrophosphate dihydrate (CPPD) or calcium hydroxyapatite, may cause a syndrome that resembles gout and that has been referred to as pseudogout.

DEVELOPMENTAL DEFECTS

TRUE CONDYLAR HYPERPLASIA

- Usually occurs after puberty and is completed by 18 to 25 years of age.
- Limitation of opening, deviation of the mandible to the side of the enlarged condyle.
- Pain is occasionally associated with the hyperplastic condyle on opening.
- Facial asymmetry often results.

HYPOPLASIA OF THE CONDYLE

- Deviation of the mandible to the affected side and facial deformities also are associated with **unilateral agenesis** and **hypoplasia** of the condyle.
- In cases of hypoplasia, there is a short wide ramus, shortening of the body of the mandible, and

antegonial notching on the affected side, with elongation of the mandibular body and flatness of the face on the opposite side.

TRAUMA

FRACTURES - often result from a blow to the chin. The patient with a condylar fracture usually presents with pain and edema over the joint area and limitation and deviation of the mandible to the injured side on opening. Bilateral condylar fractures may result in an anterior open bite. The diagnosis of a condylar fracture is confirmed by radiographic examination. Intracapsular nondisplaced fractures of the condylar head are usually not treated surgically. Early mobilization of the mandible is emphasized to prevent bony or fibrous ankylosis.

DISLOCATION - In dislocation of the mandible, the condyle is positioned anterior to the articular eminence and cannot return to its normal position without assistance. This disorder contrasts with subluxation, in which the condyle moves anterior to the eminence during wide opening but is able to return to the resting position without manipulation.

ANKYLOSIS - True bony anklyosis of the TMJ involves fusion of the head of the condyle to the temporal bone. Trauma to the chin is the most common cause of TMJ ankylosis although infections also may be involved. Children are more prone to ankylosis because of greater osteogenic potential and an incompletely formed disk. Ankylosis frequently results from prolonged immobilization following condylar fracture. Limited mandibular movement, deviation of the mandible to the affected side on opening, and facial asymmetry may be observed in TMJ ankylosis. Osseous deposition may be seen on radiographs.

QUESTIONS

1. **Unilateral TMJ ankylosis is associated with the following features except.** [AIPG 2004]
   1. Multiple carious teeth.
   2. Facial asymmetry with fullness on the normal side of mandible.
   3. Chin deviated towards the affected side.
   4. Prominent ante gonial notch on the affected side.

Ans. **1**

Because partial mouth opening is there in unilateral ankylosis, patient is able to maintain oral hygiene

2. **Which of the following is the most frequent cause of anykylosis of the temperomandibular joint?** [AIPG 91]
   1. Osteoarthritis
   2. Traumatic injury
   3. Congenital syphilis
   4. Traumatic occlusion

Ans. **2**

A traumatic injury to TMJ is the most common cause of ankylosis, followed by septic arthritis and otitis media.

3. **The most common complication of rheumatoid arthritis involving the temporomandibular joint is:** [AIPG 1989]
   1. Subluxation
   2. Fibrous Ankylosis
   3. Osteoma of the condyle
   4. Resorption of the condyle.

Ans. **2**

Rheumatoid arthritis - most common radiographic manifestation - flattening of the head of condyle & erosion of the condyle. Subluxation is seen in osteoarthritis.

NOTES

18

Cysts in Maxillofacial Region

MEDIAN ANTERIOR MAXILLARY CYST / NASOPALATINE DUCT CYST / INCISIVE CANAL CYST

- Arise from proliferation of epithelial remnants of nasopalatine duct.
- Appears as round, ovoid or *Heart shaped radiolucent area*, in midline between or above the roots of maxillary central incisors.
- Median alveolar cyst – arise anterior to incisive canal, represents primordial cyst developing from a supernumerary tooth bud.

MEDIAN PALATAL CYST

- Arise from epithelium entrapped along the line of fusion of the palatal processes of the maxilla.

GLOBULOMAXILLARY CYST

- Found within the bone at the junction of the globular portion of the median nasal process and the maxillary process, the globulomaxillary fissure, usually between the maxillary lateral incisor and cuspid.
- Appears as an inverted *"pear-shaped"* radiolucency.

MEDIAN MANDIBULAR CYST

- Arise from epithelial remnants entrapped in the median mandibular fissure during fusion of bilateral mandibular arches.

NASOALVEOLAR CYST / NASOLABIAL CYST / KLESTADT'S CYST

- Arise at the junction of globular process, the lateral nasal process and the maxillary process.
- They are not primarily central lesion and therefore may not be visible on the radiograph.
- The cyst probably originates from lower anterior part of the nasolacrimal duct.

PALATAL CYSTS OF THE NEONATE

Bohn's nodules: Scattered over hard palate, most numerous along the junction of hard and soft palate.

Epstein's pearls: Linearly along the median raphe of the hard palate.

Dental Lamina cyst of Newborn: Found on the alveolar ridges, derived from remnants of the dental lamina.

THYROGLOSSAL TRACT CYST

- Can occur anywhere along the embryonic thyroglossal tract, between foramen caecum of tongue and thyroid glands.
- Unknown etiology, infection of lymphoid tissue in the area may be a triggering factor.
- Firm, cystic, midline mass.
- Surgical excision is the treatment of choice.

BENIGN CERVICAL LYMPHOEPITHELIAL CYST / BRANCHIAL CLEFT CYST / BENIGN CYSTIC LYMPH NODE

- Occurs on lateral aspect of the neck, usually close to anterior border of sternocleidomastoid muscle, originates from remnants of the branchial arches or pharyngeal pouches.
- May contain thin watery fluid or a thick, gelatinous, mucoid material.
- Surgical excision is treatment of choice.
- Development of carcinoma from the epithelium lining the cyst has been reported.

DERMOID CYSTS

- Form of cystic teratoma derived from embryonic germinal epithelium.
- Cysts in floor of mouth, submaxillary and sublingual areas derived from enclavement of epithelial debris in the midline during closure of the mandibular and hyoid branchial arches.
- "Doughlike" feel to palpation.
- Clinical presentation
  - Bulging in floor of mouth – cysts above the geniohyoid muscle.
  - Submental bulge – cyst between geniohyoid and mylohyoid muscle or below the mylohyoid muscle.

ODONTOGENIC CYSTS

DENTIGEROUS CYST (FOLLICULAR/ PERICORONAL CYST)

- Occurs due to fluid accumulation between crown of unerupted tooth & layers of reduced enamel epithelium.
- Multiple dentigerous cysts are associated with-
  - Basal cell nevus syndrome.
  - Cleidocranial dysplasia

- Potential complication – Ameloblastomas
    - Mucoepidermoid carcinoma
- *Eruption cyst* is form of dentigerous cyst occurring when a tooth is impeded in its eruption within the soft tissues overlying the bone.

ODONTOGENIC KERATOCYST

- Highest rate of recurrence due to presence of satellite cysts.
- Associated with
    - Gorlin Goltz syndrome
    - Marfan syndrome
    - Ehlers Danlos syndrome
    - Noonan's syndrome
- Anteroporterior expansion is associated with odontogenic Keratocysts.
- Histopathology - the basal cell layer has a *'Picket fence'* or *'tomb stone'* appearance.

PRIMODIAL CYST

Originates when cystic changes take place in stellate reticulum of tooth germ before any calcified enamel or dentin has been formed.

LATERAL PERIODONTAL CYST AND GINGIVAL CYST OF ADULT

- Located in interproximal bone between apex and alveolar crest.
- Gingival cyst appears as dome shaped swelling in attached gingiva.
- Most frequent location of lateral periodontal cyst is the lateral surface of roots of vital teeth in mandibular canine & premolar region followed by anterior region of maxilla.
- Gingival cyst is an uncommon cyst.

CALCIFYING EPITHELIAL ODONTOGENIC CYST

- Also called *Gorlin's cyst* or Keratinizing & Calcifying odontogenic cyst or Dentinogenic Ghost cell Tumor.
- It has some features suggestive of cyst but also has many characteristics of solid neoplasm.
- Most common site is maxillary anterior region.

RADICULAR CYST

- Also called apical periodontal cyst, periapical cyst, or dental root end cyst.
- Inflammatory cyst.
- Associated with a non vital tooth.
- Hyaline bodies or Rushton bodies are often found in great numbers in the epithelium of apical periodontal cyst.
- Collection of cholesterol cleft with associated multinuclear giant cells is found in the wall of the lesion.

RESIDUAL CYST

- It is the cyst that either remained as such in the jaw when its associated tooth was removed or was formed in residual epithelium of cell rests from a periodontal ligament of the lost tooth.

INFLAMMATORY COLLATERAL CYST

- It arises in the periodontium on the lateral aspect of erupted tooth as a result of inflammatory process in the periodontal pocket. They arise by the proliferation of rests of Malassez in lateral periodontium.

PARADENTAL CYST

- It is a cyst of inflammatory origin occurring on the lateral aspect of the root of partially erupted mandibular third molar with an associated history of pericoronitis.
- Usually associated with third molar on the buccal surface and covers the bifurcation.
- Involved tooth is vital.
- Also called buccal bifurcation cyst.

QUESTIONS

1. **Multiple odontogenic keratocyst are associated with:** [AIPG 2004]
   1. Gardner's syndrome
   2. Gorlin- Goltz syndrome
   3. Goldenhar's syndrome
   4. Grinspan syndrome

Ans. **2**

Gardner's syndrome – Multiple osteomas, polyposis, supernumerary teeth, dermoid and epidermoid cysts.

Goldenhar syndrome – Unilateral hypoplasia of mandible, rudimentary ear, epicanthal colobomas.

Grinspan syndrome- Diabetes mellitus, hypertension & erosive lichen planus.

2. **Periodontal cyst is similar radiographically to:** [AIPG 2002]
   1. Dentigerous cyst
   2. Aneurysmal cyst
   3. Periapical cyst
   4. Stafne bone cyst.

Ans. **1**

It resembles lateral variety of dentigerous cyst.

3. **Which of the following shows the presence of cholesterol crystals?** [AIPG 2001]
   1. Keratocyst
   2. Periodontal cyst

3. Aneurysmal cyst

4. Hemorrhagic cyst

Ans. **1**

Cholesterol crystals are seen in radicular cyst and keratocyst.

4. **Ramlal, a 40-year-old patient, shows a dome shaped fluctuant non-tender swelling with discharge from the incisive papilla. Extraction of the incisors does not provide any relief. Lesion may be:** [AIPG 2001]

1. Periapical abscess

2. Periapical cyst

3. Nasopalatine cyst

4. Local osteomyelitis

Ans. **3**

The lesion described here is most probably an infective nasopalatine cyst.

5. **An empty cavity in the mandible with no lining is most likely to be:** [AIPG 2000]

1. Aneurysmal bone cyst

2. Idiopathic bone cavity

3. Stafne bone cyst

4. Keratocyst.

Ans. **2**

Idiopathic bone cavity or traumatic bone cyst or solitary bone cyst is a pseudocyst, which is not lined by epithelium and is an empty cavity in bone. Mostly located in posterior mandible, above the inferior alveolar canal.

6. **All the following are true for odontogenic keratocyst except:** [AIPG 2000]

1. The cyst is enclosed by a thin fibrous capsule and indistinct epithelium

2. Cystic fluid has a low protein content

3. Low recurrence rate

4. Extends anteriorly and posteriorly in the marrow spaces.

Ans. **3**

OKC has a high recurrence rate due to presence of satellite cysts

7. **One of them is not a true cyst:** [AIPG 97]

1. Haemorrhagic bone cyst

2. Median palatal cyst

3. Globulomaxillary cyst

4. Nasolabial cyst

Ans. **1**

A true cyst is one in which the cystic cavity is lined by epithelium. As there is no epithelial lining in hemorrhagic bone cyst, it is considered as a pseudocyst. Another example of pseudocyst is aneurysmal bone cyst.

8. Which of the following cysts are not seen on X-rays? AIPG 96]

1. Nasopalatine cyst
2. Globulomaxillary cyst
3. Midpalatine cyst
4. Nasolabial cyst

Ans. **4**

Because it is a soft tissue cyst. It may be visualized on X-rays after some contrast media in injected into the cystic cavity.

9. Keratocyst has all of the following features except: [AIPG 96]

1. It is more common in mandible
2. May be filled with thin straw coloured fluid
3. Low recurrence rate
4. Expansion of bone is clinically seen

Ans. **3**

Odontogenic keratocyst has the maximum recurrence rate among all the cysts due to presence of satellite cysts in its lining.

10. The most common cyst of the oral regions is the: [AIPG 94]

1. Dermoid inclusion cyst
2. Dentigerous cyst
3. Periapical cyst
4. Primordial cyst

Ans. **3**

Periapical cysts are sequalae of dental caries and trauma.

11. Cyst which recurs is: [AIPG 93]

1. Primordial cyst
2. Keratocyst
3. Radicular cyst
4. Ameloblastoma

Ans. **3**

Keratocyst has highest rate of recurrence due to presence of satellite cysts, scalloping and thin friable lining.

12. Which of the following is a soft tissue cyst? [AIPG 92]

1. Nasolabial cyst
2. Nasopalatine cyst

3. Palatine cyst

4. Median alveolar cyst

Ans. **1**

13. **The characteristic of primordial cyst is:** [AIPG 1990]

1. Develops in place of teeth

2. Attached to apical third of a tooth

3. Remains after the tooth is extracted

4. None of the above

Ans. **1**

2- Radicular cyst

3- Residual cyst.

14. **The odontogenic cyst having the highest recurrence rate is the:** [AIPG 1989]

1. Keratocyst

2. Radicular cyst

3. Periapical cyst

4. Dentigerous cyst

Ans. **1**

Keratocyst highest recurrence rate due to following reasons:

- Thin connective tissue wall.

- Islands of odontogenic epithelium in the cyst wall give rise to satellite microcysts.

Radicular/ periapical cyst- usually does not recur.

Dentigerous cyst - three types of neoplastic changes.

- Ameloblastoma, squamous cell carcinoma & mucoepidermoid carcinoma.

15. **A traumatic bone cyst is best treated by:**

1. Marsupilization

2. Enucleation of cyst lining

3. Opening of the cavity & packing open

4. Opening of the cavity & inducing bleeding

Ans. **4**

Opening of the cavity & inducing bleeding as the cyst lacks an epithelial lining and is often found on surgical exploration to be empty i.e. devoid of fluid.

NOTES

19 Odontogenic Tumors

AMELOBLASTOMA / ADAMANTINE EPITHELIOMA / ADAMANTINOMA

- Most common clinically significant odontogenic tumor.
- Locally aggressive tumor.
- They may arise from rests of dental lamina, from a developing enamel organ, from the epithelium of odontogenic and dentigerous cyst, oral mucosa or heterotrophic epithelium in other parts of body.
- Constitutes about 1% of all tumors and 11% of odontogenic tumors.
- Slight male predilection.
- Usually between 20-50 years of age.
- Mostly seen in molar ramus area, followed by maxillary sinus and floor of nose.
- Facial asymmetry, displacement of teeth, egg shell crackling, and paraesthesia are common features.
- *Mural Ameloblastoma* – Arise from lining of dentigerous cyst.
- *Follicular type* – Many small discrete islands of tumor cells, reverse polarity of basal cells, cystic degeneration, micro cyst formation.
- *Plexiform type* – Tumor cells arranged in irregular masses or network of interconnecting strands of cells. Exhibits stromal degeneration and cyst formation, may be filled with blood.
- *Acanthomatous type* - Stellate reticulum undergoes squamous metaplasia to form keratin pearls. May be confused with squamous cell carcinoma.
- *Granular type* - Conversion of stellate reticulum to coarse granular eosinophilic appearance. Aggressive type.
- *Basal type* - Shows basaloid pattern. Resembles basal cell carcinoma.
- *Desmoplastic type*- Usually occurs in maxillary anterior region. Stromal desmoplasia and moderately cellular fibrous connective tissue with abundant collagen formation.
- *Radiographic features*
  - Ameloblastoma causes expansion of bone rather than destruction.

- Infiltrates cancellous bone but it is largely confined by compact bone. It never infiltrates Haversian canal. Hence, actual margins are much greater than radiological margin.
- Root resorption is common (smooth manner).
- *Common appearances*
  - Cystic appearance.
  - Honeycomb appearance.
  - Soap-bubble appearance.
- *Extra osseous / peripheral Ameloblastoma* - Usually seen in males on the mandibular gingiva in molar premolar area. Pressure resorption or saucer-shaped depression beneath the tumor may be seen.
- *Pituitary Ameloblastoma / Rathke's pouch tumor / Craniopharyrgiomas* - Occurs in anterior lobe. Most common in childhood and adolescence. Often destroy pituitary gland and compress nearby cranial nerves.
- *Adamantinoma of long bones* – Occurs in tibia, ulna, and femur.
- *Malignant Ameloblastoma* – Those Ameloblastoma that metastasize but in which the metastatic lesion do not show any histologic difference from the primary tumor.
- *Ameloblastic carcinoma* – shows obvious histological malignant transformation but the metastatic lesions do not bear resemblance to the primary odontogenic tumor.
- *Ameloblastic fibrosarcoma* – very rare
  - Occurs in young adults.
  - More frequent in maxilla.
  - Odontogenic epithelium maintains its benign appearance.
  - Mesenchymal tissue exhibits malignant fibroblasts and atypical mitotic features.
  - Extensive bone destruction.

ADENOMATOID ODONTOGENIC TUMOR / ADENOAMELOBLASTOMA

- Usually associated with unerupted teeth, arise from odontogenic epithelium.
- Most common site is maxillary anterior region, especially cuspid area.
- Represents 3% of odontogenic tumors.
- 70% tumors occur in 2nd decade of life.
- Expansion of bone and fluctuation may be elicited.
- *Radiographic features*
  - Well demarcated mixed radiolucent- opaque lesion.
  - *Target appearance* – There is a radiolucent circumferential halo which envelops a dense, central radiopaque mass.
  - *Milky way lumen*
- Histological picture shows polyhedral or spindle shaped epithelial cells arranged in a duct like fashion.

AMELOBLASTIC FIBROMA / SOFT ODONTOMA / GRANULAR CELL AMELOBLASTIC FIBROMA

- May develop from the dental follicle before or after the onset of calcification of tooth.
- Usually seen before 20 years of age.
- Common site – premolar molar area in mandible.
- Enlarges by gradual expansion so that the periphery of bone often remains smooth.
- Unilocular or multilocular radiolucency associated with unerupted or missing tooth.

CALCIFYING EPITHELIAL ODONTOGENIC TUMOR / PINDBORG TUMOR / CALCIFYING AMELOBLASTOMA

- Develops from reduced enamel epithelium of the embedded tooth or from stratum intermedium.
- Mean age – 42 years.
- Mandible more commonly affected (2:1), in premolar molar area.
- Locally invasive with a high recurrence rate.
- *Radiographic features* – Initially multilocular or honeycomb pattern. Later on appear as *"Driven-snow"*.
- Histological picture: Liesgang rings, clear cells, eosinophilic cytoplasm.

ODONTOMA

- Hamartoma of odontogenic origin.
- Ectoderm origin – Enameloma.
- Mesodermal origin – 1. Dentinoma, 2. Cementoma.
- Mixed origin –
  Complex composite – Non discrete masses of dental tissues.
  Compound composite – multiple well formed teeth.
  Compound complex – contains not only multiple teeth like structure, but also calcified masses of dental tissue in a haphazard manner.
  Geminated odontoma
  Dilated odontoma with dens in dente.
- Compound odontoma mostly occurs in maxillary incisor, canine area while complex occurs in mandibular 1st and 2nd molar area.
- Slight predilection for occurrence in males.
- Histopathological features – presence of ghost cells, fibrous capsule.

SQUAMOUS ODONTOGENIC TUMOR

- Well-differentiated odontogenic tumor composed of islands or sheet of squamous epithelium that lack recognizable features of enamel organ differentiation.
- Occurs in anterior maxilla and posterior mandible.

ODONTOGENIC MYXOMA / ODONTOGENIC FIBRO MYXOMA

- Non-invasive neoplasm that arise from dental papilla, follicular mesenchyme and PDL.
- More common in females.
- Mandible more commonly affected (3:1).
- Usually associated with congenitally missing teeth.
- May cause root resorption, displacement of teeth, invasion of maxillary sinus and exopthalmos.
- *Radiographic features:*
  - Tennis racket appearance
  - Honey comb appearance
  - Soap-bubble appearance
  - Unilocular
- *Histopathology* – Loosely arranged spindle shaped and stellate cells in mucoid intercellular substance.

PERIPHERAL ODONTOGENIC FIBROMA / CALCIFYING FIBROUS EPULIS / PERIPHERAL AMELOBLASTIC FIBRO DENTINOMA

- Usually seen in young age (5-25 years).
- Occurs commonly in mandible, almost exclusively on free margin of gingiva and involves interdental papilla.

CENTRAL ODONTOGENIC FIBROMA

- Surrounds the crown of an unerupted tooth resembling a small dentigerous cyst.
- Most common in anterior maxilla.
- Radiograph reveals expansile radiolucency similar to Ameloblastoma.

PERIAPICAL CEMENTAL DYSPLASIA / PERIAPICAL OSTEOFIBROMA / SCLEROSING CEMENTUM

- Reactive fibro-osseous lesion derived from odontogenic cells in PDL.
- Located at apex of tooth.
- Female to male ratio 9:1 and 3 times more common in blacks.
- Occurs in middle age.
- Mandibular anterior region most commonly affected.
- Involved teeth are vital.
- Histopathological features shows deposition to be composed of bone, cementum or osteo cementum.
- *Radiographic features* – epicenter is at apex of tooth.
  - Stage I – well defined radiolucency with loss of lamina dura around the tooth.
  - Stage II – cementoblastic stage. Mixed opaque-lucent lesion.
  - Stage III – radiopaque shadow, well defined; lamina dura of adjacent teeth is discontinuous.

BENIGN CEMENTOBLASTOMA / TRUE CEMENTOMA

- Derived from PDL.
- Mostly seen in mandible (3:1) in relation to second premolar and first molar.
- *Radiographic features* – well defined radiopacities usually attached to the roots of premolars and molar surrounded by a radiolucent halo.
  - *Wheel-spoke pattern.*
  - Outline of tooth is obliterated due to resorption of root and fusion of the mass to tooth.
  - Expansion of jaws is common.

AMELOBLASTIC ODONTOMA

- Simultaneous occurance of an Ameloblastoma and a composite odontoma.

AMELOBLASTIC FIBRO - ODONTOMA

- Mixed epithelial – mesenchymal proliferation.
- Usually seen in children.
- Consists of elements of ameloblastic odontoma and is more aggressive than the common odontoma.

TERATOMA / TERATOBLASTOMA / TERATOID TUMOR

- It is a neoplasm of different types of tissue, which are not native to the area in which the tumor occurs.
- Present at birth or is discovered shortly thereafter.
- Can occur in ovaries, testis, anterior mediastinum, retroperitonial area presacral and coccygeal regions, pineal region, head, neck and abdominal viscera.
- They are benign lesions and grow slowly.

QUESTIONS

1. The type of ameloblastoma, considered to be the deadliest with the worst prognosis is:

[AIPGEE 2008]

1. Follicular
2. Granular
3. Plexiform
4. Acanthomatous

Ans. **2**

- **Follicular type** – many small discrete islands of tumor cells, reverse polarity of basal cells, cystic degeneration, micro cyst formation.
- **Plexiform type** – tumor cells arranged in irregular masses or network of interconnecting stands of cells. Exhibits stromal degeneration and cyst formation, may be filled with blood.

- **Acanthomatous type -** Stellate reticulum undergoes squamous metaplasia to form keratin pearls. May be confused with squamous cell carcinoma.
- **Granular type -** Conversion of stellate reticulum to coarse granular eosinophilic appearance. Aggressive type.
- **Basal type -** Shows basaloid pattern. Resembles basal cell carcinoma.
- **Desmoplastic type -** Usually occurs in maxillary anterior region. Stromal desmoplasia and moderately cellular fibrous connective tissue with abundant collagen formation.

2. **Which of the following cyst shows the maximum amount of recurrence?**   **[AIPGEE 2008]**
    1. Odontogenic Keratocyst
    2. Dentigerous cyst
    3. Calcifying Odontogenic epithelial cyst
    4. Follicular cyst

Ans. **1**

Keratocyst highest recurrence rate due to following reasons
- Thin connective tissue wall
- Islands of odontogenic epithelium in the cyst wall give rise to satellite microcysts.

3. **An odontogenic tumor with ectodermal and mesodermal elements is:**   **[AIPG 99]**
    1. Ameloblastic fibroma
    2. Ameloblastoma
    3. Cementoma
    4. Calcifying epithelial odontogenic cyst

Ans. **1**

CEOC and ameloblastoma is epithelial in origin, cementoma is mesodermal in origin.

4. **Florid osseous dysplasia is another name for:**   **[AIPG 96]**
    1. Cementoma
    2. Periapical fibrosis
    3. Gigantiform cementoma
    4. Sclerotic cemental masses

Ans. **4**

Cementoma is also known as periapical cemental dysplasia or cementifying fibroma or periapical osteofibroma or cementoblastoma.

Gigantiform cementoma is also called familial multiple cementoma.

5. **Which of the following is derived from both ectoderm and mesoderm?**   **[AIPG 1995]**
    1. Odontogenic myxoma
    2. Ameloblastic fibroma
    3. Ameloblastoma
    4. Pindborg tumour

Ans. 2

Ameloblastic fibroma is caused by simultaneous proliferation of both epithelial and mesenchymal tissues without formation of enamel & dentin.

6. Ghost cells' are seen in: [AIPG 94]

1. Noncalcifying odontogenic tumour
2. Calcifying odontogenic epidermal tumour
3. Calcifying odontogenic cyst
4. Ameloblastoma

Ans. 3

Ghost cells are pale, eosinophilic, swollen epithelial cells that have lost the nucleus, but show a faint outline of the cellular and nuclear membrane. They contain many tonofibrils. They are also seen in ameloblastic fibro-odontomas and complex and compound odontomas and craniopharyngiomas.

7. Which of the following odontogenic neoplasms is least likely to demonstrate radiopacities? [AIPG 92]

1. Pindborg tumor
2. Cementoblastoma
3. Complex odontoma
4. Ameloblastic fibroma

Ans. 4

Pindborg tumor (CEOT), cementoblastoma and complex odontoma shows radiopacity at some stage of development.

8. Which of the following tumours is most aggressive? [AIPG 91]

1. Myxoma
2. Cementoblastoma
3. Ameloblastic tumor
4. Ameloblastic fibroodontoma

Ans. 1

Myxoma is not encapsulated. So, it can invade the surrounding tissues. Others are benign lesions.

9. Of the following regions where ameloblastomas frequently occur? [AIPG 1990]

1. Mandibular molar region
2. Maxillary molar region
3. Mandibular premolar region
4. Maxillary premolar region

Ans. 1

About 70% tumours occur in this region.

10. **The odontogenic tumour frequently found in children and associated with an unerupted tooth in the anterior portion of the maxilla is:** [AIPG 1990]
    1. Odontogenic myxoma
    2. Ameloblastic fibroma
    3. Cementifying fibroma
    4. Odontogenic adenomatoid tumor

Ans. **4**

    1. Not associated with unerupted tooth. Seen in posterior mandible.
    2. Mandibular molar area
    3. Mandible.

11. **A patient with ameloblastoma of the jaw can best be treated by:** [AIPG 1989]
    1. Irradiation
    2. Excision
    3. Enucleation
    4. Surgical removal followed by cauterisation

Ans. **4**

Benign Tumors (Non Odontogenic)

PAPILLOMA

Focal dermal hypoplasia syndrome – Associated with focal dermal hypoplasia.

Cowden's syndrome (multiple hamartoma and neoplasia syndrome)

- Autosomal dominant
- Facial trichilemmomas.
- GIT, thyroid, CNS and musculoskeletal abnormalities.
- Oral lesions like papillomas.

Kerato acanthoma

- Self healing carcinoma.
- Resembles squamous cell CA closely.
- Usually occurs on exposed skin.
- Papillomas are considered as cutaneous markers of breast cancer.

PIGMENTED CELLULAR NEVUS

1. Congenital
   (a) Small – 1-5 cm
   (b) Garment - > 10cm

2. Acquired
   (a) Intradermal (Most common)
   (b) Compound nevi
   (c) Spindle cell / Epitheloid cell nevus
   (d) Junctional
   (e) Blue (Jadassohn - Tieche) nevus.

- Junctional nevus has malignant potential.
- Spindle cell nevus is more common in children.
- Blue nevus is a true Mesodermal structure.

- *Abtropfung or "dropping-off" effect* seen in junctional nevus is due to apparent crossing of overlying epithelium into the connective tissue.
- *B-K Mole syndrome* – large pigmented nevi with high risk of development of melanoma.
- Congenital nevi have a great risk for malignant transformation.

CONNECTIVE TISSUE ORIGIN

FIBROMA

Most common benign soft tissue neoplasm in oral cavity.

GIANT CELL FIBROMA

Most common site is gingiva. Multinucleated giant fibroblasts makes up bulk of the lesion.

PERIPHERAL OSSIFYING FIBROMA / PERIPHERAL CEMENTIFYING FIBROMA

- Lesion is derived from PDL
- Occurs only on gingiva.
- Occurs anterior to the molar area.
- Most commonly appears to originate from an interdental papilla.

CENTRAL OSSIFYING FIBROMA

- Common in young adults, mostly occurs in mandible; usually seen in females and blacks.
- Slow growth pattern.
- Always well circumscribed and demarcated from surrounding bone in contrast to fibrous dysplasia.
- Radiolucent in early stage, becomes flecked with opacity as the lesion matures, ultimately appears as uniform radiopaque mass.
- Histopathology – Bizarre *Chinese character shape of bony trabeculae* similar to fibrous dysplasia.

PERIPHERAL GIANT CELL GRANULOMA / OSTEOCLASTOMA / GIANT CELL EPULIS

- Trauma is usually a common etiology.
- Always occur on gingival / alveolar process.
- Most frequently in anterior region.
- Originate from PDL or mucoperiosteum.
- "Peripheral cuffing" of bone may be seen in edentulous regions.

CENTRAL GIANT CELL GRANULOMA / TUMOR

- Usually occurs in young age.
- Females commonly affected.

- Mandible is more often affected.
- More common in anterior segments of jaws and frequently cross midline.
- X-ray radiation is contraindicated.

ANEURYSMAL BONE CYST

- Seen in young age.
- There is history of traumatic injury often.
- Lesion is usually tender or painful.
- Blood *"welling up"* from the tissue is seen at the time of operation, described as *"blood - soaked sponge"* with large pores.
- Some cysts have elevated vascular pressures as high as arteriolar levels.
- *"Honey- comb" or "Soap-bubble"* appearance eccentrically ballooned.
- Radiation therapy is controvertial due to potential development of radiation sarcoma.

LIPOMA

- Differ metabolically from normal fat cells. During starvation, fat is not lost from lipoma.

LIPOBLASTOMATOSIS

- Not a true neoplasm, rather a continuation of the normal process of fetal fat development carried into postnatal life.

VERRUCIFORM XANTHOMA (HISTIOCYTOSIS "Y")

- Most common site is gingival / alveolar ridge.
- Verrucous, hyperparakeratotic surface.
- Large swollen *"FOAM-CELLS"* or Xanthoma cells are characteristically present in connective tissue papillae.

HEMANGIOMA (VASCULAR NEVUS)

- Often congenital.
- Not a true neoplasm, rather a hamartoma.
- Most common sites are lips, tongue, buccal mucosa and palate.
- Central hemangioma may appear radiographically as *"Honey-comb"* appearance or *"sun-burst"* appearance.
- *"Pumping tooth"* is often associated with central hemangioma.
- *"Diascopy"* is used for diagnosis of vascular lesion.
- Central hemangioma tends to be less invasive than peripheral counterpart.

HEREDITARY HEMORRHAGIC TELANGIECTASIA / RENDU-OSLER-WEBER DISEASE

- Congenital hereditary disease.
- Telangiectatic or angiomatous areas, mainly on face, neck and chest, and oral mucosa.

- Earliest sign, preceding telangiectasia is epistaxis.
- Differential diagnosis includes scleroderma, *CREST syndrome*, Lupus erythematosus.
- CT, BT are normal.
- Actual cause of bleeding is either a primary intrinsic defect of the endothelial cells or defect in perivascular supportive tissue bed.

ENCEPHALO TRIGEMINAL ANGIOMATOSIS / STURGE-WEBER SYNDROME

- Combination of venous angioma of leptomeninges over the cerebral cortex with ipsilateral angiomatous lesion of the face.
- Portwine nevi are generally present, confined to skin area supplied by trigeminal nerve.
- Cranial radiographs reveals intracranial convolutional calcifications *(TRAM-LINE CALCIFICATIONS)*.
- Ocular – Glaucoma, exopthalmos, angioma of the choroids.
- Neurological – Convulsive disorders, spastic hemiplegia with or without mental retardation.

NASOPHARYNGEAL ANGIOFIBROMA

- Rare neoplasm, occurring almost exclusively in the nasopharynx of adolescent males.
- Generally manifested by nasal obstruction, epistaxis and sinusitis.

LYMPHANGIOMA

- Usually congenital.
- Intraoral lymphangioma most commonly occurs on the tongue, but may be seen on the palate, buccal mucosa, gingivae and lips.
- Macroglossia is a common manifestation, anterior dorsal part is affected.
- Cystic Hygroma presents as large deep, diffuse swelling in neck.

MYXOMA

- Extremely rare.
- Histopathologically exist as loose textured tissue containing moderate number of delicate reticulin fibres and mucoid material, probably hyaluronic acid.
- Tumor is not encapsulated and may invade surrounding tissue.
- Radiographic features – *Tennis racket appearance.*

CHONDROMA

- Occurs in mandible in mental region, coronoid process and condyle, in maxilla near the malar process and premaxillary area and nasal septum.
- Radiographically appears as irregular radiolucent or mottled area.

BENIGN CHONDROBLASTOMA (CODMAN'S TUMOR)

- Primary central bone tumor.

- Usually involves long bones, rarely condyle.

OSTEOMA

- Slow growing circumscribed swelling on the jaw producing obvious asymmetry.
- *Gardner syndrome*
  Multiple Osteomas
  Multiple polyposis of large intestine.
  Multiple epidermoid or sebaceous cysts of skin.
  Occasional desmoid tumors.
  Impacted supernumerary and permanent teeth.

TORUS PALATINUS

- Usually occurs in midline of hard palate.
- Higher incidence in American Indians,Norwegians and Eskimos.
- Homogenously radiopaque.

TORUS MANDIBULARIS

- Most common site is premolar region.
- Higher incidence seen in mongoloid group, low frequency in Caucasoid group.
- Usually bilateral.

MUSCLE ORIGIN

LEIOMYOMA

- Benign tumor derived from smooth muscle.
- Common oral sites are posterior portion of tongue, palate, cheeks, gingival, lips, and salivary glands.

RHABDOMYOMA

- Most common location is tongue and floor of the mouth.

GRANULAR CELL MYOBLASTOMA: (GRANULAR CELL TUMOR / GRANULAR CELL SCHWANNOMA)

- Most common site is tongue.
- Arise from Schwann cells, stained with protein antisera to S-100.

NERVE TISSUE ORIGIN

TRAUMATIC NEUROMA (AMPUTATION NEUROMA)

- Not a true neoplasm, but rather an exuberant attempt at repair of a damaged nerve trunk.

- Site – Appears as a small nodule or swelling of mucosa, near the mental foramen, lips or tongue.
- Central lesion may also occur.
- Digital pressure cause pain.
- Derived mainly from perineurium.

MULTIPLE ENDOCRINE NEOPLASIA SYNDROMES

MEN I – Tumors or hyperplasias of pituitary, parathyroids, adrenal cortex and pancreatic islets occurring in association with peptic ulcers and gastric hypersecretion.

MEN II a or *MEN II - Sipple's syndrome.*
- Parathyroid adenoma but no tumor of pancreas.
- Pheochromocytomas of adrenal medulla.
- Medullary CA of thyroid.
- No peptic ulcers.

MEN II b or MEN III
- Mucocutaneous neuromas.
- Pheochromocytomas of adrenal medulla.
- Medullary CA of thyroid.
- Marfanoid habitus.
- GIT disorders.
- Presence of oral neuromas mostly on lips *("Bumpy lips")*, tongue.

NEUROFIBROMA / NEUROFIBROMATOSIS / VON RECKLINGHAUSEN'S DISEASE OF SKIN / FIBROMA MOLLUSCUM

- Arise from Schwann cells, fibroblasts and occasional perineural cells with, intermingled neurites or axons.
- Sessile or pedunculated, elevated smooth surfaced nodules over skin surface or deeper, more diffuse lesions (also known as *"elephantiasis neuromatosa"*).
- *"Café-au-lait" spots.*
- Axillary freckling.
- Pigmentation.
- Hirsuitism.
- Intra oral non-ulcerated nodules may be seen on buccal mucosa, palate, alveolar ridge, vestibule and tongue.
- Macroglossia.
- Central lesions appear as fusiform enlargement of the mandibular canal.
- May undergo malignant transformation.
- Radioresistant.

NEUROLEMMOMA (NEURILEMMOMA / SCHWANNOMA)

- Derived from Schwann cells.
- Usually painless.
- Composed of 2 types of tissues.
    - Antoni type A
    - Antoni type B

 Antoni type A tissue is composed of cells with elongated or spindle shaped nuclei, aligned in palisading pattern. Antoni type B is disorderly arrangement of cells and fibers with areas of what appears to be edema fluid and with formation of microcysts.

- Well encapsulated.

MELANOTIC NEUROECTODERMAL TUMOR OF INFANCY / MELANOTIC AMELOBLASTOMA / RETINAL ANLAGE TUMOR.

- High urinary excretion of vanillyl mandelic acid (VMA)
- Neural crest tumor.
- Rapidly growing darkly pigmented lesion.
- Radiographic appearance is suggestive of an invasive malignant neoplasm.

NOTES

21 Malignant Tumors

BASAL CELL CARCINOMA (RHODENT ULCER)

- Mostly develops on exposed surfaces of skin, the face and scalp in middle-aged or elderly persons.
- Also known as *"BENIGN CARCINOMA"*. There is no tendency for metastasis, but spreads by direct invasion.
- Relatively rare in blacks.
- Most frequently seen in the middle 3rd of face.
- Nests, islands and sheets of cells with palisade appearance of basal layer are seen on histopathology.
- Basal cells are pluripotent. So this CA can form adenoid BCC, cystic BCC, keratotic BCC or primordial BCC.
- Treatment of choice is surgery or radiation.
- Multiple BCC are characteristic feature of *"Gorlin Goltz syndrome"*.

SQUAMOUS CELL CARCINOMA

- Most common malignant neoplasm of oral cavity.
- Can occur at any intraoral site.
- Most common site in India is mucobuccal fold.
- Predisposing factors include tobacco, alcohol, syphilis, sunlight sepsis, trauma, Plummer Vinson syndrome, viruses like EBV, CMV, HSV, and VZV.
- Lesions of base of tongue and postero lateral border have poorest prognosis.
- Radiographically, it appears as a radiolucent lesion with invasive, erosive or infiltrative borders. Pathological fracture may occur with sharpened thinned bone ends and displacement. There is destruction of adjacent cortices.
- Causes spiked root resorption.

- Floating tooth appearance
- *TNM categories:*

  T – Primary tumor

  T_{is} – CA in situ.

  T_1 – Tumor 2 cm or less in greatest diameter.

  T_2 – Tumor greater than 2 cm but not greater than 4 cm in greatest diameter.

  T_3 – Tumor greater than 4 cm in greatest diameter.

  N – Regional lymph nodes

  N_0 – No clinically palpable cervical lymph nodes.

  N_1 – Clinically palpable ipsilateral LN that are not fixed, metastasis suspected.

  N_2 – Clinically palpable contralateral or bilateral cervical LN that are not fixed.

  N_3 – Clinically palpable LN that are fixed.

  M – Distant metastasis.

  M_0 – No distant metastasis.

  M_1 – Clinical / radiographic evidence of metastasis other than to cervical lymph modes.

- **Staging**

  Stage   I – $T_1 N_0 M_0$

         II – $T_2 N_0 M_0$

        III – $T_3 N_0 M_0$

            $T_1 N_1 M_0$

            $T_2 N_1 M_0$

            $T_3 N_1 M_0$

       IV – $T_{1,2,3} N_2 M_0$

            $T_{1,2,3} N_3 M_0$

  Any T or N category with M1.

VERRUCOUS CARCINOMA

- Form of SCC, slow-growing, chiefly exophytic and only superficially invasive.
- Lesions commonly have rugae like folds with deep cleft between them.
- Generally shows a marked epithelial proliferation with downgrowth of epithelium into connective tissue but usually without a pattern of true invasion.
- Parakeratin plugging is also seen.
- May cause invasion of bone.

SPINDLE CELL CARCINOMA / LANE TUMOR / CARCINOSARCOMA

- Chiefly occurs in upper respiratory and alimentary tracts.
- It is either a SCC associated with an atypical, benign, reactive connective tissue process, a combination of collision growth of a carcinoma and a sarcoma or a SCC with spindle cell anaplasia.

ADENOID SQUAMOUS CELL CARCINOMA / ADENOACANTHOMA

- Originates from pilosebaceous structures or areas of senile keratosis.
- Aggressive tumor.
- Most common site is lip.

MALIGNANT MELANOMA

- 3rd most common cancer of skin.
- Sunlight is an important etiologic factor.
- Most common types are:
  (a) Superficial spreading melanoma.
  (b) Nodular melanoma.
  (c) Lentigo melanoma.
- Superficial spreading melanoma:
  (a) Most common cutaneous melanoma in caucasians.
  (b) Chiefly occurs in 5th –7th decade of life, mainly in males.
  (c) Exists in radial-growth pattern.
  (d) Also called *pre-malignant melanoma or pagetoid melanoma in situ*.
  (e) Vertical growth pattern is marked by increase in size, change in color, nodularity and ulceration.
- Nodular melanoma:
  (a) Exist solely in a vertical growth phase.
  (b) May be amelanotic or black.
- Lentigo maligna melanoma (melanotic freckle of Hutchinson)
  (a) Radial growth pattern.
- Oral melanoma is one of the most common sites of this neoplasm in Japanese.
- Most common sites are palate, maxillary gingiva/ridge.
- Radiographically, indistinguishable from osteomyelitis.
- Treatment is surgical excision, cryosurgery, radiation, chemotherapy, immunotherapy.
- Melanoma of BANS (back, posterolateral arm, neck and scalp) tend to have higher metastatic rate.

CONNECTIVE TISSUE ORIGIN

FIBRO SARCOMA

- Occurs in relatively young persons.
- Metastasize through blood stream, producing more widespread foci of 2^0 tumor growth.
- Common sites- cheek, maxillary sinus, pharynx, palate, lip, periosteum of maxilla and mandible.
- Treatment of choice is surgery. Radiation is usually not helpful.

- Locally aggressive fibrous lesions:
  - Nodular fascitis.
  - Aggressive fibromatosis.
  - Proliferative myositis
  - Fibrous histiocytoma
  - Atypical fibroxanthoma.
  - Desmoplastic fibroma of bone.

HEMANGIOENDOTHELIOMA

- Most commonly found in the skin and subcutaneous tissues.
- More common in females.
- Clinically similar to hemangioma.
- A silver reticulin stain best demonstrates this vascularity.

HEMANGIOPERICYTOMA

- Characterized by proliferation of capillaries surrounded by masses of round or spindle-shaped cells.
- Tumor may appear encapsulated at operation, but this is often not confirmed microscopically.

KAPOSI'S SARCOMA / ANGIORETICULOENDOTHELIOMA

- Common malignancy in Africa (10%)
- Etiology is unknown.
- Most common malignancy in AIDS.
- Patients with Kaposi's sarcoma usually develop second primary cancer including lymphoma, myeloma, CA of colon, breast, prostate, tongue, tonsil and pancreas.
- 85-90% cases occur in males.
- Multiple lesions involve skin, many visceral organs and lymph nodes and sometimes oral cavity.
- 3 Stage of desease – inflammation, granuloma and neoplasia.
- X-ray irradiation is the treatment of choice.

EWING'S SAROMA / "ROUND CELL" SARCOMA

- Primary destructive lesion of bone arises from undifferentiated cells of reticulo endothelial system.
- Occurs predominantly in children and young adults.
- Intermittent pain and swelling are the earliest clinical signs. Facial neuralgia and lip paraesthesia may also occur.
- May involve the extra skeletal tissue also.
- *Radiographic appearance – "onion peel"* appearance or *"sun-ray"* appearance.
- Radio-sensitive tumor, treatment of choice is a combination of surgery, radiation and chemotherapy.

- Highly malignant.

CHONDROSARCOMA

- May occur in mandible or maxilla with primary involvement of the alveolar ridge or near antrum.
- Slowly increasing diastemma may be the 1st sign.
- May resemble chondroma histologically and radiographically.
- Cause expansion of bone, rather than its destruction.
- Surgery is the treatment of choice.

OSTEOSARCOMA

- Exists in 2 forms – Osteoblastic or sclerosing type and Osteolytic type
- Bimodal peak – 2nd and 5th decade.
- Chiefly occurs in young age.
- Predominantly involves long bones.
- Can occur in bones affected by osteitis deformans, X-ray radiation of jaws for fibrous dysplasia, giant cells.
- Genetic mutation and viral infection have also been implicated as the etiological agents.
- Usually proceeded by trauma.
- More commonly occurs in males.
- Mandible involvement more common than maxilla.
- Radiographic features.
- *"Sun-ray"* appearance, *"Onion peel"* appearance and *"Codman's triangle"* are seen in sclerotic form.
- Irregular radiolucency, expansion of cortical plates and destruction can occur in osteolytic form.
- Widening of PDL space around one or more teeth is usually the 1st sign *(Garrington's sign)*
- Radio resistant.
- Adjuvant chemotherapy in combination with surgery is the treatment of choice.

MALIGNANT LYMPHOMA

- Derived from lymphocytes and histiocytes.
- Radiographically, may have osteolytic, mixed or osteoblastic appearance.

NON-HODGKIN'S LYMPHOMA

- Involve lymph nodes, lymphoid organs and extra nodal organs and tissues including CNS, GIT, kidneys, testes, bone and skin.
- Mycosis fungoides – A form of cutaneous T-cell lymphoma.
- Lymphoproliferative disease of hard palate usually presents as non-Hodgkin's lymphoma.
- Histological picture is either diffuse or nodular.
- Nodular type has more favourable prognosis than diffuse type.

- Treatment of choice is radiation & chemotherapy.

PRIMARY LYMPHOMA OF BONE / PRIMARY RETICULUM CELL SARCOMA OF BONE

- More frequent in mandible.
- Diagnosis is usually based upon histopathology and difficult.
- Treatment – surgical excision or X-ray irradiation.

BURKITT'S LYMPHOMA / AFRICAN JAW LYMPHOMA

- Constitute 50% of all malignant tumors seen in African children.
- It is a non-Hodgkin's lymphoma (B-cell type).
- EBV is causally related.
- Primarily involves extra nodal tissues like jaws, sinuses, orbit, visceral organs.
- Histology – *"starry sky" effect.*
- Chemotherapy is treatment of choice.

HODGKIN'S DISEASE

- Primarily involves lymph nodes and lymphoid tissue, often the initial site is cervical nodes.
- Bimodal age incidence peak one in young adults and 2nd in 5th decade.
- There is painless lymph node enlargement, node are firm and *rubbery* in consistency.
- Diagnosis is usually made by lymph node biopsy and *Gordon's biologic test.*
- Histological features: Multinucleated Reed-Sternberg cells in an appropriate cellular background. These cells are considered to be malignant, have lymphocytic origin. *"Lacunar cells"* are seen in nodular sclerosis type.
- Radiotherapy & chemotherapy is the treatment of choice.

MULTIPLE MYELOMA / PLASMA CELL MYELOMA / PLASMACYTOMA

- Originates from plasma cells of bone narrow.
- Pain is usually an early feature.
- Swelling over the involved area and pathological fractures are common.
- Mandible more commonly involved than maxilla.
- *Radiographic features* – Numerous *sharply punched-out areas* in a variety of bones like skull, ribs, vertebrae, jaws and ends of long bones. May show multilocular appearance, opaque teeth, loss of lamina dura.
- *Laboratory findings* – Reversal of serum albumin globulin ratio.
  - Increase in total serum proteins to a level of 16 gm%.
  - Presence of *Bence-Jones proteins in urine*, which coagulates when the urine is heated to $40 - 60^0C$ and disappears when the urine is boiled.
  - Anaemia.
- *Histologic features – "cart-wheel" or "Checker board" pattern*.
  - Russell bodies are also found.

- Chemotherapy is the treatment of choice.

SOLITARY PLASMA CELL MYELOMA / PLASMACYTOMA

- Criteria for diagnosis of plasmacytoma.
    - Presence of solitary bone tumor.
    - Biopsy showing plasma cell histology.
    - Absence of myeloma cells in bone marrow examination.
    - Absence of anemia, hypercalcemia or renal involvement.
    - Absence of or a low monoclonal component on serum electrophoresis.
    - Normal levels of Immunoglobulins after treatment.
- Extramedullary plasmacytoma may be situated on the gingiva, palate, floor of mouth, tongue, tonsils and pillar as well as nasal cavity, nasopharynx and paranasal sinuses.
- *Radiographic features*: Purely destructive intramedullary lesions resembling carcinoma or expansile lesion resembling giant cell tumor.
- *Laboratory findings:*
    - Bence-Jones protein in urine.
    - Hyperglobulinemia and anaemia are absent.
- *Histologic features – "Cart wheel" or "Checker board" pattern.*
- Treatment of choice is surgery and radiotherapy.

MUSCLE TISSUE ORIGIN

LEIOMYOSARCOMA

- Very rare malignant tumor of smooth muscle origin.
- Cheek and floor of mouth are most common sites.

RHABDOMYOSARCOMA

- 4 forms
    - (a) Pleomorphic
    - (b) Alveolar
    - (c) Embryonal
    - (d) Botryoid
- Embryonal form is more common in head & neck region. Sites of occurrence include orbit, inner canthus, tonsil, soft palate, mastoid, internal ear, parotid, zygoma, temporal and cervical regions.
- *Histologic features*

    Pleomorphic type – "Racquet" cells, "Strap" and "Ribbon" cells.

    Alveolar type – "dropping off" appearance of cells from collagen trabecular. Cells "floating" in alveolar space.

Embryonal type – Eosinophilic spindle cells and round cells.

- Treatment of choice is surgical excision followed by radiotherapy.

NERVE TISSUE ORIGIN

MALIGNANT SCHWANNOMA / NEUROGENIC SARCOMA / NEUROFIBROSARCOMA

- In peripheral malignant schwannomas, lip, gingiva, palate & buccal mucosa are commonly involved.
- In central tumors, the mandible or mandibular nerve is more frequently affected than maxilla.
- Radiographic features – diffuse radiolucency resembling malignant infiltrating neoplasm or dilatation of mandibular canal.

OLFACTORY NEUROBLASTOMA / ESTHESIONEUROBLASTOMA

- Originates from olfactory apparatus. Involves nasal cavity and nasopharynx.
- Appears as a painful swelling in area of nasal fossae.

METASTATICS TUMORS OF JAWS

- Various primary tumors which metastasize to jaws are:

Breast 31%	Lung 18%
Kidney 15%	Thyroid 6%
Prostate 6%	Colon 6%
Stomach 5%	Malanocarcinoma 5%

- Mandible more commonly involved than maxilla, mainly molar area due to rich deposit of hematopoietic tissue.

QUESTIONS

1. **Punched out radiolucencies on the radiograph with the presence of Bence Jones proteins in urine is indicative of:** [AIPGEE 2008]
   1. Multiple myeloma
   2. Hodgkin's lymphoma
   3. Hand-Schuller-Christian disease
   4. Hyperparathyroidism

Ans. **1**

Other radiographic features of multiple myeloma are multilocular appearance, opaque teeth, loss of lamina dura. Laboratory findings may include Reversal of serum albumin globulin ratio, increase in total serum proteins to a level of 16 gm% and anaemia. Bence Jones proteins in urine are also seen in plasmacytoma, Leukaemia, Polycythemia.

2. Features of dysplasia are hyperchromatism, abnormal mitotic figures &: [AIPGEE 2008]

1. Hyperkeratosis
2. Decreased nuclear cytoplasmic ratio
3. Test tube rete pegs
4. Balloon shaped cells

Ans. **1**

Features of dysplasia are

- Increased abnormal mitosis.
- Individual cell keratinization.
- Epithelial pearls within spinous layer.
- Alteration in nuclear cytoplasmic ratio.
- Loss of polarity and disorientation of cells.
- Hyperchromatism of cells.
- Large, prominent nucleoli.
- Dyskaryosis or nucleus atypism.
- Poikilokaryocytosis or division of nuclei without division of cytoplasm.
- Basilar hyperplasia.

3. Syndrome associated with predisposition to development of oral cancer is termed as:
[AIPGEE 2008]

1. Plummer Vinson syndrome
2. Rendu-Osler-Weber syndrome
3. Sturge Weber syndrome
4. Gardener's syndrome

Ans. **1**

Sturge-weber Syndrome

- Angiomatosis of face (nevus flammeus) and leptomeningeal angiomas.
- There is also intracranial calcifications and contralateral hemiplegia.
- Massive growth of gingiva and asymmetrical jaw growth and tooth eruption sequence

Plummer-vinson Syndrome

- Cracks or fissures at the corner of mouth (angular cheilitis).
- Dysphagia due to esophageal webs.
- Atrophy of filiform papillae and koilonychia.
- Predisposition to oro- oesophagial carcinomas

Gardner's Syndrome

- *Systemic* features—multiple polyposis of large intestine and polyp of colon and rectum.

- Tumors—osteomas of bone including long bones, skull and jaws. There may be occasional occurrence of desmoid tumors. Other tumors which can occur are lipoma, leiomyoma and adenocarcinoma of colon.
- Cysts—multiple epidermoid or sebaceous cyst of skin particularly of scalp and back.
- Oral features—hypercementosis, multiple unerupted supernumerary teeth and compound odontoma.

Osler – Rendu – Weber Syndrome (Hereditary Hemorrhagic Telangiectasia)

- Autosomal dominant condition characterized by telangiectasia on skin and mucosa, IgA deficiency and rarely Von Willebrand's disease
- Telangiectases may be seen in any part of mouth and may be conspicuous on lips

4. Rodent ulcer is also referred to as: [AIPGEE 2008]
1. Squamous cell carcinoma
2. Basal cell carcinoma
3. Malignant melanoma
4. Verrucous carcinoma

Ans. **2**

Also known as BENIGN CARCINOMA. May be associated with *Gorlin Goltz syndrome.*

5. The most common benign tumor occurring in oral cavity is: [AIPG 2005]
1. Papilloma.
2. Fibroma.
3. Adenoma.
4. Epulis.

Ans. **2**

6. On clinical examination a 60-years-old female had a tumor in the right buccal mucosa. The size of the tumor was about 2 cm in diameter. There was no involvement of regional lymph nodes and also had no distant metastasis. The TNM stage of the tumor is: [AIPG 2004]
1. Tl N0 M0
2. Tl Nl M0
3. Tl N2 M0
4. T2 Nl M0

Ans. **1**

T1 = < 2 cm.
T2 = 2-4 cm.
T3 = < 4 cm.
T4 = > 4 cm with local infiltration.

7. The commonest site of oral cancer among Indian population is: [AIPG 2004]
1. Tongue

2. Floor of mouth.

3. Alveobuccal complex

4. Lip

Ans. **3**

Because of placing the tobacco in vestibule.

8. **A 70-year old male who has been chewing tobacco for the past 50 years presents with a six-month history of a large, fungating and soft papillary lesions in the oral cavity. The lesion has penetrated into the mandible lymph nodes are not palpable. Two biopsies taken from the lesion proper show benign appearing papillomatosis with hyperkeratosis and acanthosis infiltrating the subjacent tissues. The most likely diagnosis is:** [AIPG 2004]

1. Squamous cell papilloma

2. Squamous cell carcinoma

3. Verrucous carcinoma

4. Malignant mixed tumour

Ans. **3**

Veracious CA usually doesn't metastatize but cause local infiltration.

9. **The most common malignant tumor of adult males in India is:** [AIPG 2004]

1. Oropharyngeal carcinoma

2. Gastric carcinoma

3. Colo-rectal carcinoma

4. Lung cancer

Ans. **1**

10. **The photomicrograph represents an excisional biopsy of and pink, painless, elevated well demarcated mass of the buccal mucosa. The condition is:** [AIPG 2003]

1. Fibroma

2. Lipoma

3. Lipofibroma

4. Papilloma

Ans. **1**

Lipoma is soft, papilloma has verrucous surface.

11. **Common benign bone tumour:** [AIPG 2002]

1. Osteoid osteoma

2. Osteochondroma

3. Chondromyxoid fibroma

4. Euchondroma.

Ans. **1**

Osteoma is the most common benign tumor of bone and frontal sinus is the most common site.

12. Which of the following regress spontaneously? [AIPG 2002]

1. Osteosarcoma
2. Retinoblastoma
3. Choriocarcinoma
4. Malignant melanoma.

Ans. 3

13. Osteosarcoma of the jaw: [AIPG 2001]

1. Occurs mostly in the maxilla
2. Seen in old age
3. Highly malignant tumour which shows early metastasis
4. Shows a soap bubble type of radiolucency in radiographs

Ans. 3

Osteosarcoma can also develop from Paget's decrease on fibrous dysplasia. It has high rate of metastasis. Treated by combination of surgery, radiotherapy and chemotherapy.

14. Which of the following conditions gives a starry sky appearance? [AIPG 2001]

1. Non Hodgkin's lymphoma
2. Hodgkin's lymphoma
3. Burkitt's lymphoma
4. Leukemia

Ans. 3

"Starry- sky" appearance is seen on histological picture of Burkett's lymphoma due to macrophages with an abundant clear cytoplasm, containing cellular debris.

15. A distinct clinical entity occurring as a proliferative reaction to local irritants on the gingiva is: [AIPG 2000]

1. Pyogenic granuloma
2. Eosinophilic granuloma
3. Hemangioma
4. Giant cell granuloma.

Ans. 1

Pyogenic granuloma is an inflammatory reactive lesion, which is thought to occur due to chronic irritation by calculus or overhanging restoration. Most commonly seen in pregnant women.

16. A patient is diagnosed of oral cancer of stage $T_3N_{2a}M_O$. The treatment indicated is: [AIPG 2000]

1. Surgery
2. Surgery + radiotherapy
3. Chemotherapy alone
4. Surgery + chemotherapy.

Ans. 2

Large tumor with regional lymph node involvement is usually treated by combination of surgery and radiotherapy.

17. **Which of the following is a malignant neoplasm of the oral cavity?** [AIPG 2000]
    1. Lipoma
    2. Chondroma
    3. Liposarcoma
    4. Haemangioma.

Ans. 3

Other three are benign tumors.

18. **In carcinoma of the prostate with mandibular secondaries which of the following will be seen?** [AIPG 2000]
    1. Increase in the serum acid phosphatase
    2. Decrease in the serum acid phosphatase
    3. Increase in the serum alkaline phosphatase
    4. Decrease in the serum alkaline phosphatase.

Ans. 1

An elevated level of serum acid phosphatase is diagnostic test for prostate carcinoma.

19. **Early change seen in multiple myeloma is:** [AIPG 2000]
    1. Multiple punched-out lesions in the mandible
    2. Single punched-out lesions in the mandible
    3. No changes
    4. Alveolar-crest bone loss.

Ans. 3

No bony changes are evident in early stages of multiple myeloma.

20. **A symmetric widening of the periodontal ligament in one or two teeth can be most probably due to:** [AIPG 2000]
    1. Paget's disease
    2. Osteosarcoma
    3. Florid osseous dysplasia
    4. Osteomalacia.

Ans. 2

Initial radiographic appearance of osteosarcoma is PDL space widening.

21. **Increased incidence of squamous cell carcinoma of the skin is due to all except:** [AIPG 99]
    1. Ultraviolet radiation
    2. Fair skin

3. Alcohol

4. Actinic keratitis

Ans. 3

Squamous cell carcinoma is usually seen in fair people who are exposed to sunlight (UV light) for prolonged time

22. **Squamous cell carcinoma with best prognosis is:** [AIPG 96]

1. Lip

2. Tongue

3. Palate

4. Floor of the mouth

Ans. 1

Because CA of lip is generally slow to metastasize.

23. **Sarcoma of the soft tissues spread by:** [AIPG 96]

1. Blood vessels

2. Lymphatics

3. Direct invasion

4. Local infiltration

Ans. 1

Sarcomas usually spread by hematogenous route while carcinomas spread via lymphatics.

24. **Hamartoma is:** [AIPG 96]

1. An abnormal collection of blood vessels caused by irritation

2. A malignant growth

3. A developmental malformation

4. A growth containing tissues from all 3 germ layers

Ans. 3

Hamartoma is an abnormal proliferation of tissues of structure native to the part. They are considered as developmental anomaly.

25. **Which of the following malignancies has the best prognosis?** [AIPG 1995]

1. Osteosarcoma

2. Multiple myeloma

3. Basal cell carcinoma

4. Carcinoma of the breast

Ans. 3

Basal cell carcinoma is a locally invasive, slowly spreading primary epithelial malignancy. Metastasis is exceptionally rare.

26. Which of the following lesions metastasizes through blood stream? [AIPG 1995]

1. Basal cell carcinoma
2. Malignant melanoma
3. Squamous cell carcinoma
4. Verrucous carcinoma

Ans. 2

Metastasis through blood vessels is a common route for sarcoma but certain carcinomas also frequently metastasize by this mode especially those of lung, breast, thyroid, kidney and prostate.

Important example of this type of spread are seen is vertebral metastasis in cancers of thyroid & prostate.

27. Kaposi's sarcoma is a tumour of: [AIPG 1995]

1. Blood vessels
2. Reticuloendothelial system
3. Striated muscles
4. Smooth muscles

Ans. 1

Kaposi's sarcoma is an unusual and uncommon disease of blood vessels, which occasionally manifest in oral cavity. They appear as reddish or brownish red nodules which may vary is size from a few mm to a cm or more in diameter and are usually tender or painful. It is normally seen in AIDS patients.

28. Malignant tumour of striated muscles is called: [AIPG 94]

1. Leiomyosarcoma
2. Rhabdomyosarcoma
3. Leiomyoma
4. Rhabdomyoma

Ans. 2

Leiomyosarcoma- malignant tumor of smooth muscles

Leiomyoma- benign tumor of smooth muscles

Rhabdomyoma- benign tumour of striated muscles.

29. Reed-Sternberg cells are characteristically seen in: [AIPG 94]

1. Alpha-thalassaemia
2. Glandular fever
3. Hansen's disease
4. Hodgkin's disease

Ans. 4

These are multinucleated cells, which are thought to be derived from B-lymphocytes or monocytes. They represent the malignant cells of Hodgkin's disease.

30. Irritational fibroma which is asymptomatic is best treated by:　　　**[AIPG 93]**

　1. No treatment is necessary because it is asymp-tomatic

　2. Simple excision

　3. Radiation therapy

　4. Wide excision followed by chemotherapy

Ans. **2**

Irritational fibroma is a benign tumor where simple excision is the treatment of choice. It rarely recurs after excision.

31. Pyogenic granuloma:　　　**[AIPG 93]**

　1. Bleeds on touch

　2. Painless

　3. Soft in consistency

　4. All of the above

Ans. **4**

32. Maximum chances of recurrence are in:　　　**[AIPG 93]**

　1. Lipoma

　2. Haemangioma

　3. Giant cell granuloma

　4. Pyogenic granuloma

Ans. **4**

During the excision of the lesion, any chronic source of irritation like calculus should also be removed, because the lesion can recur.

33. Treatment for cementoma is:　　　**[AIPG 93]**

　1. No treatment

　2. Extraction of tooth

　3. Surgical removal of mass while saving the tooth

　4. None of the above

Ans. **1**

No treatment is required for cementoma as it is an innocuous lesion. Extraction of the involved tooth should be considered in case of benign cementoblastoma.

34. All of the following predispose to oral cancer except:　　　**[AIPG 93]**

　1. Infective hepatitis

　2. Leukoplakia

　3. OSF and submucous fibrosis

　4. Carcinoma in situ

Ans. **1**

Leukoplakia, OSMF and carcinoma in situ, all have a definite premalignant potential.

35. **A 24-year old man suffers from loose tooth and gingivitis in one quadrant. Radiograph shows irregular bone loss. Blood chemistry is normal. Biopsy shows diffuse proliferation of histiocytes and an infiltrate containing many eosinophils. Most appropriate diagnosis is:**
[AIPG 92]

1. Apical granuloma
2. Chronic periodontitis
3. Eosinophilic granuloma
4. Parasitic infection

Ans. **3**

Eosinophilia granuloma is marked by destructive, well-demarcated lesions of bone, which are replaced by a soft tissue. Radiograph shows irregular radiolucent areas involving superficial alveolar bone with destruction of cortex and sometimes-pathological fractures.

36. **If multiple myeloma is suspected in a patient's history and intraoral radiograph, which of the following radiographs should be taken to confirm the diagnosis:** [AIPG 92]

1. Lateral skull
2. Anterior posterior view
3. Lateral oblique
4. Posterior anterior view

Ans. **2**

Anteroposterior view of skull shows the typical punched out radiolucencies of skull and jaws.

37. **The most common metastatic lesion of jaw bones is from a primary tumour located in:**
[AIPG 92]

1. Lung
2. Stomach
3. Breast
4. Large intestine

Ans. **1**

38. **A blue nodular mass on the lateral border of the tongue is soft, smooth and blanches upon pressure. It is most likely to be:** [AIPG 92]

1. Lymphoma
2. Hemangioma
3. Epulis fissuratum
4. Epithelioma

Ans. **2**

Blanching on pressure in a characteristic feature of hemangioma. Lymphoma in oral cavity is usually seen as ulcerative lesion. Epulis fissuratum occurs in vestibule due to denture irritation and is firm in consistency.

39. A 1.5 cm suspicious looking ulcer on the floor of the mouth is to be studied microscopically. A specimen is best obtained by: [AIPG 92]

1. Needle biopsy
2. Excisional biopsy
3. Incisional biopsy
4. None of the above

Ans. 3

Incisional biopsy is the modality of choice when size of lesion is > 1 cm.

40. The usual radiographic appearance of an osteosarcoma is a: [AIPG 91]

1. Discrete radiolucency with regular borders.
2. Multicystic radiolucency with a soap-bubble appearance.
3. Cotton-wool appearance with an irregular peripheral border.
4. Sunburst pattern with radiopaque strands extending from the cortical plates.

Ans. 4

Discrete radiolucency with regular borders is a feature of cysts. Soap bubble appearance is seen in ameloblastoma, giant cell lesion, aneurysmal bone cyst and central hemangioma. Cotton-wool appearance is a feature of Paget's disease.

41. Which of the following signs or symptoms is most suggestive of metastatic disease? [AIPG 91]

1. Paraesthesia
2. Sudden swelling
3. Root resorption
4. Diffuse radiolucency

Ans. 1

Paraesthesia is the most common feature of metastatic disease due to neural invasion, although other features like sudden swelling, root resorption and diffuse radiolucency are also found.

42. A nonpainful, slowly enlarging, benign neoplasm appears as a submucosal lump and exhibits pseudoepitheliomatous hyperplasia in the overlying epithelium, is most probably: [AIPG 91]

1. Fibroma
2. Rhabdomyoma
3. Granular cell tumour
4. Papilloma

Ans. 1

Granular cell tumor caries from schwann cells and forms a submucosal nodule. Most common site is tongue. Rhabdomyoma arises from muscles.

43. The most common malignancy of the oral cavity is: [AIPG 91]

1. Basal cell carcinoma

2. Transitional cell carcinoma

3. Melanoma

4. Squamous cell carcinoma

Ans. **4**

44. **The most common malignancy found in bone is:** [AIPG 1990]

1. Osteosarcoma

2. Multiple myeloma

3. Malignant lymphoma

4. Metastatic carcinoma

Ans. **4**

Metastasis to bone from different primaries is the most common malignancy of bone.

45. **Rodent ulcer (or) Basal cell carcinoma is usually present in the:** [AIPG 1990]

1. Intraorally lateral border of the tongue

2. Upper third of the face

3. Middle third of the face

4. Lower third of the face

Ans. **3**

Seen in persons exposed to sunlight. It is not seen intraorally, but may infiltrate through skin to intraoral sites.

46. **Which of the following is most likely to be fatal?** [AIPG 1990]

1. Osteochondroma

2. Giant cell tumour

3. Paget's disease

4. Multiple myeloma

Ans. **4**

Due to multiple systems of the body involved and infection.

47. **The most reliable single histologic criteria for a diagnosis of oral squamous cell carcinoma is:**
[AIPG 1989]

1. Invasion

2. Degeneration

3. Pleomorphism

4. Encapsulation

Ans. **1**

Invasion

Dysplastic lesions – mild, moderate, severe dysplasia are limited to epithelium.

Carcinoma in situ – abnormal cells involve the entire epithelium without invasion of basement membrane.

Carcinoma- is diagnosed when there is disruption of basement membrane & invasion into connective tissue.

48. **Which of the following conditions is characterized by café-au-lait spots, non-encapsulation and potential for malignant transformation?** [AIPG 1989]

    1. Neurilemmoma
    2. Neurofibroma
    3. Traumatic neuroma
    4. Solitary plasmacytoma

Ans. **2**

Neurofibroma or Von-Recklinghausen's Neurofibromatosis

– Potential for malignant transformation

– Malignant neurilemmona (5% of cases)

– Pheochromocytoma

– Astrocytoma & glioma.

49. **A man who suffered a displaced mandibular fracture sometime ago complains of pain. The pain is in the old fracture site, near the mental foramen, exquisitely tender mass in the described area. The best preoperative diagnosis is:** [AIPG 1989]

    1. Neurolemmoma
    2. Neurofibroma
    3. Traumatic neuroma
    4. Von Recklinghausen's disease

Ans. **3**

50. **Which of the following is most malignant?** [AIPG 1989]

    1. Neurolemmoma
    2. Traumatic neuroma
    3. Neurofibroma
    4. Neurogenic fibroma

Ans. **3**

Neurofibroma

- Most malignant tumor of nerve sheaths.
- High risk into malignant neurofibrosarcoma

Traumatic neuroma

- Benign, formed after injury to nerve due to an attempt to repair of the nerve .

Neurilemmona / schwanoma

- Benign tumor arising from axon sheath.
- Capsulated tumor with two types of tissues Antony A & B.
- Antony B - verocay bodies. (Hyaline bodies)

22 Red and White Lesions of the Oral Mucosa

BASIS FOR A WHITE LESION

- Increased the thickness of the keratin layer, or hyperkeratosis.
- An increase in the amount of edema fluid in the epithelium (i.e, leukoedema),
- Reduced vascularity in the underlying lamina propria.
- Deposits on the surface of mucosa.
- Chemical and thermal injury.

LEUKOEDEMA

- The incidence is more in black
- The most frequent site is the buccal mucosa bilaterally, may be seen rarely on the labial mucosa, soft palate, and floor of the mouth.
- It usually has a *faint, white, diffuse, and filmy appearance*, with numerous surface folds resulting in wrinkling of the mucosa, cannot be scraped off, and *disappears on stretching* the mucosa.
- *"Velvet like veil"*appearance.
- *"Mother of pearl appearance"*.
- Intracellular edema of the stratum spinosum.
- No treatment indicated. No malignant change reported.

WHITE SPONGE NEVUS

- A rare autosomal dominant disorder.
- Predominantly affects noncornified stratified squamous epithelium of buccal mucosa.
- May be present at birth or may first manifest or become more intense at puberty.
- Genetic analyses showed a missense mutation in one allele of keratin 13 that leads to proline substitution for leucine within the keratin gene cluster on chromosome 17.
- *Soft, "spongy," or velvety thick plaques* of the buccal mucosa, other sites involved are the ventral tongue, floor of the mouth, labial mucosa, soft palate, and alveolar mucosa.
- Histopathology shows large cells with poorly stained "washed out" or empty cytoplasm.

- No treatment needed.

HEREDITARY BENIGN INTRAEPITHELIAL DYSKERATOSIS (Witkop's Disease/ Witkop- Von Sallman Syndrome)

- Thick, corrugated, asymptomatic, white "spongy" plaques involving the buccal and labial mucosa. Other intraoral sites include the floor of the mouth, the lateral tongue, the gingiva, and the palate.
- The most significant aspect of HBID involves the bulbar conjunctiva, where thick, gelatinous, foamy, and opaque plaques form adjacent to the cornea, chronic relapsing ocular irritation and photophobia. May lead to blindness.
- Ultrastructural findings in patients with HBID reveal the the presence of numerous vesicular bodies in immature dyskeratotic cells, densely packed tonofilaments within the cytoplasm of these cells, and the disappearance of cellular bridging in mature dyskeratotic cells *(tobacco cells or cells within the cells)*.
- No treatment required.

DYSKERATOSIS CONGENITA (Zinssner Engman Cole Syndrome)

- Unusual due to the high incidence of oral cancer in young affected adults.
- Oral changes occur in association with severely dystrophic nails and a prominent reticulated hyperpigmentation of the skin of the face, neck, and chest.
- Many cases also exhibit hematologic changes including pancytopenia hypersplenism, and an aplastic or Fanconi's anemia.
- Oral lesions commences before 10 years of age as crops of vesicles.

LINEA ALBA (WHITE LINE)

- It is a horizontal streak on the buccal mucosa at the level of the occlusal plane extending from the commissure to the posterior teeth.
- It is a very common finding and is most likely associated with pressure, frictional iritation, or sucking trauma from the facial surfaces of the teeth.
- Is usually present bilaterally and may be pronounced in individuals with reduced overjet of the posterior teeth. It is often restricted to dentulous areas.
- No treatment indicated.

FRICTIONAL (TRAUMATIC) KERATOSIS

- White plaque with a rough and frayed surface that is clearly related to an identifiable source of mechanical irritation and that will usually resolve on elimination of the irritant.
- Upon removal of the offending agent, the lesion should resolve within 2 weeks. Biopsies should be performed on lesions that do not heal to rule out a dysplastic lesion.

CHEEK CHEWING (Morsicatio Buccarum)

- Result from chronic irritation due to repeated sucking, nibbling, or chewing.

- Chronic chewing of the labial mucosa (*morsicatio labiorum*) and the lateral border of the tongue (*morsicatio linguarum*) may be seen with cheek chewing or may cause isolated lesions.
- The lesions are most frequently found bilaterally on the posterior buccal mucosa along the plane of occlusion.
- The occurrence is twice as prevalent in females.

CHEMICAL INJURIES OF THE ORAL MUCOSA

- Transient nonkeratotic white lesions of the oral mucosa are often a result of chemical injuries caused by a variety of agents-
  - *Aspirin Burn* -the tissue is damaged when aspirin is held in the mucobuccal fold area for prolonged periods of time for the relief of common dental pain.
  - *Silver Nitrate*- commonly used as a chemical cautery agent for the treatment of apthous ulcers. It can destroy tissue around the immediate area of application.
  - *Hydrogen Peroxide*- often used as an intraoral rinse for the prevention of periodontal disease. At concentrations of 3%, hydrogen peroxide is associated with epithelial necrosis.
  - *Sodium Hypochlorite*- or dental bleach is commonly used as a root canal irrigant and may cause serious ulcerations due to accidental contact with oral soft tissues.
  - *Dentifrices and Mouthwashes*- an unusual sensitivity reaction with severe ulcerations and sloughing of the mucosa can occur due to cinnamon-flavored dentifrice Caustic burns of the lips, mouth, and tongue are seen with mouthwashes containing alcohol and chlorhexidine.
- Lesion is irregular in shape, white, covered with a pseudomembrane, and very painful. A superficial white and wrinkled appearance without resultant necrosis is seen. Long-term contact can cause severe damage and sloughing of the necrotic mucosa.
- The unattached nonkeratinized tissue is more commonly affected than the attached mucosa.

ACTINIC KERATOSIS (CHEILITIS)

- A premalignant epithelial lesion related to long-term sun exposure, classically found on the vermilion border of the lip.
- Small percentage of these lesions will transform into squamous cell carcinoma.
- The mainstay of treatment of actinic keratosis is surgery. Chemotherapeutic agents such as topical 5-fluorouracil have been used with some success.

SMOKELESS TOBACCO–INDUCED KERATOSIS (Snuff Dipper's Keratosis, Or Tobacco Pouch Keratosis)

- Accepted as precancerous, but have a much lower risk of malignant transformation.
- Smokeless tobacco contains several known carcinogens, including N-nitrosonornicotine (NNN), which causes mucosal alterations.
- Leads to development of root surface caries and, to a lesser extent, coronal caries.
- The most common area of involvement is the anterior mandibular vestibule, followed by the posterior vestibule.

NICOTINE STOMATITIS (Stomatitis Nicotina Palatii, Smoker's Palate)

- White lesion on the hard and soft palate in heavy cigarette, pipe, and cigar smokers, restricted to areas that are exposed to a relatively concentrated amount of hot smoke during inhalation.
- Areas covered by a denture are usually not involved.
- The lesion is not considered to be premalignant.
- Found in older males with a history of heavy long-term cigar, pipe, or cigarette smoking.
- The palatal mucosa becomes diffusely gray or white. Numerous slightly elevated papules with punctate red centers that represent inflamed and metaplastically altered minor salivary gland ducts are noted.
- Nicotine stomatitis is completely reversible once the habit is discontinued.

SANGUINARIA-INDUCED LEUKOPLAKIA

- Sanguinaria extract, used in oral rinses and toothpaste can cause leukoplakia of the maxillary vestibule in patients who used sanguinaria-based products on a routine basis.
- Typically, patients present with a white, velvety, wrinkled or corrugated patch of leukoplakia involving both the attached gingiva and vestibular mucosa, usually very distinct and sharply demarcated from surrounding tissue.
- No appropriate treatment has been established for sanguinaria-induced leukoplakia. However, an initial biopsy is mandatory.

ORAL HAIRY LEUKOPLAKIA

- A corrugated white lesion that usually occurs on the lateral or ventral surfaces of the tongue in patients with severe immunodeficiency (HIV infection).
- Epstein-Barr virus (EBV) is implicated as the causative agent.
- Hairy leukoplakia has also occasionally been reported in patients with other immunosuppressive conditions, such as patients undergoing organ transplantation and patients undergoing prolonged steroid therapy.
- No treatment is indicated. The condition usually disappears when antiviral medications such as zidovudine, acyclovir, or gancyclovir are used in the treatment of the HIV infection. Topical application of podophyllin resin or tretinoin has led to short-term resolution of the lesions, but relapse is often seen.

CANDIDIASIS

- *Candida* is predominantly an opportunistic infectious agent.
- *Candida* may be a carcinogen or promoting agent, rather than only an innocuous opportunistic infectious entity.
- The typical lesions in infants are described as soft white adherent patches on the oral mucosa, generally painless and can be removed with little difficulty. In the adult, inflammation, erythema, and painful eroded areas are more often associated with this disease.

- *Classification of Oral Candidiasis*
  Acute
  > Pseudomembranous
  > Atrophic (erythematous)
  > Antibiotic stomatitis

  Chronic
  > **Atrophic**
  > Denture sore mouth
  > Angular cheilitis
  > Median rhomboid glossitis

  > **Hypertrophic/hyperplastic**
  > Candidal leukoplakia
  > Multifocal
  > Mucocutaneous

  > **Syndrome associated**
  > Familial +/– endocrine candidiasis syndrome
  > Myositis (thymoma associated)
  > Immunocompromise (HIV) associated.

  Diffuse or localized
- *Candida* species are normal inhabitants of the oral flora of many individuals, but are present in the mouth of the healthy carrier in a low concentration of 200 to 500 cells per milliliter of saliva and cannot be identified by microscopic examination.
- *Predisposing Factors-*
  - Marked changes in oral microbial flora (due to the use of antibiotics [especially broad-spectrum antibiotics], excessive use of antibacterial mouth rinses, xerostomia).
  - Chronic local irritants (dentures and orthodontic appliances).
  - Administration of corticosteroids (aerosolized inhalant and topical agents are more likely to cause candidiasis than systemic administration).
  - Poor oral hygiene.
  - Pregnancy
  - Immunologic deficiency
  - Congenital or childhood (chronic familial mucocutaneous candidiasis ± endocrine candidiasis sydrome [hypoparathyroidism, hypoadrenocorticism], and immunologic immaturity of infancy).
  - Acquired or adult (diabetes, leukemia, lymphomas, and AIDS).
  - Iatrogenic (from cancer chemotherapy, bone marrow transplantation, and head and neck radiation).
  - Malabsorption and malnutrition.

- Candidal leukoplakia is considered a chronic form of oral candidiasis in which firm white leathery plaques are detected on the cheeks, lips, palate, and tongue. The differentiation of candidal leukoplakia from other forms of leukoplakia is based on finding periodic acid Schiff (PAS)–positive hyphae in leukoplakic lesions.
- Localized CMC is a variant associated with chronic oral candidiasis and lesions of the skin and nails.
- Antibiotics nystatin and amphotericin B. An imidazole derivative (clotrimazole) is for topical use. Systemic therapy includes the use of any one of these three: ketoconazole, itraconazole, and fluconazole. Fluconazole and amphotericin B may be used intravenously for the treatment of the resistant lesions of CMC and systemic candidiasis.

PARULIS (gumboil)

- Localized accumulation of pus in gingival tissues, originates from either an acute periapical abscess or an occluded periodontal pocket.

IDIOPATHIC "TRUE" LEUKOPLAKIA

- Leukoplakia is a white oral precancerous lesion with a recognizable risk for malignant transformation.
- The most commonly encountered and accepted precancerous lesions in the oral cavity are leukoplakia and erythroplakia.
- Risk of malignant transformation varies according to the histologic and clinical presentation, but the total lifetime risk of malignant transformation is estimated to be 4 to 6%.
- A number of locally acting etiologic agents, including tobacco, alcohol, candidiasis, electrogalvanic reactions, and (possibly) herpes simplex and papillomaviruses (particularly subtypes HPV-16 and HPV-18) have been implicated as causative factors for leukoplakia. True leukoplakia is most often related to tobacco usage.
- Smokeless tobacco is also a well-established etiologic factor for the development of leukoplakia; however, the malignant transformation potential of smokeless tobacco–induced lesions is much lower than that of smoking-induced lesions.
- Many varieties of leukoplakia have been identified-
  A. *"Homogeneous leukoplakia" (or "thick leukoplakia")* refers to a usually well -defined white patch, localized or extensive, that is slightly elevated and that has a fissured, wrinkled, or corrugated surface. On palpation, these lesions may feel leathery to *"dry, or cracked mud-like", fine lines (cristae), pumice pattern, ebbing tide appearance.*
  B. *Nodular (speckled) leukoplakia (granular or nonhomogeneous)* refers to a mixed red-and-white lesion in which keratotic white nodules or patches are distributed over an atrophic erythematous background. This type is associated with a higher malignant transformation rate.
  C. *"Verrucous leukoplakia" or "verruciform leukoplakia"* is a thick white lesion with papillary surfaces in the oral cavity. These lesions are usually heavily keratinized and are most often seen in older adults in the sixth to eighth decades of life. Some of these lesions may exhibit an exophytic growth pattern.

    D. *Proliferative verrucous leukoplakia (PVL)* **extensive** papillary or verrucoid white plaques that tend to slowly involve multiple mucosal sites in the oral cavity and to inexorably transform into squamous cell carcinomas PVL has a very high risk for transformation to dysplasia, squamous cell carcinoma or verrucous carcinoma.

- Characterized by variable patterns of hyperkeratosis and chronic inflammation. The lesions represent benign hyperkeratosis (ortho or parakeratin) with or without a thickened spinous layer (acanthosis).
- Definitive diagnosis is established by tissue biopsy. Adjunctive methods such as vital staining with toluidine blue and cytobrush techniques are helpful in accelerating the biopsy and/or selecting the most appropriate spot at which to perform the biopsy.
- *Toluidine blue staining* uses a 1% aqueous solution of the dye that is decolorized with 1% acetic acid. The dye binds to dysplastic and malignant epithelial cells with a high degree of accuracy.
- The cytobrush technique uses a brush with firm bristles that obtain individual cells from the full thickness of the stratified squamous epithelium; this technique is significantly more accurate than other cytologic techniques used in the oral cavity.
- Definitive treatment involves surgical excision although cryosurgery and laser ablation are often preferred because of their precision and rapid healing. Total excision is aggressively recommended when microscopic dysplasia is identified.
- The use of antioxidant nutrients and vitamins A, C, and E; beta carotene; analogues of vitamin A; and diets that are high in antioxidants and cell growth suppressor proteins (fruits and vegetables) have been tried.
- Speckled leukoplakia carries the highest average transformation potential, followed by verrucous leukoplakia; homogeneous leukoplakia carries the lowest risk.

BOWEN'S DISEASE

- Bowen's disease is a localized intraepidermal squamous cell carcinoma of the skin that may progress into invasive carcinoma over many years.
- Bowen's disease also occurs on the male and female genital mucosae and (rarely) in the oral mucosa as an erythroplakic, leukoplakic, or papillomatous lesion.
- Bowen's disease occurs most commonly on the skin, as a result of arsenic ingestion.

ERYTHROPLAKIA (ERYTHROPLASIE DE QUEYRAT)

- Erythroplakia has been defined as a "bright red velvety plaque or patch that cannot be characterized clinically or pathologically as being due to any other condition."
- It has been proposed that most erythroplakic lesions are precursors of oral squamous cell carcinoma.
- Classified as "homogeneous erythroplakia, erythroplakia interspersed with patches of leukoplakia, and granular or speckled erythroplakia".
- Erythroplakia occurs predominantly in older men, in the sixth and seventh decades of life.
- Erythroplakias are more commonly seen on the floor of the mouth, the ventral tongue, the soft palate, and the tonsillar fauces, all prime areas for the development of carcinoma.

- The treatment of erythroplakia should follow the same principles outlined for that of leukoplakia.

ORAL LICHEN PLANUS

- Oral lichen planus (OLP) is a *common chronic immunologic inflammatory mucocutaneous disorder* that varies in appearance from keratotic (reticular or plaquelike) to erythematous and ulcerative.
- The etiology of lichen planus involves a cell-mediated immunologically induced *degeneration of the basal cell layer* of the epithelium.
- Lichen planus is one variety of a broader range of disorders of which an immunologically induced lichenoid lesion is the common denominator. Other factors proposed for causation are stress, diabetes, hepatitis C, trauma, and hypersensitivity to drugs and metals.
- Lichenoid reaction can occur due to reactions to dental restorations, mouth rinses, antibiotics, gold injections for arthritis, and immunocompromised status such as graft-versus-host disease.
- The mean age of onset is the fifth decade of life, and there is clearly a female predominance.
- The *buccal mucosa* is the most common site.
- OLP is classified as *reticular* (lacelike keratotic mucosal configurations), *atrophic* (keratotic changes combined with mucosal erythema), or *erosive* (pseudomembrane-covered ulcerations combined with keratosis and erythema) and *bullous* (vesiculobullous presentation combined with reticular or erosive patterns).
- The reticular form consists of (a) slightly elevated fine whitish lines (*Wickham's striae*) that produce either a lacelike pattern or a pattern of fine radiating lines or (b) annular lesions. This is the most common and most readily recognized form of lichen planus. Most patients with lichen planus at some time exhibit some reticular areas.
- *Koebner phenomenon-* fresh lesions may appear at the site of trauma or on scratch marks
- The most common sites include the buccal mucosa (often bilaterally), followed by the tongue; lips, gingivae, the floor of the mouth, and the palate are less frequently involved.
- Whitish elevated lesions, or papules, usually measuring 0.5 to 1.0 mm in diameter, may be seen on the well-keratinized areas of the oral mucosa.
- Atrophic or erosive lichen planus involving the gingivae results in desquamative gingivitis.
- Three features are considered essential for the histopathologic diagnosis of lichen planus:
  1. areas of hyperparakeratosis or hyperorthokeratosis, often with a thickening of the granular cell layer and a *saw-toothed* appearance to the rete pegs;
  2. *"liquefaction degeneration,"* or necrosis of the basal cell layer, which is often replaced by an eosinophilic band; and
  3. a dense subepithelial band of lymphocytes.
- Isolated epithelial cells, shrunken with eosinophilic cytoplasm and one or more pyknotic nuclear fragments *(Civatte bodies),* are often scattered within the epithelium and superficial lamina propria. These represent cells that have undergone apoptosis.
- Direct immunofluorescence demonstrates a *shaggy band of fibrinogen in the basement membrane zone* Patients also may have multiple mainly IgM-staining cytoid bodies, usually located in the dermal papilla or in the peribasillar area.

- The status of OLP as a premalignant condition is controvertial.
- There is no known cure for OLP; therefore, the management of symptoms guides therapeutic approaches. Corticosteroids have been the most predictable and successful medications for controlling signs and symptoms.
- Retinoids are also useful, usually in conjunction with topical corticosteroids as adjunctive therapy for OLP. Systemic and topically administered beta all-*trans* retinoic acid, vitamin A acid, systemic etretinate, and systemic and topical isotretinoin are all effective.
- Other topical and systemic therapies reported to be useful, such as dapsone, doxycycline, and antimalarials, require additional research.
- Topical application of cyclosporine appears to be helpful in managing recalcitrant cases of OLP.

LICHENOID REACTIONS

- Lichenoid reactions and lichen planus exhibit similar histopathologic features.
- Associated with the administration of a drug, contact with a metal, the use of a food flavoring, or systemic disease and resolution occurs when the drug or other factor was eliminated or when the disease was treated.
- Drug-induced lichenoid reactions may resolve promptly when the offending drug is eliminated. However, many lesions take months to clear; in the case of a reaction to gold salts, 1 or 2 years may be required before complete resolution. Gold therapy, nonsteroidal anti-inflammatory drugs (NSAIDs), diuretics, other antihypertensives, and oral hypoglycemic agents of the sulfonylurea type are all important causes of lichenoid reactions.

GRAFT-VERSUS-HOST DISEASE

- Immunologic phenomenon characterized by the interaction of immunocompetent cells from one individual (the donor) to a host (the recipient) who is not only immunodeficient but who also possesses transplantation isoantigens foreign to the graft and capable of stimulating it.
- Occur in up to 70% of patients who undergo allogenic bone marrow transplantation, usually for treatment of refractory acute leukemia.
- There may be both acute (< 100 days after bone marrow transplantation) and Chronic (after day 100 days post transplantation) forms of the condition.
- The epidermal lesions of acute GVHD range from a mild rash to diffuse severe sloughing. This may include toxic epidermal necrolysis *(Lyell's disease)*.
- Oral lesions occur in 1/3 rd of cases.
- Chronic GVHD is associated with lichenoid lesions that affect both skin and mucous membranes; salivary and lacrimal gland epithelium may also be involved.
- Because of the potential involvement of salivary glands in chronic GVHD, biopsy of minor salivary glands is a useful diagnostic procedure in some cases.
- The histopathologic features of chronic GVHD may resemble those of OLP.
- Topical corticosteroids and palliative medications may facilitate the healing of the ulcerations. Ultraviolet A irradiation therapy with oral psoralen has also been shown to be effective in treating resistant lesions.

ORAL SUBMUCOUS FIBROSIS

- Oral submucous fibrosis (OSF) is a slowly progressive chronic fibrotic disease of the oral cavity and oropharynx, characterized by fibroelastic change and inflammation of the mucosa, leading to a progressive inability to open the mouth, swallow, or speak.
- These reactions may be the result of either direct stimulation from exogenous antigens like *Areca* alkaloids or changes in tissue antigenicity that may lead to an autoimmune response.
- It occurs almost exclusively in inhabitants of Southeast Asia, especially the Indian subcontinent.
- The inflammatory response releases cytokines and growth factors that promote fibrosis by inducing the proliferation of fibroblasts, up-regulating collagen synthesis and down-regulating collagenase production.
- Even though the etiopathology is incompletely understood, several factors are believed to contribute to the development of OSF, including general nutritional and vitamin deficiencies and hypersensitivity to certain dietary constituents such as chill peppers, chewing tobacco, etc. However, the primary factor is the habitual use of betel and its constituents, which include the nut of the areca palm *(Areca catechu)*, the leaf of the betel pepper *(Piper betle)*, and lime (calcium hydroxide).
- OSF is regarded as a premalignant condition.
- The disease presents as burning sensation of the mouth, particularly during consumption of spicy foods, vesicles, ulcers, altered taste sensation, dysphagia, and dysphonia.
- The mucosa appears blanched and opaque with the appearance of fibrotic bands that can easily be palpated. The bands usually involve the buccal mucosa, soft palate, posterior pharynx, lips, and tongue.
- Histologic examination reveals severely atrophic epithelium with complete loss of rete ridges. Varying degrees of epithelial atypia may be present. The underlying lamina propria exhibits severe hyalinization, with homogenization of collagen. Cellular elements and blood vessels are greatly reduced.
- OSF is very resistant to treatment. Many treatment regimens have been proposed to alleviate the signs and symptoms, without much success; including Submucosal injected steroids and hyaluronidase, oral iron preparations, and topical vitamin A and steroids, surgical intervention.
- Malignant transformation rate for submucous fibrosis is 4 to 13%.

QUESTIONS

1. Which of the following epithelial changes commonly signify precancerous?   [AIPG 2001]
1. Dyskeratosis
2. Hyperkeratosis
3. Parakeratosis
4. Acanthosis

Ans. **1**

2 and 3 are seen in white lesion. 4 is seen in vesiculobullous disease.

2. Leukoplakia with the worst prognosis is seen on the: [AIPG 2001]

1. Dorsum of tongue
2. Floor of mouth
3. Buccal mucosa
4. Palate

Ans. 2

Leukoplakia in floor of mouth has a higher malignant potential. Also the rate of metastasis is also high if cancer develops.

3. Grinspan's syndrome is associated with: [AIPG 97]

1. Hypertension, diabetes, lichen planus
2. Oral, ocular, genital lesions
3. Hypertension with oral lesions
4. Pemphigus, CHF, diabetes

Ans. 1

Grinspan syndrome is characterized by hypertension, diabetes & lichen planus.

(2) Choice constitutes the features of Behchet syndrome.

4. Which of the following lesions has the greatest malignant potential? [AIPG 97]

1. Leukoedema
2. Lichen planus
3. Actinic cheilitis
4. White sponge nevus

Ans. 3

Actinic chelitis is a common premalignant alteration of the lower lip vermilion that occurs due to prolonged exposure to UV light. More commonly seen in light complexioned people.

Premalignant status of lichen planus is controvertial. Leukoedema occurs due to masticatory forces or smoking. It is a benign lesion and regress when the etiology is removed white sponge nevus is a developmental anomaly.

5. Dermokeratosis refers to: [AIPG 97]

1. Lichen planus
2. Leukoplakia
3. Leukocytosis
4. All of the above

Ans. 1

6. Which of the following is a premalignant lesion? [AIPG 96]

1. Leukoplakia
2. Bowen's disease
3. Leukoedema

    4.   White sponge nevus

Ans.   **2**

Bowen's disease or carcinoma in situ is more appropriate choice because if left untreated, it eventually progresses to carcinoma. Leukoplakia is also a premalignant lesion but frequency of malignant transformation is less as compared to Bowen's disease.

7. **The oral mucosa becomes rigid, blanched and opaque in which of the following conditions?**
   [AIPG 1995]
   1. Pemphigus vulgaris
   2. Lupus erythematosis
   3. Ehlers-Danlos syndrome
   4. Submucous fibrosis

Ans.   **4**

OSMF is characterized by restricted mouth opening, stiffening of oral mucosa, blanching of mucosa caused by impairment of local vascularity

Blanched mucosa is opaque & white, vertical fibrous bands appear, mobility of soft palate is restricted, uvula has shrunken appearance, tongue is depapillated & protrusion of tongue is impaired.

8. **Liquefaction degeneration is seen in:**   **[AIPG 94]**
   1. Lichen planus
   2. Psoriasis
   3. Pemphigus
   4. Darier's disease

Ans.   **1**

Liquifaction degeneration is a common feature in lichen planus.

9. **Which of the following lesions have the most malignant potential?**   **[AIPG 94]**
   1. Leukoplakia
   2. Aspirin burn
   3. Submucous fibrosis
   4. Leukoderma

Ans.   **1**

Malignant conversion of leukoplakia forms 69% of oral cancers.

10. **Which white lesion stains darker in iodine test?**   **[AIPG 93]**
    1. Aspirin burn
    2. Lichen planus
    3. White sponge nevus
    4. Leukoplakia

Ans.   **1**

Iodine stains normal tissue more intensely than dysplastic tissue.

11. Oral hairy leukoplakia is seen in which of the following conditions: [AIPG 92]

1. AIDS
2. Hepatitis B
3. Smoker's keratitis
4. Candidiasis

Ans. 1

Oral hairy leukoplakia is a velvety appearance of lateral border of tongue seen in HIV positive patients

12. During oral examination of a 57-year-old-man a large keratotic patch that covers the entire palate is noted. Some 'Red spots' are also seen in the patch. The patient most likely is a: [AIPG 91]

1. Pipe smoker
2. Cigar smoker
3. Snuff chewer
4. Tobacco chewer

Ans. 1

The features described here are that of smoker's palate where there is white keratotic patch with red umbilicate areas which denotes the opening of minor salivary glands. It is usually seen in patients with habit of reverse smoking. It has a very low malignant potential.

13. Parakeratosis may be absent in: [AIPG 1990]

1. Leukoplakia
2. Erythroplakia
3. Lichen planus
4. Psoriasis

Ans. 2

All others are which lesions with ortho or parakeratosis. In erythroplakia, usually there is atrophy of epithelium or thinning of keratin layer of keratin layer (red lesion).

14. Sloughing of necrotic epithelium is characteristic of: [AIPG 1990]

1. Aspirin burn
2. Denture sore mouth
3. Traumatic ulcer
4. Contact dermatitis

Ans. 1

2, 4 – erosive areas

3 – ulcers

15. A 14- years old boy has bilateral. Pearly-white thickening of the buccal mucosa. The boy has had the lesions since the birth. His younger brother also has similar lesions. History and clinical findings are consistent with a diagnosis of: [AIPG 1989]

1. Leukoedema
2. Lichen planus
3. Mucous patches
4. White sponge nevus

Ans. **4**.

White sponge nevus - Autosomal dominant missense mutation in one allele of keratin 13 that leads to praline substitution for leucine within keratin gene cluster on chromosome 17.

Leukoedema presents as faint, white, diffuse filmy appearance with numerous folds resulting in wrinkling of mucosa, and fades upon stretching the mucosa. Not familial

Lichen planus appears as slightly elevated five whitish lines or Wicham's striae – in a lace like or annular pattern, Age 4-5 decades.

Mucous patches - superficial grayish area of mucosal necrosis seen in secondary syphilis within 6 weeks after the primary lesion. Diffuse maculopapular eruption of the skin & mucous membrane.

15. Which of the following is a characteristic histologic feature of lichen planus? [AIPG 1989]

1. Blunted retepegs
2. Acantholysis
3. Saw tooth retepegs
4. True dyskeratosis

Ans. **3**

Histologic features

1. Hyper para/ortho keratosis with saw tooth rate pegs & thickening of granular cell layers.

2. Liquefaction degeneration of the basal cell layer replaced often by eosinophilic band.

3. A dense subepithelial band of lymphocytes.

23 Ulcerative, Vesicular, and Bullous Lesions

- Dermatologic lesions are classified according to their clinical appearance and include the following basic lesions:
    1. **Macules**. Well-circumscribed, flat lesions that are noticeable because of their change from normal skin color. They may be red due to the presence of vascular lesions or inflammation, or pigmented due to the presence of melanin, hemosiderin, and drugs.
    2. **Papules**. Solid lesions raised above the skin surface that are smaller than 1 cm in diameter. Papules may be seen in a wide variety of diseases including erythema multiforme simplex, rubella, lupus erythematosus, and sarcoidosis.
    3. **Plaques.** Solid raised lesions that are over 1 cm in diameter; they are large papules.
    4. **Nodules**. These lesions are present deep in the dermis, and the epidermis can be easily moved over them.
    5. **Vesicles**. Elevated blisters containing clear fluid that are under 1 cm in diameter.
    6. **Bullae**. Elevated blisterlike lesions containing clear fluid that are over 1 cm in diameter.
    7. **Erosions**. Moist red lesions often caused by the rupture of vesicles or bullae as well as trauma.
    8. **Pustules**. Raised lesions containing purulent material.
    9. **Ulcers**. A defect in the epithelium; it is a well-circumscribed depressed lesion over which the epidermal layer has been lost.
    10. **Purpura**. Reddish to purple flat lesions caused by blood from vessels leaking into the subcutaneous tissue. Classified by size as petechiae or ecchymoses, these lesions do not blanch when pressed.
    11. **Petechiae**. Purpuric lesions 1 to 2 mm in diameter. Larger purpuric lesions are called **ecchymoses.**

HERPES VIRUS INFECTIONS

- There are 80 known herpes viruses, and eight of them are known to cause infection in humans.
- All herpes viruses contain a *deoxyribonucleic acid (DNA)* nucleus.
- In immuno-compromised patients, HHV6 can cause interstitial pneumonitis and bone marrow suppression.
- HHV8 has been closely associated with Kaposi's sarcoma in human immunodeficiency virus (HIV) infected patients. There is also evidence-linking HHV8 to forms of lymphoma and Castleman's disease.
- HSV1, HSV2, and varicella-zoster are viruses that are known to cause oral mucosal disease.
- Cytomegalovirus is an occasional cause of oral ulceration in immunosuppressed patients, and it is suspected as a cause of salivary gland disease in HIV-infected patients.
- Classically, HSV1 causes a majority of cases of oral and pharyngeal infection, meningioencephalitis, dermatitis above the waist; HSV2 is implicated in most genital infections. However, changing sexual habits are making that distinction less important. Both types can cause primary or recurrent infection of either the oral or the genital area, and both may cause recurrent disease at either site. Primary infection may also occur concurrently in both oral and genital sites from either HSV1 or HSV2.

- Humans are the only natural reservoir of HSV infection, and spread occurs by direct intimate contact with lesions or secretions from an asymptomatic carrier.
- Latency, a characteristic of all herpes viruses, occurs when the virus is transported from mucosal or cutaneous nerve endings by neurons to ganglia where the HSV viral genome remains present in a nonreplicating state. During the latent phase, herpes DNA is detectable, but viral proteins are not produced. Reactivation of the latent virus occurs when HSV switches to a replicative state; this can be due to number of factors including peripheral tissue injury from trauma or sunburn, fever, or immunosuppression.
- Reactivation of HSV is the most common cause of Bell's palsy.
- There is evidence-linking HSV to carcinogenesis.

PRIMARY HERPES SIMPLEX VIRUS INFECTION

- Primary HSV may also be spread by asymptomatic shedders with HSV present in salivary secretions.
- Infection of the fingers and thumbs (**herpetic whitlows or herpetic paronychia**) of health professionals may occur during treatment of infected persons.
- **Geometric glossitis**- chronic herpes on tongue.
- Infection of the newborn result in viremia and disseminated infection of the brain, liver, adrenals, and lungs. Newborns of mothers with antibody titers are protected by placentally transferred antibodies during the first 6 months of life. After 6 months of age, the incidence of primary HSV1 infection increases. The incidence of primary HSV1 infection reaches a peak between 2 and 3 years of age.
- Significant percentage of cases of primary herpes are subclinical.
- Incubation period is most commonly 5 to 7 days but may range from 2 to 12 days.
- Patients with primary oral herpes have a history of generalized prodromal symptoms that precede the local lesions by 1 or 2 days.
- Small vesicles appear on the oral mucosa; these are thin-walled vesicles surrounded by an inflammatory base .The vesicles quickly rupture, leaving shallow round discrete ulcers. The lesions occur on all portions of the mucosa.
- An important diagnostic criterion in this disease is the appearance of generalized acute marginal gingivitis.
- Primary HSV in otherwise healthy children is a self-limiting disease.
- Cytology from a fresh vesicle stained with *Giemsa, Wright's, or Papanicolaou's stain* shows multinucleated giant cells, syncytium, and ballooning degeneration of the nucleus. **Lip Schultz bodies** *(intranuclear inclusions, Cowdry type A).*
- HSV Isolation and neutralization of a virus in tissue culture is the most positive method of identification and has a specificity and sensitivity of 100%.
- Conclusive evidence of a primary HSV infection includes testing for complement-fixing or neutralizing antibody in acute and convalescent sera.
- Acyclovir has been shown to be effective in the treatment of primary oral HSV in children when therapy was started in the first 72 hours. Newer anti-herpes drugs are now available, including

valacyclovir and famciclovir. Milder cases can be managed with supportive care only. A topical anesthetic (Dyclonine hydrochloride 0.5%) may be administered prior to meals.

- Antibiotics are of no help in the treatment of primary herpes infection, and use of *corticosteroid is contraindicated.*

COXSACKIE VIRUS INFECTIONS

- Coxsackieviruses are ribonucleic acid (RNA) enteroviruses. These viruses cause hepatitis, meningitis, myocarditis, peri-carditis, and acute respiratory disease.
- Three clinical types of infection of the oral region that have been described are usually caused by group A coxsackieviruses: herpangina, hand-foot-and-mouth disease, and acute lymphonodular pharyngitis. Types of coxsackievirus A have also been described as causing a rare mumps like form of parotitis.

HERPANGINA

- Caused by **Coxsackievirus A4** mainly, but types A1 to A10 as well as types A16 to A22 have also been implicated.
- After a 2-10-day incubation period, the infection begins with generalized symptoms of mild fever, chills, and anorexia, sore throat, dysphagia, and occasionally sore mouth.
- Within 24 to 48 hours, the vesicles rupture, forming small 1 to 2 mm ulcers. The disease is usually mild and heals without treatment in 1 week.
- Herpangina may be clinically distinguished from primary HSV infection by several criteria:
  - Herpangina occurs in epidemics; HSV infections do not.
  - Herpangina tends to be milder than HSV infection.
  - Lesions of herpangina occur on the pharynx and posterior portions of the oral mucosa, whereas HSV primarily affects the anterior portion of the mouth.
  - Herpangina does not cause a generalized acute gingivitis like that associated with primary HSV infection.
  - Lesions of herpangina tend to be smaller than those of HSV.
- Cytology smear from the base of a fresh vesicle and stained with Giemsa will not show ballooning degeneration or multinucleated giant cells. This helps to distinguish herpangina from herpes simplex and herpes zoster, which do show these changes.
- Herpangina is a self-limiting disease, and treatment is supportive, including proper hydration and topical anesthesia when eating or swallowing is difficult. Specific antiviral therapy is not available.

ACUTE LYMPHONODULAR PHARYNGITIS

This is a variant of herpangina caused by coxsackievirus A10. The distribution of the lesions is the same as in herpangina, but yellow-white nodules appear that do not progress to vesicles or ulcers.

HAND-FOOT-AND-MOUTH DISEASE

- Caused by infection with *coxsackievirus A16* in a majority of cases, although instances have been described in which A5, A7, A9, A10, B2, or B5 or enterovirus 71 has been isolated.

- The disease is characterized by low-grade fever, oral vesicles and ulcers, and nonpruritic macules, papules, and vesicles, particularly on the extensor surfaces of the hands and feet. The oral lesions are more extensive than are those described for herpangina, and lesions of the hard palate, tongue, and buccal mucosa are common.

- Severe cases with central nervous system involvement, myocarditis, and pulmonary edema have been reported in epidemics caused by enterovirus.

- Treatment is supportive.

VARICELLA-ZOSTER VIRUS INFECTION

- Varicella zoster (VZV) is a herpesvirus, and remains latent in neurons present in sensory ganglia. VZV is responsible for two major clinical infections of humans: *chickenpox (varicella)* and shingles *(herpes zoster [HZ])*.

- Chickenpox is a generalized primary infection, analogous to the acute herpetic gingivostomatitis of herpes simplex virus. After the primary disease is healed, VZV becomes *latent in the dorsal root ganglia of spinal nerves* or extramedullary ganglia of cranial nerves. VZV becomes reactivated, causing lesions of localized herpes zoster.

- The incidence of HZ increases with age or immunosuppression and these lesions may be deep-seated and disseminated, causing pneumonia, meningoencephalitis, and hepatitis.

- Chickenpox is a childhood disease characterized by mild systemic symptoms and a generalized intensely pruritic eruption of maculopapular lesions that rapidly develop into vesicles on an erythematous base. Oral vesicles that rapidly change to ulcers may be seen.

- HZ commonly has a prodromal period of 2 to 4 days, when shooting pain, paresthesia, burning, and tenderness appear along the course of the affected nerve. Unilateral vesicles on an erythematous base then appear in clusters, chiefly along the course of the nerve, giving the characteristic clinical picture of single dermatome involvement. Some lesions spread by viremia outside the dermatome. The vesicles turn to scabs in 1 week, and healing takes place in 2 to 3 weeks. The nerves most commonly affected with HZ are C3, T5, L1, L2, and the first division of the trigeminal nerve.

- Pain caused by VZ virus without lesions developing along the course of the nerve is known as *zoster sine herpete* or zoster sine.

- HZ may also occasionally affect motor nerves. HZ of the sacral region may cause paralysis of the bladder. The extremities and diaphragm have also been paralyzed during episodes of HZ.

- The most common complication of HZ is *postherpetic neuralgia*, which is defined as pain remaining for over a month after the mucocutaneous lesions have healed, although some clinicians do not use the term postherpetic neuralgia unless the pain has lasted for at least 3 months after the healing of the lesions. The overall incidence of postherpetic neuralgia is 12 to 14%.

- Involves one of the divisions of the trigeminal nerve in 18 to 20% of cases, but the ophthalmic branch is affected several times more frequently than are the second or third divisions. HZ of the first division can lead to blindness secondary to corneal scarring.

- HZ has been associated with dental anomalies and severe scarring of the facial skin when trigeminal HZ occurs during tooth formation. Pulpal necrosis and internal root resorption have also been related to HZ.

- HZ of the geniculate ganglion *(Ramsay Hunt syndrome)*, is a rare form of the disease characterized by Bell's palsy, unilateral vesicles of the external ear, and vesicles of the oral mucosa.
- Although the histopathology is not specific, two major histologic patterns have been described: an epidermal pattern characterized by lichenoid vasculitis and intraepidermal vesicles, and a dermal pattern characterized by lymphocytic vasculitis and subepidermal vesiculation.
- Fluorescent antibody stained smears using fluorescein conjugated monoclonal antibodies is more reliable than is routine cytology and is positive in over 80% of cases. The most accurate method of diagnosis is viral isolation in tissue culture.
- Acyclovir or famciclovir accelerate healing and reduce acute pain, but they do not reduce the incidence of postherpetic neuralgia. The use of systemic corticosteroids to prevent postherpetic neuralgia in patients over 50 years of age is controversial.
- Effective therapy for postherpetic neuralgia includes application of capsaicin; a substance extracted from hot chili peppers. Use of a tri-cyclic antidepressant or gabapentin is indicated.

ERYTHEMA MULTIFORME (ECTODERMOSIS EROSIVA PLURIORIFICIALIS)

- Erythema multiforme (EM) is an acute inflammatory disease of the skin and mucous membranes that causes a variety of skin lesions—hence the name *"multiforme."*
- EM has several clinical presentations:
  - Milder self-limiting form.
  - Severe life-threatening form that may present as either *Stevens-Johnson syndrome or toxic epidermal necrolysis (TEN).*
- EM is an immune-mediated disease. Many cases of EM are labeled idiopathic. Precipitating factors include:

  Herpes simplex infection

  Bacterial infection

  Fungal infection

  Drugs (barbiturates, phenylbutazone, digitalis, iodides, mercurials, penicillin, salicylates, sulfonamides, oral contraceptives.)

  Vaccination

  Radiation

  Crohn's disease

  Ulcerative collitis
- EM is seen most frequently in children and young adults.
- It has an acute or even an explosive onset; characterized by macules and papules 0.5 to 2 cm in diameter, appearing in a **symmetric distribution.**
- The most common cutaneous areas involved are the hands, feet, and extensor surfaces of the elbows and knees. The face and neck are commonly involved, but only severe cases affect the trunk. The pathognomonic lesion is the **Bull's eye, target or iris lesion**, which consists of a central bulla or pale clear area surrounded by edema and bands of erythema.

- The more severe vesiculobullous forms of the disease, Stevens-Johnson syndrome and TEN have a significant mortality rate.
- **Stevens-Johnson syndrome** manifests as generalized vesicles and bullae involving the skin, mouth, eyes, and genitals.
- The most severe form of the disease is **TEN (toxic epidermal necrolysis OR Lyell's disease)**, which is usually secondary to a drug reaction and results in sloughing of skin and mucosa in large sheets. Patients with this form of the disease are most successfully managed in burn centers, where necrotic skin is removed under general anesthesia and healing takes place under sheets of porcine xenografts.
- Oral lesions commonly appear along with skin lesions in approximately 70% cases.
- The finding of a perivascular lymphocytic infiltrate and epithelial edema of spinous layer producing sub epidermal vesicle and hyperplasia is considered suggestive of EM.
- Mild cases of oral EM may be treated with supportive measures only, including topical anesthetic mouthwashes. Adults treated with short-term systemic steroids Patients with severe cases of recurrent EM have been treated with dapsone, azathioprine, levamisole, or thalidomide.

CONTACT ALLERGIC STOMATITIS

- Contact allergy results from a delayed hypersensitivity reaction that occurs when antigens of low molecular weight penetrate the skin or mucosa of susceptible individuals.
- Contact stomatitis may result from contact with dental materials, oral hygiene products, or foods. Common causes of contact oral reactions are cinnamon or peppermint, which are frequently used flavoring agents in food, candy, and chewing gum, as well as oral hygiene products such as toothpaste, mouthwash and dental floss, dental materials including mercury in amalgam, gold in crowns, free monomer in acrylic, and nickel in orthodontic wires.
- Lesions may appear as *lichenoid lesion, plasma cell gingivitis.*
- Contact allergy is most accurately diagnosed by the use of a patch test by placing the suspected allergens in small aluminum disks, called *Finn chambers*, which are taped onto hairless portions of the skin. The disks remain in place for 48 hours. A positive response to a contact allergen is identified by inflammation at the site of the test, which is graded on a scale of 0 to 3.
- Management depends on the severity of the lesions. In mild cases, removal of the allergen suffices. In more severe symptomatic cases, application of a topical corticosteroid is helpful.

ORAL ULCERS SECONDARY TO CANCER CHEMOTHERAPY

- Anticancer drugs may cause oral ulcers directly or indirectly. Drugs that cause stomatitis indirectly depress the bone marrow and immune response, leading to bacterial, viral, or fungal infections of the oral mucosa. Others, such as methotrexate, cause oral ulcers via direct effect on the replication and growth of oral epithelial cells by interfering with nucleic acid and protein synthesis, leading to thinning and ulceration of the oral mucosa.

ACUTE NECROTIZING ULCERATIVE GINGIVITIS

- ANUG became known notoriously as **"trench mouth"** during World War I because of its prevalence in the combat trenches, and it was incorrectly considered a highly contagious disease.

- Organisms that cause the lesions are the fusiform bacillus and spirochetes.
- Tissue destruction is thought to be caused by endotoxins that act either directly on the tissues or indirectly by triggering immunologic and inflammatory reactions.
- It is associated with three major factors:
    Poor oral hygiene with pre-existing marginal gingivitis or faulty dental restorations
    Smoking
    Emotional stress
- Systemic disorders associated with ANUG are diseases affecting neutrophils (such as leukemia or aplastic anemia), marked malnutrition, and HIV infection.
- A fulminating form of ulcerative stomatitis related to ANUG is **noma (cancrum oris)**, characterized by extensive necrosis that begins on the gingiva and then progresses from the mouth through the cheek to the facial skin. The major risk factors associated with noma include malnutrition, poor oral hygiene, and concomitant infectious diseases such as measles.
- The onset of acute forms of ANUG is usually sudden, with pain, tenderness, profuse salivation, a peculiar metallic taste, and spontaneous bleeding from the gingival tissues, loss of the sense of taste and a diminished pleasure from smoking. The teeth are frequently thought to be slightly extruded, sensitive to pressure, or to have a **"woody sensation."**
- The typical lesions of ANUG consist of necrotic punched-out ulcerations, developing most commonly on the interdental papillae and the marginal gingivae.
- The therapy of ANUG uncomplicated by other oral lesions or systemic disease is local débridement, followed by complete gingival curettage and root planning.
- Antibiotics are usually not necessary for routine cases, should be prescribed for patients with extensive gingival involvement, lymphadenopathy, or other systemic signs. Metronidazole and penicillin are the drugs of choice.

RECURRENT APHTHOUS STOMATITIS (CANKER SORES)

- Immunologic disorders, hematologic deficiencies, and allergic or psychological abnormalities have all been implicated in cases of RAS.
- RAS is classified according to clinical characteristics:
    Minor ulcers
    Major ulcers (Sutton's disease, periadenitis mucosa necrotica recurrens, Miculicz's scarring)
    Herpetiform ulcers.
- **Minor ulcers** - comprise over 80% of cases
    Less than 1 cm in diameter
    Heal without scars.
- **Major ulcers** - over 1 cm in diameter
    Take longer to heal
    Often scars
- **Herpetiform ulcers** are considered a distinct clinical entity that manifests as recurrent crops of dozens of small ulcers throughout the oral mucosa.

- The current concept is that RAS is a clinical syndrome with several possible causes. The major factors identified include heredity, hematologic deficiencies, immunologic abnormalities, nutritional deficiency, such as celiac disease. Other factors that have been suggested as being etiologic in RAS include trauma, psychological stress, anxiety, and allergy to foods such as milk, cheese, wheat, and flour and detergent present in toothpaste, sodium lauryl sulfate (SLS).
- The individual lesions are round, symmetric, and shallow (similar to viral ulcers), but no tissue tags are present from ruptured vesicles (this helps to distinguish RAS from disease with irregular ulcers such as EM, pemphigus, and pemphigoid).
- The buccal and labial mucosae are most commonly involved. Lesions are less common on the heavily keratinized palate or gingiva.
- Most patients with RAS have between two and six lesions at each episode and experience several episodes a year.
- Histology- **Anitschkow cells** (epithelial cells with elongated nuclei containing a linear bar of chromatin with radiating processes of chromatin extending towards the nuclear membrane). Also seen in – sickle cell anaemia, megaloblastic anaemia, iron deficiency anaemia, cancer chemotherapy.
- In mild cases with two or three small lesions, use of a protective emollient is all that is necessary. Pain relief of minor lesions can be obtained with use of a topical anesthetic agent or topical diclofenac. In more severe cases, the use of a high-potency topical steroid preparation, such as fluocinonide, betamethasone or clobetasol, placed directly on the lesion shortens healing time and reduces the size of the ulcers. Other topical preparations that have been shown to decrease the healing time of RAS lesions include amlexanox paste and topical tetracycline. Drugs that have been reported to reduce the number of ulcers in selected cases of major aphthae include colchicine, pentoxifylline, dapsone, short bursts of systemic steroids, and thalidomide.

Behçet's Syndrome

- Triad of recurring oral ulcers, recurring genital ulcers, and eye lesions. The concept of the disease has changed from a triad of signs and symptoms to a multisystem disorder.
- Positive pathergy reaction.
- Arthritis occurs in greater than 50% of patients.
- Central nervous system involvement is the most distressing component of the disease.
- Thrombophlebitis, intestinal ulceration, venous thrombosis, and renal and pulmonary disease.
- A variant of Behçet's syndrome, **MAGIC syndrome**, has been described. It is characterized by Mouth and Genital ulcers with Inflammed Cartilage.
- A new set of diagnostic criteria was developed that includes recurrent oral ulceration occurring at least three times in one 12-month period plus two of the following four manifestations:
  - Recurrent genital ulceration.
  - Eye lesions including uveitis or retinal vasculitis.
  - Skin lesions including erythema nodosum, pseudofolliculitis, papulopustular lesions, or acneform nodules in postadolescent patients not receiving corticosteroids.
  - A positive pathergy test.

- The management of Behçet's syndrome depends on the severity and the sites of involvement. Azathioprine combined with prednisone has been shown to reduce ocular disease as well as oral and genital involvement. Pentoxifylline, which has fewer side effects than do immunosuppressive drugs or systemic steroids.

RECURRENT HERPES INFECTION

- RIH lesions in otherwise normal patients are similar in appearance to RHL lesions, but the vesicles break rapidly to form ulcers. The lesions are typically a cluster of small vesicles or ulcers, 1 to 2 mm in diameter, clustered on a small portion of the heavily keratinized mucosa of the gingiva, palate, and alveolar ridges.
- Smears from herpetic lesions show cells with *ballooning degeneration and multinucleated giant cells;* those from RAS lesions do not. For more accurate results, *cytology smears* may also be tested for HSV using fluorescein-labeled HSV antigen.
- Viral cultures also are used to distinguish herpes simplex from other viral lesions, particularly varicella-zoster infections.

RECURRENT HERPES INFECTION OF THE MOUTH (Recurrent Herpes Labialis, Common Cold Sore or Fever Blister [RHL]

- Recurrent herpes is not a re-infection but a reactivation of virus that remains latent in nerve tissue between episodes in a non-replicating state.
- RHL, may be precipitated by fever, menstruation, ultraviolet light, and perhaps emotional stress.
- Acyclovir and newer antiviral drugs such as valacyclovir, a prodrug of acyclovir, and famciclovir, are highly effective in preventing genital recurrences. The use of antiherpes nucleoside analogues to prevent and treat RHL in otherwise normal individuals is controversial.
- Foscarnet has been effective therapy for immunocompromised patients.

HERPES GLADIATORUM/ SCRUMPOX

Recurrent herpes infection in players at areas of abrasion.

THE PATIENT WITH CHRONIC MULTIPLE LESIONS

PEMPHIGUS

- Pemphigus is a potentially life-threatening disease that causes blisters and erosions of the skin and mucous membranes. These epithelial lesions are a result of autoantibodies that react with desmosomal glycoproteins that are present on the cell surface of the keratinocyte. The immune reaction against these glycoproteins causes a loss of cell-to-cell adhesion, resulting in the formation of intraepithelial bullae.
- Pemphigus occurs more frequently in the Jewish population.
- The major variants of pemphigus are:
  Pemphigus vulgaris (PV)

Pemphigus vegetans

Pemphigus foliaceous

Pemphigus erythematosus

Paraneoplastic pemphigus (PNPP)

Drug-related pemphigus.

- Pemphigus vegetans is a variant of pemphigus vulgaris, and pemphigus erythematosus is a variant of pemphigus foliaceous.

- Each form of this disease has antibodies directed against different target cell surface antigens, resulting in a lesion forming in different layer of the epithelium. In pemphigus foliaceus, the blister occurs in the superficial granular cell layer, whereas, in pemphigus vulgaris, the lesion is deeper, just above the basal cell layer. Mucosal involvement is not a feature of the foliaceus and erythematous forms of the disease.

PEMPHIGUS VULGARIS

- PV is the most common form of pemphigus, accounting for over 80% of cases. The underlying mechanism responsible for causing the intraepithelial lesion of PV is the binding of IgG autoantibodies to desmoglein 3, a transmembrane glycoprotein adhesion molecule present on desmosomes. The separation of cells, called acantholysis, takes place in the lower layers of the stratum spinosum.

- Pemphigus has been reported coexisting with other autoimmune diseases, particularly myasthenia gravis, thymoma, lymphoma.

- The classical lesion of pemphigus is a thin-walled bulla arising on otherwise normal skin or mucosa. The bulla rapidly breaks but continues to extend peripherally, eventually leaving large areas denuded of skin.

- In patients with PV, the bulla enlarges by extension to an apparently normal surface.

- Another characteristic sign of the disease is that pressure to an apparently normal area results in the formation of a new lesion. This phenomenon, called the *Nikolsky sign*, results from the upper layer of the skin pulling away from the basal layer. The Nikolsky may also occur in epidermolysis bullosa.

- Eighty to ninety percent of patients with pemphigus vulgaris develop oral lesions sometime during the course of the disease, and, in 60% of cases, the oral lesions are the first sign. Most commonly the lesions start on the buccal mucosa, often in areas of trauma along the occlusal plane. The palate and gingiva are other common sites of involvement. Lesions are similar to skin lesions.

- In some cases, the lesions may start on the gingiva and be called desquamative gingivitis.

- Biopsy from the advancing edge of the lesion shows areas of characteristic *suprabasilar acantholysis*. This study is best performed on a biopsy specimen that is obtained from clinically normal-appearing perilesional mucosa or skin.

- **TZANCK CELLS**- Clumps of epithelial cells often found lying free within the vesicular space, have swollen nuclei and hyperchromatic staining.

- In cases of PV, the technique will detect antibodies, usually IgG and complement, bound to the surface of the keratinocytes.
- The mainstay of treatment remains high doses of systemic corticosteroid, usually given in dosages of 1 to 2 mg/kg/d. When steroids must be used for long periods of time, adjuvants such as azathioprine or cyclophosphamide are added to the regimen to reduce the complications of long-term corticosteroid therapy. One new immuno-suppressive drug, mycophenolate, has been effective when managing patients resistant to other adjuvants. Other therapies that have been reported as beneficial are parenteral gold therapy, dapsone, tetracycline, and plasmapheresis and administration of 8-methoxypsoralen

PEMPHIGUS VEGETANS

- Pemphigus vegetans, which accounts for 1 to 2% of cases.
- Is a relatively benign variant of pemphigus vulgaris.
- Two forms of pemphigus vegetans are recognized:
    The Neumann type; and
    The Hallopeau type.
- *Neumann type* is more common, and the early lesions are similar to those seen in pemphigus vulgaris, with large bullae and denuded areas. Heal by developing vegetations of hyperplastic granulation tissue.
- In the *Hallopeau type*, which is less aggressive, pustules, not bullae, are the initial lesions. These pustules are followed by verrucous hyperkeratotic vegetations.
- Biopsy show *suprabasilar acantholysis*.In older lesions, hyperkeratosis and pseudoepitheliomatous hyperplasia become prominent. Immunofluorescent study shows changes identical to those seen in PV.
- Oral lesions are common in both forms of pemphigus vegetans and may be the initial sign of disease. Gingival lesions may be lace-like ulcers with a purulent surface on a red base or have a *granular or cobblestone appearance*.
- Serpenginous pattern in mouth with surface resembling pus is seen. Often contains many eosinophils.
- Oral lesions that are associated with inflammatory bowel disease and resemble pemphigus vegetans both clinically and histologically are referred to as pyostomatitis vegetans.
- Treatment is the same as that for PV.

PEMPHIGUS ERYTHEMATOSUS (SENEAR- USHER SYNDROME)

- Skin lesions resemble seborrhoeic dermatitis.

FAMILIAL BENIGN CHRONIC PEMPHIGUS (HAILEY- HAILEY DISEASE)

- Epidermal defect, either a fault in the synthesis or maturation of the tonofilaments and desmosome complex.
- Positive Nikolsky's sign.
- Lesions enlarge peripherally, but heal in the center.

- More extensive acantholysis than PV.
- *"DELAPIDATED BRICK WALL"* effect of adjacent epithelial cells on histologic studies.

PARANEOPLASTIC PEMPHIGUS

- PNPP is a severe variant of pemphigus that is associated with an underlying neoplasm-most frequently non-Hodgkin's lymphoma, chronic lymphocytic leukemia, or thymoma.
- Castleman's disease and Waldenströms macroglobulinemia are also associated with cases of PNPP.
- Treatment of this disease is difficult, and most patients die from the effects of the underlying tumor, respiratory failure due to acantholysis of respiratory epithelium, or the severe lesions that do not respond to the therapy successful in managing other forms of pemphigus.
- Histopathology of lesions of PNPP includes inflammation at the dermal-epidermal junction and keratinocyte necrosis in addition to the characteristic acantholysis seen in PV. The results of direct and indirect immunofluorescence also differ from those in PV. DIF shows deposition of IgG and comple-ment along the basement membrane as well as on the keratinocyte surface. Indirect immunofluorescence demonstrates antibodies that not only bind to epithelium but to liver, heart, and bladder tissue as well.

SUBEPITHELIAL BULLOUS DERMATOSES

Subepithelial bullous dermatoses are a group of mucocutaneous autoimmune blistering diseases that are characterized by a lesion in the basement membrane zone. The diseases in this group include bullous pemphigoid (BP), mucous membrane (cicatricial) pemphigoid (MMP), linear IgA disease (LAD), chronic bullous dermatosis of childhood (CBDC), and erosive lichen planus.

BULLOUS PEMPHIGOID (parapemphigus)

- BP is the most common of the *subepithelial blistering* diseases.
- It is *self-limiting* and may last from a few months to 5 years.
- In pemphigoid, the initial defect is not intraepithelial as in PV, but it is subepithelial in the lamina lucida region of the basement membrane. There is no acantholysis, but the split in the basement membrane is accompanied by an inflammatory infiltrate that is characteristically rich in eosinophils. Primary change occurs in connective tissue.
- Indirect immunofluorescence studies show circulating antibodies against basement membrane.
- The characteristic skin lesion of BP is a blister on an inflamed base that chiefly involves the scalp, arms, legs, axilla, and groin. Pruritic macules and papules may also be a presenting sign.
- The bullae do not continue to extend at the periphery to form large denuded areas, although death may occur from sepsis or cardiovascular disease secondary to long-term steroid use.
- Oral involvement is common in BP.The oral lesions of pemphigoid are smaller, form more slowly, and are less painful than those seen in pemphigus vulgaris, and the extensive labial involvement seen in pemphigus is not present. Desquamative gingivitis is also a manifestation of BP.

- Patients with localized lesions of BP may be treated with high-potency topical steroids or combined with immunosuppressive drugs such as azathioprine, cyclophosphamide, or mycophenolate or dapsone or a combination of tetracycline and nicotinamide.

BENIGN MUCOUS MEMBRANE PEMPHIGOID (CICATRICIAL PEMPHIGOID OR OCULAR PEMPHIGUS)

- MMP is a chronic autoimmune subepithelial disease that primarily causes ulceration and scarring. The primary lesion of MMP occurs when autoantibodies directed against proteins in the basement membrane zone, acting with complement (C3) and neutrophils, cause a subepithelial split and subsequent vesicle formation. The antigens associated with MMP are most frequently present in the lamina lucida portion of the basement membrane.
- The majority of cases of MMP demonstrate IgG directed against antigens on the epidermal side of the salt-split skin, which have been identified as BP180 (also called type XVII collagen); however, cases of MMP have also been identified where the antigen is present on the dermal side of the split. This latter antigen has been identified as epiligrin (laminin 5).
- The lesions of MMP most frequently involve the oral mucosa. The conjunctiva is the second most common site of involvement and can lead to scarring and adhesions developing between the bulbar and palpebral conjunctiva called **symblepharon**. Corneal damage is common, and progressive scarring leads to blindness.
- Lesions may also affect the genital mucosa, Larynx, esophagus. Skin lesions, usually of the head and neck region, are present in 20 to 30% of patients.
- Oral lesions occur in over 90% of patients with MMP. Desquamative gingivitis is the most common manifestation. The erosions typically spread more slowly than pemphigus lesions and are more self-limiting.
- Routine histopathology shows **subbasilar cleavage** and no acantholysis.
- Direct immunofluorescent technique demonstrates positive fluorescence for immunoglobulin and complement in the basement membrane zone. Only 10% of MMP patients demonstrate positive indirect immunofluorescence for circulating antibasement membrane-zone antibodies.
- Management of MMP depends on the severity of symptoms. When the lesions are confined to the oral mucosa, systemic corticosteroids will suppress their formation. Patients with mild oral disease should be treated with topical and intralesional steroids. When topical or intralesional therapy is not successful, dapsone therapy may be attempted.

LINEAR IgA DISEASE

- LAD is characterized by the deposition of IgA rather than IgG at the basement membrane zone.
- The clinical manifestations may resemble either dermatitis herpetiformis or pemphigoid presents as pruritic papules and blisters at sites of trauma.
- Minorities of cases have been drug induced.
- Antigens associated with LAD are heterogeneous and may be found in either the lamina lucida or lamina densa portions of the basement membrane.
- Oral lesions may be seen in up to 70% of patients. These lesions are clinically indistinguishable

from the oral lesions of MMP, with blisters and erosions of the mucosa frequently accompanied by desquamative gingivitis.

- The oral lesions of LAD may be managed with the use of topical steroids, but dapsone is effective therapy for more severe cases. Resistant cases may require systemic corticosteroids.

CHRONIC BULLOUS DISEASE OF CHILDHOOD:

- Chiefly affects children below the age of 5 years.
- It is characterized by the deposition of IgA antibodies in the basement membrane zone, which are detected by direct immunofluorescence on the epidermal side of skin or mucosa.
- The characteristic lesion of CBDC is a cluster of vesicles and bullae on an inflamed base. The genital, conjunctival, rectal, and oral lesions may also be present.
- Oral mucosal involvement is present in up to 50% of cases, and the oral lesions are similar to those observed in patients with MMP.
- Diagnosis is made by biopsy demonstrating a subepithelial lesion on routine histology and by deposition of IgA in the basement membrane zone on direct immunofluorescence. Indirect immunofluorescence demonstrates circulating IgA in 80% of cases.

EROSIVE LICHEN PLANUS

- An erosive and bullous form of this disease presents as chronic multiple oral mucosal ulcers. The erosive form of lichen planus has been associated with drug therapy, underlying medical disorders, and reactions to dental restorations.
- The drugs most commonly associated with severe lichenoid reactions include NSAIDs, hydrochlorothiazide, penicillamine, and angiotensin-converting enzyme inhibitors. Contact allergic reactions to flavoring agents such as cinnamon and peppermint and to dental materials such as mercury in amalgam, Graft-versus-host disease due to bone marrowtransplantation may also result in lichenoid reactions of the oral mucosa.
- The most frequently reported underlying disease associated with oral lichenoid reactions is chronic hepatitis caused by hepatitis C.
- Biopsy of the erosive lesions shows *hydropic degeneration of the basal layer* of epithelium. This can help to distinguish it from *mucous membrane pemphigoid*, which is also a subepithelial lesion but which shows an *intact basal layer*, or from pemphigus vulgaris, in which acantholysis is demonstrated.
- Patients with severe lichen planus should have drug therapy and underlying disease ruled out as possible causes.. The treatment of choice is topical corticosteroids. Cyclosporine rinses may be effective for patients with severe erosions resistant to topical steroids. Tacrolimus, another immunosuppressive drug, in a topical form is also useful. Systemic etretinate, dapsone, or photochemotherapy have also been reported to be effective in severe resistant case.
- patients with oral lichen planus appear to be in a higher risk group for development of squamous cell carcinoma.

THE PATIENT WITH SINGLE ULCERS

The deep mycoses were rare causes of oral lesions prior to HIV infection and immunosuppressive drug therapy. The dentist must consider this group of diseases in the differential diagnosis whenever isolated ulcerative lesions develop in known or suspected immunosuppressed patients.

HISTOPLASMOSIS

- Histoplasmosis is caused by the fungus Histoplasma capsulatum and rarely H. duboisii.
- Infection results from inhaling dust contaminated with droppings, particularly from infected birds or bats.
- In most cases, particularly in otherwise normal children, primary infection is mild, manifesting as a self-limiting pulmonary disease. In a small percentage of cases, progressive disease results in cavitation of the lung and dissemination of the organism to the liver, spleen, adrenal glands, bone marrow and meninges.
- Oral involvement is usually secondary, may appear as a papule, a nodule, an ulcer, or vegetation.
- The cervical lymph nodes are enlarged and firm. The clinical appearance of the lesions, as well as the accompanying lymphadenopathy, often resembles that of squamous cell carcinoma or even Hodgkin's disease.
- Mild to moderate cases of histoplasmosis can be treated with ketoconazole or itraconazole for 6 to 12 months. Immunosup-pressed patients or patients with severe disease require intra-venous amphotericin B for up to 10 weeks.

BLASTOMYCOSIS (NORTH AMERICAN BLASTOMYCOSIS)

- Blastomycosis is caused by Blastomyces dermatitidis, a dimorphic organism.
- The organism is found as a normal inhabitant of soil; therefore, the highest incidence of this infection is found in agricultural workers.
- Infection occurs by inhalation and leads to pulmonary involvement. Infection of the skin, mucosa, and bone may also occur, resulting from metastatic spread of organisms from the pulmonary lesions through the lymphatic system.
- Oral lesions occur secondary to pulmonary symptoms .The most common appearance of the oral lesions of blastomycosis is a nonspecific painless *verrucous ulcer* with indurated borders, often *mistaken for squamous cell carcinoma*.
- Other oral lesions include hard nodules and radiolucent jaw lesions.
- Treatment is similar to that of histoplasmosis.

MUCORMYCOSIS (PHYCOMYCOSIS)

- Usually seen with poorly controlled diabetes or hematologic malignancies or those undergoing cancer chemotherapy or immunosuppressive drug therapy.
- In the debilitated patient, mucormycosis may appear as a pulmonary, gastrointestinal, disseminated, or rhinocerebral infection.

- *Rhinomaxillary form* invades arteries and causes damage secondary to thrombosis and ischemia leading to nasal discharge, ptosis, proptosis secondary to invasion of the orbit, fever, swelling of the cheek, and paresthesia of the face.
- The most common oral sign of mucormycosis is *ulceration of the palate*, which results from necrosis due to invasion of a palatal vessel.
- The histopathologic specimen shows necrosis and nonseptate hyphae, which are best demonstrated by a periodic acid–Schiff stain.
- Cured by a combination of surgical débridement of the infected area and systemic administration of amphotericin B for up to 3 months.

QUESTIONS

1. **Auspitz sign is seen in:**   [AIPGEE 2008]
   1. Pemphigus
   2. Herpes simplex
   3. Psoriasis
   4. Varicella zoster

Ans.   **3**

Auspitz sign - If the deep scales are removed, one or more tiny bleeding points are disclosed.

2. **25-year old male shows ulcerations in the oral cavity surrounded by an erythematous halo, they are called:**   [AIPG 99]
   1. Pemphigus vulgaris
   2. Aphthous ulcers
   3. Herpes simplex
   4. Lichen planus

Ans.   **2**

Pemphigus appears as vesicles or ulcers with attached tissue tags at periphery. Lichen planus is usually surrounded by Wickhem's stria. Herpes simplex infection occurs as vesicles or gingivitis.

3. **Clinical features of which of the following include conjunctivitis, urethritis, mucocutaneous lesions and arthritis?**   [AIPG 1995]
   1. Behcet's syndrome
   2. Hodgkin's disease
   3. Greenspan syndrome
   4. Ehler-Danlos syndrome

Ans.   **1**

Behcet's syndrome is characterized by
Recurrent oral ulceration
Recurrent genital ulceration

Skin lesions – pustular

Ocular lesions – uveitis, retinal vasculitis, optic atrophy, keratitis, recurrent conjunctivitis.

4. Oral ulcers, which occur in groups, persist for about 6 weeks and leave scars on healing are:
[AIPG 1995]

1. Recurrent aphthous major
2. Recurrent aphthous minor
3. Recurrent herpetiform ulcers
4. Acute herpetic gingivostomatitis

Ans. 1

Recurrent aphthous major ulcers are characterized by occurrence of large painful ulcers which persist for upto six weeks and leave a scar upon healing.

5. Of the following conditions, gingival involvement would be unusual in: [AIPG 2003]

1. Pemphigoid
2. Primary herpes
3. Recurrent aphthae
4. Pyogenic granuloma

Ans. 3

Recurrent aphthae usually involves non-keratinised mucosa.

6. Which of the following is true of herpangina? [AIPG 2002]

1. It begins with sore throat and high fever
2. Dysphagia
3. Dyspepsia
4. Extremely painful ulcers on the buccal mucosa and tongue.

Ans. 2

7. Which of the following is a difference between herpangina and primary herpetic stomatitis?
[AIPG 2001]

1. It is preceded by prodromal symptoms
2. It is unilateral in nature
3. Ulcers seen on the anterior faucial pillars
4. Viral etiology

Ans. 3

Ulcers in herpangina are mainly seen on soft palate, tonsils and faucial pillars while in primary herpetic stomatitis, gingiva and hard palate is the most common site.

8. A 60 year-old male has fever of 3 days duration and bullous lesions with an erythematous halo and multiple target lesions. He is most probably suffering from: [AIPG 2000]

1. Herpes zoster
2. Chicken pox

3. Steven-Johnson syndrome

4. Pemphigus.

Ans. 3

Target lesions are hallmark of erythema multiforme or Steven Johnson syndrome. Also, the acute onset of bullae confirms the diagnosis.

9. **Steven-Johnson syndrome involves:** [AIPG 98]

1. Type I hypersensitivity reaction

2. Type II hypersensitivity reaction

3. Type III hypersensitivity reaction

4. Type IV hypersensitivity reaction

Ans. 3

Steven- Johnson syndrome or Erythema Multiforme is initiated by deposition of immune complexes in superficial vasculature of skin and mucosa or by cell- mediated immunity.

10. **Primary herpetic lesions involving the gingiva are most likely to occur during ages:**
[AIPG 97]

1. 1-5 years

2. 6-12 years

3. 13-16 years

4. They are likely to occur equally at any age

Ans. 1

Because body's immune mechanism are weak during the age of 1-5 years.

11. **A 46-year-old man has a painful 1.5 cm ulcerated buccal lesion, which has been present for one month. Numerous mucosal scars are present when similar ulcers have healed. He states that he has suffered from such lesions for years. Which of the following conditions is most suspected?** [AIPG 97]

1. Pemphigus

2. Erythema multiforme

3. Recurrent herpes

4. Periadenitis mucosa necrotica recurrence

Ans. 4

The typical history is of recurrent aphthous ulcers. The size of 1.5 cm is suggestive of aphthae major which usually heals with scaring of the mucosa.

12. **Intraepithelial vacuolation with formation of vesicle or bulla intraepithelially above the basal layer is characteristically seen in:** [AIPG 1995]

1. Candida albicans

2. Bullous pemphigoid

3. Pemphigus

    4. Lichen planus

Ans. 3

Pemphigus is an autoimmune disease involving the skin & mucosa and characterized by intra-epidermal bulla formation. Separation of cells takes place in lower layer of stratum spinosum.

Nikolsky's sign is positive in pemphigus.

13. Recurrent ulcers occurring on gingiva and palate are most probably: [AIPG 1995]

    1. Aphthous ulcers

    2. Herpes simplex

    3. Koplik's spots

    4. Lesions of Behcet's syndrome

Ans. 2

Recurrent ulcers occurring or gingiva and palate are most probably caused by herpes simplex. Ulcers reversibly develop on oral mucosa that is tightly bound to periosteum.

The most common sites of occurrence of apthous ulcers are buccal and labial mucosa, tongue, soft palate, pharynx & gingiva, all locations of labile mucosa not bound to periosteum.

14. Erythema multiforme is seen in: [AIPG 94]

    1. Behcet's syndrome

    2. Sutton's disease

    3. Trotter's syndrome

    4. Eagle's syndrome

Ans. 1

Behcet's syndrome is marked by a triad of oral lesions, urethritis and conjunctivitis.

Sutton's disease or Mikulicz's scarring aphthae are associated with recurrent aphthous major.

Trotter's syndrome is associated with nasopharyngeal tumor.

Eagle's syndrome is associated with enlarged, calcified stylohyoid ligament.

15. Multiple acute ulcerations of oral mucosa are seen in: [AIPG 94]

    1. White sponge nevus

    2. Stomatitis medicamentosa

    3. Pernicious anemia

    4. Lupus erythematosus

Ans. 2

Stomatitis medicamentosa is an acute allergic reaction due to use of certain medications or drugs. White sponge nevus result in white, folded, thickened bilateral buccal mucosa and is a hereditary condition. Main feature of pernicious anemia is glossitis and atrophic mucosa. Lupus erythematosus shows red lesions with central atrophic areas, surrounded by white radiating stria.

16. Pemphigus is characterized by: [AIPG 94]

    1. Acanthosis

2. Acantholysis

3. Hyperorthokeratosis

4. Hyperparakeratosis

Ans. **2**

There is oedema of the spinous layer, which results in acantholysis and suprabasilar split. This gives rise to positive Nikolsky's sign.

17. **Tzanck cells are characteristic of:** [AIPG 94]

1. Lichen planus

2. Pemphigus

3. Erythema multiforme

4. Lupus erythematosus

Ans. **2**

Tzanck cells are clumps of epithelial cells, which are often found living free within the vesicular space. They show degenerative changes like swelling of the nuclei and hyperchromatic staining, which are more obvious in cytological smears taken from early, freshly opened vesicles.

18. **Immunofluorescence test is positive in:** [AIPG 91]

1. Psoriasis

2. Pemphigus vulgaris

3. Lupus erythematosus

4. Scleroderma

Ans. **2**

19. **Inflammation of the dorsal root ganglion and vesicular eruption of the skin and mucous membrane in area supplied by a sensory nerve that is affected is characteristic of:**
[AIPG 91]

1. Herpes zoster

2. Herpes simplex

3. Uveoparotid fever

4. Aphthous stomatitis

Ans. **1**

Varicella zoster virus lies dormant in dorsal root ganglia of spinal nerves and may get reactivated in immunocompromised situation to cause vesicular eruption along the entire dermatome.

20. **Each of the following disease causes desquamative gingivitis except:** [AIPG 1990]

1. Pemphigus

2. Pemphigoid

3. Lichen planus

4. Herpes simplex

Ans. **4**

In herpes simplex, besides vesicles and ulcers, acute marginal gingivitis is seen.

1, 2, and 3 are marked by desquamative gingivitis due to intraepithelial or subepithelial oedema and loss of cell to cell adhesion.

21. **Acantholytic cells may be seen in all except:**   [AIPG 1990]
    1. Keratotic follicularis
    2. Warty dyskeratoma
    3. Pemphigus
    4. White sponge nevus

Ans.   **4**

There is intracellular edema but no loss of adhesiveness.

22. **"Corps ronds" may be seen in:**   [AIPG 1990]
    1. Pemphius
    2. Keratosis follicularis
    3. Lichen planus
    4. Leukoplaka

Ans.   **2**

They are round, homogeneous cells with basophilic nucleus and dark eosinophilic cytoplasm and distinct cells membrane.

23. **The presence of which the following condition is not a contraindication to the use of corticosteroids?**   [AIPG 1989]
    1. Peptic ulcer
    2. Herpes simplex
    3. Aphthous ulcer
    4. Latent tuberculosis

Ans.   **3**

Aphthous ulcer: topical or sy6stemic steroids for major ulcers

Herpes simplex: is of viral etiology use of corticosteroid can aggravate the lesions.

Peptic ulcer: Caused by H. pylori, exogenous steroids may be a causative factor also cause increase in acid production

NERVOUS SYSTEM

CEREBRAL PALSY

Types of cerebral palsy

1. **Spastic**

Monoplegic	-	Involves only one limb
Paraplegic	-	Lower extremities
Hemiplegic	-	One upper & lower limb on same side.
Double hemiplegic	-	All limbs, but mainly arms.
Diplegic	-	All limbs, but mainly legs
Quadriplegic	-	All limbs equally.

2. **Athetoid**

Athetosis	-	All limbs equally
Chorea		
Choreoathetosis		

3. **Ataxic**
4. **Rigid**
5. **Mixed**

DENTAL ASPECTS

1. Access problems: Patient may have to be treated in wheel chairs. Patient may become apprehensive in dental chair.
2. Uncontrolled movements, especially is athetosis make treatment difficult.
3. Bruxisms, attrition, spontaneous dislocation or sublocation of TMJ are common.
4. Communication difficulties due to low intelligence.

5. Concentration is often poor.

6. Epilepsy

7. Abnormal swallowing and drooling of saliva is common.

8. Anxiety may worsen athetosis and spasticity. So premedication is needed.

9. Poor manual dexterity, which leads to periodontal diseases and caries. So, parental counselling about diet, oral hygiene and fluoride use is needed.

10. Delayed eruption of primary dentition and enamel hypoplasia is common.

11. Malocclusion is common due to abnormal muscle behaviour. Palate is usually ovoid, high arched. Upper teeth are labially inclined due to abnormal swallowing patterns.

EPILEPSY

Causes of fits at different ages: -

Age of onset		Common causes
Young child	-	Birth trauma, fevers, metabolic disease, congenital disease or idiopathic
Adolescent	-	Idiopathic or traumatic
Young adult	-	Traumatic, neoplastic, idiopathic, alcoholism, barbiturate abuse, AIDS
Middle age	-	Neoplastic, traumatic, cerebrovascular disease, AIDS or drug abuse.
Elderly	-	Cerebrovascular disease or neoplasm.

DENTAL ASPECTS

1. When carrying out dental treatment in a known epileptic, a strong mouth prop should be kept in position and the oral cavity kept as free as possible of debris.

2. As much apparatus as possible should be kept away from the area around the patient.

3. Few drugs can be epileptogenic or interfere with anticonvulsant therapy or can themselves be changed by anticonvulsants and may therefore, be contraindicated.

4. Gingival hyperplasia can occur especially with phenytoin. Carbamazepine or Gabapentin obviate this problem.

5. Large doses of lidocaine given i/v for severe dysrhythmias; may occasionally cause convulsions.

6. Conscious sedation in epilepsy should be safe.

7. Electronic dental analgesia should be avoided.

8. Behaviour problems may be encountered especially in temporal lobe epilepsy.

9. Convulsions frequently lead to maxillofacial injuries, especially with grand-mal epilepsy

10. Acrylic is probably better used for prosthesis than porcelain as it is more resilient.

Common Oral adverse effects of anticonvulsant drugs:

1. Carbamazepine - Xerostomia

                                  Erythema multiforme

                                  Dyskinesia

2. Sodium valproate - Purpura

3. Phenytoin   - Gingival swelling
                          - Osteomalacia
                          - Dental anomalies
                          - Erythema multiforme
                          - Lupoid syndrome or ulcer
                          - Folic acid deficiency
                          - Cervical lymphadenopathy

4. Primidone   - Megaloblastic anaemia

5. Ethosuximide   - Lupoid syndrome.

Drugs contraindicated in Epilepsy (Epileptogenic)

1. Lidocaine (large doses)
2. Alcohol
3. Chlorpromazine
4. Enflurane
5. Flumazenil
6. Fluoxetine
7. Ketamine
8. Metronidozole
9. Tricyclic antidepressants
10. Quinolones
11. Tramadol

Drug problems in Epilepsy

1. Acetaminophen- Hepatotoxicity may be increased by anti convulsants.
2. Doxycycline- Metabolism may be increased by carbamazepine.

Dentistry drugs that can increase anticonvulsant activity:

1. Aspirin   - Can increase the bleeding tendency induced by valproate.
2. Azole antifungals - Can interfere with phenytoin, carbamazepine.
                          - Can increase the bleeding tendency induced by valproate.
3. Metronidazole - Can interfere with phenytoin.
                          - Can increase valproate induced bleeding tendency.
4. Propoxyphene - Can interfere with carbamazepine.

CEREBROVASCULAR ACCIDENTS

Dental aspects

1. Since a person who has had a stroke is at greater risk of another, elective dental care should be deferred for 6 months.
2. Usually access is a problem due to impaired mobility.

3. Communication may be a problem due to dysarthria, aphasia, confusion, memory loss and emotional distress.

4. There can be loss of swallowing and gag reflexes in brainstem lesions. So, patients with stroke are best treated sitting upright and extra care must be taken to avoid foreign bodies entering the pharynx. Good suction must at hand.

5. Use of norepinephrine in LA should be avoided as it can cause fatal subarachnoid haemorrhage.

6. Cerebral haemorrhage can also occur from MAO inhibitors and pethidine.

7. Opioids are avoided as they may cause severe hypotension.

8. Short, morning appointments are preferred.

9. BP monitoring is necessary.

10. Minimum use of epinephrine in L.A

11. Avoid use of epinephrine containing gingival retraction cords.

12. Avoid electronic dental analgesia.

13. Unilateral lower facial palsy (upper motor neuron) may be present.

14. Oral hygiene tends to deteriorate on the paralysed side due to impaired manual dexterity.

15. Calcified atherosclerotic plaques may sometimes be detected on dental OPG.

CRANIAL NERVE INJURIES

Cranial nerves	Main features	Causes
I	- Anosmia - Hyposmia	- Trauma - Infections - Neoplasm
II	- Visual defect or blindness - Diplopia - Paralysis of internal upward and downward movement of eye - Divergent squint	- Trauma - Infection - Neoplasm - Cerebrovascular accident - Multiple sclerosis - Fixed pupil
III	- Ptosis - Diplopia - Paralysis of internal upward and downward movement of eye - Divergent squint - Fixed pupil	- Trauma - Diabetes - Orbital apex diseases - Cavernous sinus disease
IV	- Diplopia, maximal on looking downwards and inwards - Normal pupils - Head tilted away from the affected side. - Orbital apex syndrome.	- Trauma - Vascular disease - Diabetes - Cavernous sinus disease

V	- Hypoaesthesia - Loss of corneal reflex due to involvement of opthamic division - Damage to taste perception - Jaw may deviate towards the affected side, when patient opens the jaw against resistance.	- Trauma - Infection - Neoplasm - Multiple sclerosis - Connective tissue disease
VI	- Diplopia, maximum on looking laterally - Normal pupils - Paralysis of abduction of eye.	- Trauma - Neoplasm - CVA - Raised Intracranial pressure.
VII	- Facial palsy - Epiphora - Xeropthalmia - Taste is diminished - Multiple sclerosis	- Trauma - Infection - Neoplasm - CVA
VII	- Impaired hearing or deafness - Vertigo - Tinnitus - CVA - Bone disease	- Trauma - Infection - Neoplasm
IX	- Impaired gag reflex - Neoplasm	- Trauma
X	- Impaired gag reflex - Hoarse voice - Bovine cough - Movement of soft palate towards unaffected side on saying 'aah'	- Trauma - Neoplasm - CVA
XI	- Weakness on shrugging shoulders (trapezius) - Weakness on turning the head away from the affected side (Sternocleidomastoid)	- CVA - Trauma - Infection (polio)
XII	- Dysarthria (difficulty in speaking) - Deviation of the tongue towards the affected side on protrusion - Bone tumours - Radiation damage.	- Trauma - Neoplasm - Paget's disease

FACIAL PALSY

Bells palsy- LMN facial palsy-

1. Caused by ischaemia of facial nerve near the stylohyoid foramen, resulting in edema and compression of nerve.
2. Mask like expressionless face.

3. Bell's phenomenon is positive.

4. *Melkerson-Rosenthal syndrome*- Recurrent attacks of facial palsy and multiple episodes of non-pitting, non- inflammatory painless edema of face, cheilitis granulomatosa and fissured tongue.

5. *Ramsay- Hunt syndrome*- Facial palsy and herpes zoster of geniculate ganglion.

6. *Bogorad syndrome (Crocodile tears)*- Generally follows Bell's palsy, result in herpes zoster or head injury, leading to a salivary, lacrimal reflex arc. Manifested as lacrimation on eating.

Differentiation of upper and lower motor nervous lesions.

	UMN lesions	LMN lesions
Emotional movements of face	Retained	Lost
Blink reflex	Retained	Lost
Ability to wrinkle forehead	Retained	Lost
Drooling from commissures	Uncommon	Common
Lacrimation, test, hearing	Unaffected	May be affected
Tongue protrusion	Normal	Deviates to unaffected side.

PARKINSON'S DISEASE

Dental aspects

1. Patient must often be treated in an upright position, making access to certain areas of oral cavity difficult.

2. Anxiety can increase both the tremors and degree of muscle rigidity.

3. Gag reflex is impaired, so special precautions must be taken to avoid the aspiration of water or materials.

4. Sialorrhea- So, maintenance of dry field may be a problem.

5. Xerostomia can occur as a side effect of antiparkinsonism medication.

6. Oral hygiene maintenance is a problem.

7. Orthostatic hypotension can occur when patient stands from supine position due to effect of levadopa.

8. Taste disturbances due to dopamine.

9. Hypotension makes them poor candidates for G.A.

10. Involuntary movements *("Flycatcher tongue")* and lip pursing may make the use of rotary instrument difficult.

MULTIPLE SCLEROSIS

1. Differentiation from trigeminal neuralgia is important especially in young patients.

2. Sensory neuropathy can lead to numbness of lower lip and chin

3. Facial paralysis appear later in course of disease

4. Patients are under steroid therapy. So, adrenal insufficiency should be considered.

5. Nitrous oxide is base avoided.

6. Abnormal perioral sensations, such as extreme hypersensitivity or facial anaesthesia.

SPINA BIFIDA (NEURAL TUBE DEFECTS)

1. Bowel and bladder are best emptied before dental treatment.

2. Postural hypotension is likely.

3. Care should be taken not to traumatize the patient.

4. High prevalence of latex allergy in such patients.

5. Patient may be on anticoagulant therapy.

ALZHEIMER'S DISEASE

1. Behavioural problems.

2. Destructions of dentition due to caries and periodontal disease along with hypo salivation occurs.

3. Maxillofacial injuries are common in demented patients.

4. Xerostomia is a common side effect of phenothiazine used for treatment.

POLIOMYELITIS

1. Patients with bulbar palsy or a high level spinal lesion may have impaired gag and cough reflexes.

2. Those with quadriplegia may benefit from the dentist constructing a mouth stick or bite stick appliance with which they can perform manual functions.

AMYOTROPHIC LATERAL SCLEROSIS

1. Because of declined function of respiratory muscles, patient may not be able to cough and chances of aspiration increases.

2. Hyperactive gag reflex.

3. Topical anaesthesia should be avoided.

4. Patient should be NPO for 12 hours prior to treatment.

5. Topical fluoride may induce nausea.

6. Poor oral hygiene due to poor manual dexterity.

MYASTHENIA GRAVIS

1. Facial muscles are commonly involved giving the patient an immobile and expressionless appearance.

2. Tongue edema.

3. Difficulty in chewing.

4. Respiratory crisis from disease itself or overmedication.

5. Narcotics should be avoided.

6. Antibiotics like tetracycline, streptomycin, sulphonamides, clindamycin may reduce neuromuscular activity. So, should be avoided.

7. L.A. is the option of choice.

8. i/v sedation and G.A. should be avoided.

NEURALGIA

1. **Trigeminal neuralgia (Tic Douloureux, Fothergill's disease)**
   - Frequently found in multiple sclerosis.
   - Common in older adults.
   - Trigger zone are often elicited.
   - Carbamazepine is the treatment of choice.

2. **Trigeminal neuritis or trigeminal neuropathy**
   - Differs from trigeminal neuralgia by nature of pain.
   - It is burning, boring, pulling, drawing or pressure sensation, continues for hours to weeks.

3. **Raeder's syndrome (paratrigeminal syndrome)**
   - Severe headache in area of trigeminal distribution.
   - Ocular sympathetic paralysis.

4. **Sphenopalatine neuralgia (Horton's syndrome, sluder headache)**
   - A symptom complex referable to nasal ganglion and vidian nerve.
   - Alarm clock headache.
   - No trigger zone.
   - Usually associated with epiphora, sneezing, swelling of nasal mucosa.

5. **Auriculotemporal syndrome (Frey's syndrome, Gustatory sweating)**
   - Occurs due to damage to auriculotemporal nerve and subsequent innervation of sweat glands by parasympathetic salivary fibres.
   - Flushing and sweating from temporal area during eating.

6. **Glossopharyngeal neuralgia**
   - Sharp shooting pain in ear, pharynx, nasopharynx, tonsil and posterior part of tongue.
   - Trigger zone located in tonsillar fossa.

7. **Causalgia**
   - Arise after injury to or sectioning of a peripheral sensory nerve.
   - Usually follows tooth extraction of multi rooted tooth.

8. **Horner's syndrome**
   - Miosis + ptosis + anhidrosis + vasodilatation
   - Atypical facial pain and sweating.

DISORDERS OF TASTE

1. Temporary disturbance can be due to chemicals like chlorhexidine, amiloride.

2. Infections like herpes zoster, otitis media, mastoiditis, cholesteatoma.
3. Other causes of hypogeusia or ageusia includes aging, xerostomia, irradiation of oral cavity, drugs like antihistaminics, antidepressants, antihypertensives, neurological disorders, nutritional deficiencies, endocrinopathies, metabolic disorders, viral infections.

MISCELLANEOUS

1. Botulinum type A toxin (Botox) is used to treat blepharospasm, masseteric hypertrophy, TMJ disc derrangements.
2. *Gilles de La Tourette syndrome*: Associated with vocal tics, swearing, lip smacking, tongue thrusting, TMJ or other oral pain, self mutilation habits.
3. Torticollis (Twisted neck): May cause difficulty in dental treatment due to abnormal patient positioning.
4. Dyskinesia: abnormal movement of tongue, facial muscles and jaw may lead to bruxism or dysphagia, involuntary tongue protrusion and facial grimacing.

DISEASES OF CARDIOVASCULAR SYSTEM

CONGENITAL AND ACQUIRED HEART DISEASES

1. Minimally stressful appointments.
2. Patients are best treated in the morning hours. However, endogenous epinephrine levels peak during morning hours and adverse cardiac events are more likely in early morning. So, late morning appointments are recommended.
3. Cardiac monitoring is desirable.
4. Effective painless L.A. is essential.
5. An aspirating syringe should be used to prevent intravascular injection of epinephrine containing L.A.
6. Epinephrine containing L.A. should not be used in excessive doses to patients taking beta-blockers as it may induce hypertension and cardiovascular complications.
7. Gingival retraction cord containing epinephrine should be avoided.
8. G.A. should be avoided, whenever possible.
9. Aspirin may cause sodium and fluid retention and may be contraindicated.
10. COX-II inhibitors increase the risk of myocardial infarction.
11. Conscious sedation should be deferred for at least 3 months for patients with myocardial infarction, recent onset angina, and unstable angina.
12. Angina can rarely cause pain in the mandible, teeth or other oral tissues.
13. Patients with ischaemic heart disease appear to have more severe dental caries and periodontal disease than the general population, the relationship is still controversial.

ANGINA PECTORIS

1. Preoperative glycerol trinitrate and sometimes oral sedation are advised.
2. Dental treatment should be stress free, oxygen saturation, BP and pulse monitoring is necessary.
3. Effective L.A. is essential.
4. Ready access to medical help, oxygen and GTN.
5. If a patient with H/O angina, experiences chest pain in dental surgery, dental treatment should be stopped, patient should be given GTN 0.3-0.6 mg sublingually and oxygen and should be kept sitting upright. Vital signs should be monitored, the pain should be relieved in 2-3 minutes, and the patient should then rest.
6. If chest pain is not relieved within about 3 minutes, myocardial infarction is a possible cause and medical help should be summoned. Pain that persists after 3 doses of GTN given every five minutes. That lasts more than 15-20 min or that is associated with nausea, vomiting, syncope or hypertension is highly suggestive of myocardial infarction.
7. If pain persists, the patient should continue oxygen and chew 300 mg of aspirin and an intravenous cannula should be inserted. In addition, nitrous oxide- oxygen or 5-10 mg of morphine sulphate given intravenously is important to relieve pain and anxiety.
8. Tricyclic antidepressants are base avoided as they can disturb cardiac rhythm. Sumatriptan may cause coronary artery vasoconstriction.
9. Elective dental care should be deferred for 6 months; emergency dental care should be in a hospital setting.
10. Patients with bypass grafts do not require antibiotic cover against infective endocarditis.
11. Patients with grafts should not receive epinephrine containing L.A.
12. While dealing with patients with vascular stents. Antibiotic prophylaxis is usually not needed. However, it may be prudent if emergency dental treatment is required in first six weeks postoperatively. Patients may require long-term anticoagulants. Appropriate action is required to deal with any bleeding tendencies.

MYOCARDIAL INFARCTION

1. Dental intervention can precipitate dysrhythmias. So, elective procedures should be deferred for six months. Simple emergency dental treatment under L.A. may be given after physician's consent.
2. Asymptomatic patients 6-12 months after MI can normally have elective dental care carried out safely. High-risk procedures such as elective surgery may be deferred.
3. Symptomatic previous MI (more than 12 months) can normally have elective dental care. But major surgery may cause reinfarctions.
4. Elective L.A. possibly supplemented with relative analgesia and monitoring of BP, ECG, pulse and oxygen saturation are indicated.
5. Dental treatment should be stopped if there are.
   (a) Chest pain
   (b) Dyspnoea

(c) A rise in heart rate of above 40 beats/min.

(d) A rise in ST segment displacement of above 0.2 mv on ECG.

(e) Dysrhythmias

(f) Rise in septolic BP > 20 mm Hg.

6. Use of G.A. should be deferred, as far as possible.

7. Management is usually complicated by a combination of anticoagulant and antiplatelet medication and sometimes-increased risk of thromboembolic events and infection.

HYPERTENSION

1. BP should be controlled before elective dental treatment.

ASA grading and dental management considerations

B.P (mm Hg)	ASA grade	Consideration
SBP< 140, DBP< 90	I	Routine dental care
SBP 140-159 DBP 90-99	II	Recheck BP before starting Routine dental care.
SBP 160-179 DBP 95-109	III	Recheck BP before starting Medical advice before routine dental care. Restrict use of epinephrine Conscious sedation may help.
SBP > 180, DBP >110	IV	Recheck BP after five min. quiet rest. Only emergency care until BP is controlled. Medical advice before routine dental care. Avoid vasoconstrictors.

2. Minimal stressful appointments.

3. Preoperative reassurance and sedation may be helpful.

4. Patients are best treated in the late morning.

5. Postural hypotension may occur after patient gets up from dental chair, if he is using antihypertensive drugs such as thiazides, furosemide or CCB.

6. Systemic corticosteroids may raise the BP.

7. Some NSAIDs (indomethacin, ibuprofen) can reduce the efficacy of antihypertensive agents.

8. Adequate L.A. must be provided.

9. An aspirating syringe should be used to give a L.A., since epinephrine should not be injected intravenously under most circumstances, the use of epinephrine in combination with L.A. is not contraindicated in hypertensive patients unless the systolic BP is over 200 mm of Hg and/ or the diastolic is over 115 mm of Hg.

10. G.A. can potentiate the effect of antihypertensive drugs, which can lead to hypotension. Intravenous barbiturates in particular can be dangerous, but halothane, enflurane and isoflurane may also cause hypotension. Antihypertensive drugs should not be stopped, since rebound hypertension can occur. G.A. is contraindicated if complicated by cardiac failure, coronary or cerebral artery insufficiency or renal insufficiency.

11. Facial palsy is an occasional complication of malignant hypertension.

12. Clonidine can cause Xerostomia.

Oral adverse affects from antihypertensive and other cardioactive drugs

Alpha adrenergic blockers (Doxazosin, terazosin)	Xerostomia
ACE inhibitors (Captopril, enalapril etc.)	Burning sensation
	Ulceration
	Loss of taste
	Angioedema
	Sinusitis with guinapril
	Lichenoid reactions.
Angiotensin II receptor blockers (Digitalis, losartan, Amiodarone)	Facial flushing
	Taste disturbance
	Gag reflex
	Dry mouth
	Lupoid reaction
Beta blockers (Atenolol, acebutolol labetalol, propanolol)	Xerostomia
	Lichenoid reaction
	Paraesthesia
Calcium channel blocker (Amlodipine, Diltiazem, felodipine)	Gingival hyperplasia (Most with nifedipine)
	Xerostomia with nicardipine
Potassium channel blockers (Nicorandil)	Ulcerations
Other (Diazoxide, minoxidil)	Lupoid reactions with hydralazine

CONGENITAL CARDIAC DEFECTS

1. Antimicrobial prophylaxis is mandatory before dental surgery in such patients. Susceptibility to infection is unrelated to severity of disease.

2. There may be bleeding tendencies caused by platelet dysfunction and excessive fibrinolytic activity.

3. Occasionally, thrombotic tendency can be there.

4. Cerebral abscess can occur as a complication of dental infection; leukopenia may be a factor in some right to left shunt.

5. Congestive cardiac failure may complicate management.

6. Associated problems like cleft palate; Down's, Turner's or William's syndrome may affect dental management.

7. Oral abnormalities can include delayed eruption of both dentitions, enamel hypoplasia, malocclusion. Teeth often have a bluish- white 'skimmed-milk' appearance and there is gross vasodilatation in pulp. Caries activity and periodontal disease activity is high.

8. An aspirating syringe should be used to give L.A.

9. Anaesthesia should be adequate.

10. Gingival retraction cord containing epinephrine should be avoided.

11. Conscious sedation with Nitrous oxide can be given. G.A. is generally avoided.

NOONAN SYNDROME

1. Short stature, unusual facies, congenital heart disease, chest deformity, and mild learning disability, cryptorchidism in males.

2. Facial features include an elongated mid face height, hypertelorism, retrognathia, lower nasal bridge, a wider mouth. More prominent upper lip and apparently lower set ears than normal control individuals.

3. Bleeding tendencies due to deficiency of factor XI and XII.

4. Associated with cherubism, giant cells lesions in jaws and neuro fibromatosis.

WILLIAM'S SYNDROME

1. Infantile hypocalcaemia.

2. Elfin facies.

3. Congenital heart defects.

4. Hypercalcaemia leads to growth deficiency, osteosclerosis and craniostenosis.

5. Dental defects include hypodontia, microdontia, hypoplasia, and wide upper arch.

6. Masseter spasm can occur with halothane.

RHEUMATIC FEVER

1. No special precautions are needed in acute stage, as there appears to be little risk of infective endocarditis at this stage.

2. Antimicrobial prophylaxis should be given in asymptomatic phase.

3. L.A. is generally safe.

4. Conscious sedation with nitrous oxide may be given if cardiac function is good.

5. G.A. should be avoided.

KAWASAKI'S DISEASE (MUCOCUTANEOUS LYMPHNODE SYNDROME)

Oral changes include:

1. Strawberry tongue

2. Labial oedema

3. Crusting of lips

4. Pharyngitis

5. Oro pharyngeal erythema

6. Cervical lymphadenopathy

7. Facial palsy occasionally

HEART FAILURE

1. It is dangerous to lay any patient with left heart failure in supine position. It can worsen dyspnoea. Dental chair should be kept in a partially reclining or erect position.
2. Dental treatment may precipitate dysrhythmias, angina or heart failure.
3. Bupivacaine should be avoided, as it is cardiotoxic.
4. NSAIDs other than aspirin should be avoided in those patients taking ACE inhibitors since they increase the risk of renal damage.
5. Erythromycin and tetracycline should be avoided as they may induce digitalis toxicity, by impairing gut flora metabolism of the digitalis.
6. Conscious sedation can be safely used usually.
7. G.A. is contraindicated in cardiac failure until it is under control.
8. ACE inhibitor can sometimes cause Erythema multiforme, angioedema or burning mouth. Procainamide can cause leucopenia or lupus-like reaction and acetazolamide can cause facial paresthesia.

CARDIOMYOPATHIES

1. Enlargement of heart muscles may restrict movements of mitral valve, leading to valvular insufficiency, making the patient susceptible to infective endocarditis.
2. Nitro-glycerine or similar drugs are contraindicated.
3. Epinephrine should be used in limited amounts.
4. Conscious sedation with nitrous oxide may be used if necessary.
5. Poor risk for G.A.

DYSRHYTHMIAS

1. Late morning or early afternoon appointments are preferred.
2. Syncope can result from dysrhythmias, which has to be distinguished from a simple fainting attack by the slowness or irregularity of pulse.
3. Patients with atrial fibrillation may be taking anticoagulants, which influence operative care.
4. Dysrhythmias may be induced by manipulation of neck, carotid sinus or eyes (Vagal reflex), rarely by L.A., G.A (halothane), preoperative digitalization, erythromycin or azole antifungal.
5. Mepivacaine 3% is thought to be preferable to lidocaine.
6. In patients with pacemakers, MRI, electro surgery, diathermy and transcutaneous nerve stimulation are contraindicated.
7. Pacemaker single beat inhibition of little consequence may occasionally be caused by dental equipments like peizoelectric ultrasonic scaler, ultrasonic baths, pulp testers, apex locators, dental induction casting machines, belt-driven motors in dental chairs, older x-ray machines.

Anticoagulant therapy and dental care

1. Aspirin irreversibly decrease platelet aggregation and consequently increase the bleeding time. Most patients taking 40-325 mg/day aspirin does not have impact on bleeding. If the patient

has other underlying medial conditions that predispose to impaired Hemostasis, then aspirin should be discontinued 3-7 days prior to surgery.

2. If emergency surgery needs to be performed and the patients bleeding time is higher than 15-20 min. DDAVP is administered parenterally at 0.3 mg/kg body weights with a maximum dose of 20-24 mg within one hour of surgery.

3. There is no need to discontinue or alter anticoagulation therapy prior to minor oral surgical procedures for patients taking other types of antiplatelet medication.

4. The efficacy of warfarin therapy is monitored by the prothrombin time or International normalized ratio (INR). The therapeutic level of INR is kept at a range of 2.0 to 4.5. There is no need to discontinue anticoagulant therapy if INR is < 3.0, within 24 hours of surgery.

   If INR > 3.0, 3 protocols can be used:

   (a) Warfarin is not discontinued. If localized haemostatic measures are inadequate, vitamin K injections and antifibrinolytic mouth rinses can be administered.

   (b) Warfarin is discontinued and the patient is not placed on any alternative anticoagulant. Warfarin is discontinued 2-3 days before surgery because the effect of warfarin lasts for 36-72 hrs.

   (c) Warfarin is discontinued, but the patient is placed on an alternative anticoagulant. Warfarin therapy is discontinued and vitamin K is administered. Patient is started on parenteral Heparin therapy, which is continued until 6 hrs before surgery, and is continued after surgery in combination with oral anticoagulant therapy until a desired INR has been reached.

INFECTIVE ENDOCARDITIS – DENTAL ASPECTS

Prevalence of bacteraemia following various oral manipulations:

1. Scaling and root planning, periodontal prophylaxis 0-25 %
2. Tooth-brushing 0-25 %
3. Extraction, periodontal surgery 25-50 %
4. Use of interdental sticks, floss, chewing, irrigants 25-50%
5. Multiple extractions 50-80%

Risk of infective Endocarditis after dental treatment

1. High risk (Antimicrobial prophylaxes considered essential)

   (a) Prosthetic valves.

   (b) Previous infective endocarditis.

   (c) Cyanotic congenital heart disease.

   (d) Mitral valve prolapse with regurgitation or thickened leaflets.

2. Intermediate or moderate risk (Prophylaxis considered necessary)

   (a) Any uncorrected cardiac valve disease or some other congenital defects

   (b) Septal defect.

   (c) Patent ductus arteriosus.

   (d) Bicuspid aortic valve.

(e) Coarctation of aorta.

(f) Rheumatic heart disease.

(g) Hypertrophic cardiac myopathy.

(h) Various systemic disorders like syphilitic heart disease, SLE, ankylosing spondylitis, Marfan syndrome, Osteogenesis imperfecta, Hurler syndrome, Kawasaki disease.

3. Negligible risk (Prophylaxis considered not needed)

(a) After myocardial infarction.

(b) Isolated secundum atrial septal defect.

(c) After coronary artery bypass graft.

(d) For implanted cardiac pacemakers, stents or defibrillators.

(e) Mitral valves prolapse without regurgitation.

(f) Pulmonary stenosis.

(g) Innocent cardiac murmurs.

Treatment needing antimicrobial prophylaxis in patients at risk

(a) Extractions.

(b) Subgingival procedures including probing scaling or cord placement.

(c) Oral or periodontal or implant surgery or raising mucogingival flap for any other purpose.

(d) Endodontics beyond the root apex.

(e) Sialography.

(f) Intraligamentary L.A.

(g) Rubber dam, matrix and wedge placement.

Procedure for which antimicrobial prophylaxis is not a requirement in persons at risk

(a) Dental radiography.

(b) Endodontics not beyond the apex.

(c) Exfoliation of primary teeth.

(d) Impression making.

(e) Non- surgical procedures that do not induce bleeding.

(f) Abscess incision and drainage.

(g) Suture removal.

(h) Orthodontic band removal.

(i) Biopsy.

DISEASES OF RESPIRATORY SYSTEM

COMMON COLD SYNDROME

- Elective dental care is best deffered.
- G.A. should be avoided as there is often some respiratory obstruction and infection can also be spread down to the lungs.
- Antibiotic prophylaxis is indicated.
- Use of xylitol chewing gum can reduce the risk of otitis media by inhibiting pneumococci.

VIRAL INFECTION

- Most common oral manifestation is the presence of small round erythmatous macular lesions on the soft palate.
- Treatment with decongestants may cause xerostomia.
- Mouth breathing may be associated with altered dentofacial morphology.

PHARYNGITIS AND TONSILLITIS

- Dysphagia is common problem.
- Sometimes, quinsy (peritonsillar abscess) can occur which has to be differentiated from odontogenic space infection of lateral pharyngeal wall.
- Streptococcal sore throats may lead to rare complications such as scarlet fever, acute glomerulonephritis, rheumatic fever.
- Elective dental care is best deffered.
- G.A. should be avoided.
- Antimicrobial prophylaxis may be indicated.
- Small round erythematous macules can be seen on hard and soft palate.

ALLERGIC RHINITIS AND CONJUNCTIVITIS

- Patients have a genetic susceptibility to allergic hypersensitivity reactions (atopy).
- Associated with pruritis, lacrimation, crusting and burning of eyes.
- Sneezing, pruritis, clear rhinorrhea and nasal congestion.
- Laboratory investigations like serum IgE levels, ESR, RAST (radioallergosorbent test) and skin testing may be helpful.
- Treatment with decongestants may cause xerostomia.
- Increased incidence of candidiasis due to use of corticosteroid sprays.

SINUSITIS

- Maxillary sinusitis may manifest as pain in maxillary molars and cheek which is worsened by biting and stomp positive.
- Dental treatment should be deferred in acute stage.

- G.A. should be avoided.
- Antimicrobial prophylaxis is indicated.
- Inhalational sedation may be impeded if the nasal airway is obstructed.
- Various mycoses may affect the paranasal sinuses in immunocompromised patients.
- Use of decongestants may cause xerostomia.
- Increased incidence of candidiasis due to use of corticosteroid sprays.
- Frequent use of antibiotics can lead to antibiotic resistance and candidiasis.
- Increased incidence of gingivitis.
- Periorbital cellulitis is a common complication in children.
- Frontal sinusitis can extend through the anterior wall and present as Pott's puffy tumor.

LUNG ABSCESS

- Inhalation of a tooth or fragment, a restoration or an endodontic instrument can frequently lead to lung abscess.
- Aspiration of oral bacteria, particularly anaerobes, especially in elderly patients or those who are intubated, can also lead to lung abscess.
- A rubber dam or other protective device should always be used to avoid danger of aspiration of instruments and prosthesis.
- Patients who aspirate tooth fragments or instruments must have chest radiograph done, and if necessary bronchoscopy.
- G.A. can also be a danger, particularly if inadequate throat packs have been used.

SEVERE ACUTE RESPIRATORY SYNDROME (SARS)

- SARS can be a severe illness and all but emergency dental treatment should be deferred until recovery.
- G.A. is hazardous and absolutory contraindicated.
- For all contents with suspect SARS patients, careful hand hygiene is urged, including hand washing with soap and water or alcohol based handrubs.

BACTERIAL PNEUMONIA

- All but emergency dental treatment should be deferred until recovery.
- G.A. is hazardous and absolutely contraindicated.
- Aspiration of salivary secretions containing oral bacteria into lower respiratory tract can cause pneumonia.

TUBERCULOSIS

- T.B. is unlikely to be transmitted to staff during oral health care unless the patient has active pulmonary infection or the dental staff is immuno compromised.
- If patients with open pulmonary TB must be treated, special precautions should be used to prevent the release of mycobacteria into the air.

- Reduction of splatter and aerosols by minimizing coughing and avoiding ultrasonic instruments, and use of rubber dam are important.
- Improved ventilation, ultraviolet germicidal light, new masks and personal respirators and other pressure protective devices, such as high efficiency particulate air filters (HGPA) are indicated.
- Heat sterilization should be used wherever possible.
- L.A. is safe and satisfactory.
- Relative analgesia is contraindicated because of the risk of contamination of the anaesthetic apparatus.
- G.A. is also contraindicated because of impaired pulmonary function and contamination of anaesthetic apparatus.
- Clearance of diazepam is enhanced by rifampicin.
- Acetaminophen should be avoided in patients on rifampicin or isomerised because of enhanced hepatotoxicity.
- Azole antifungals, clarithromycin, benzodiazepine interact with rifampicin.
- Aspirin should be avoided in patients on streptomycin, amikacin, kanamycine.
- Streptomycin may enhance the activity of some neuromuscular blocking drugs and in large doses may alone cause a myasthenic syndrome.
- Oral complications of anti-tubercular drugs are rare but rifampicin and rifabutin can cause red saliva.

Management of patients with T.B.		
H/O T.B.	**Infectivity potential**	**Comment**
1. Acid sputum positive T.B., Recent H/O T.B.	High	Defer elective dental care until T.B. treatment is complete.Use special infection control precaution.
2. Past H/O T.B.	Needs confirmation	Defer elective dental care until medical advice received
3. No H/O T.B. but signs and symptoms suggestive.	Needs confirmation	Defer elective dental care until medical advice received. Use special infection control precautions for emergency dental care.
4. No H/O T.B. but positive tuberculin test	Needs confirmation	Defer elective dental care until medical advice received.Use special infection control precautions.

ATYPICAL MYCOBACTERIA (NON TUBERCULOUS MYCOBACTERIA)

- Mycobacterium avium complex (MAC) involves lungs, skin or lymph nodes.
- M. kansasii- Lung disease.
- M. fortuitum and M. chelonae- skin, wound infections, abscesses.

- M. marinum- 'Swimming pool granuloma'.
- M. ulcerans- chronic ulcerative lesions.
- MTB, MAC, M. serofulaceum, M. kanasaii - Tuberculous cervical lymphadenitis.
- NTM is the most common cause of unilateral cervical lymphadenopathy in children and may form a 'cold abscess'.
- Most NTM are resistant to standard anti-tubercular medication.
- Examination of water from dental units has revealed NTM species.

CHRONIC OBSTRUCTIVE LUNG DISEASE (COPD)

- Patients with COPD are treated in an upright position
- Use of rubber dam may be difficult as they may not tolerate the additional obstruction to breathing
- Patients are frequently taking corticosteroids treatment, so adrenal insufficiency is a concern.
- Interactions of theophylline with drugs such as epinephrin, erythromycin, clindamycin, erythromycin or ciprofloxacin may result in dangerously high levels of theophylline.
- L.A. is preferred for dental treatment.
- Bilateral mandibular or palatal injections should be avoided
- Relative analgesia and G.A. should be given only if absolutely necessary.
- Diazepam and imidazolem are mild respiratory depressants and should not be used.
- Intravenous barbiturates are totally contraindicated.
- Postoperative respiratory complications are more prevalent.
- The most important factor in preoperative care is cessation of smoking for at least one weak preoperatively.
- Ipratropium can cause Xerostomia.

ASTHMA

- Patients should be asked to bring their usual medication with them, when coming for dental treatment.
- Elective dental care should be deferred in severe asthamatics until they are in a better phase.
- Allergy to penicillin may be more frequent.
- Interaction of theophylline with epinephrine, erythromycin, clindamycin, azithromycine, clarithromycin, ciprofloxacin may result in dangerously high levels of theophylline.
- Patients on leukotriene modifying drugs may have a prolonged INR and bleeding tendency because of impaired liver metabolism.
- Patients may be on systemic corticosteroid therapy and the risks from steroid complications should be taken care of.
- Due to nasal obstruction, patients can have long face syndrome.
- Asthmatic attacks may occasionally be precipitated by anxiety. So patient should be stress-free during dental treatment.

- **List of drugs, which should be avoided:**
  - Aspirin and other NSAIDs.
  - Sulphites in L.A.
  - L.A. containing vasoconstrictors should be avoided.
  - Epinephrine is contraindicated in patients using theophylline as it may precipitate dysrhythmias.
  - Sedatives in general are better avoided as in acute asthmatics attack; even benzodiazepines can precipitate respiratory failure.
  - G.A. is least avoided because it may be complicated by hypoxia and hypercapnia, which can cause pulmonary oedema, and cardiac failure. The risk of postoperative collapse of lung or pneumothorax is also increased.
  - An asthamatic attack may be precipitated by drugs causing histamine release directly, therefore morphine and some other opioids, methohexitone, thiopentone, Suxamethonium tubocurarine and pancuronium should be avoided.
  - Use of corticosteroid inhalers can cause oral and pharyngeal thrush, rarely bullous haemorrhages.
  - β 2 agonist like ipratropium bromide can cause Xerostomia.
  - Antiasthamatic drugs can lower the salivary pH.
  - Periodontal inflammation is greater in asthmatics.
  - Gasto-esophageal reflux is not uncommon with occasional tooth erosions.
  - L.A. is best used for dental treatment.
  - Relative analgesia with nitrous oxide and oxygen is preferable to intravenous sedation and gives more immediate control of the asthmatic patient.
  - Halothane or better, enflurane, isoflurane, desflurane or sevoflurane are the preferred anaesthetics, but ketamine may be useful in children.
  - Acrylic monomer, toothpaste, fissure sealants, tooth enamel diet, cotton rolls and cyanoacrylates may occasionally precipitate an attack.
- **Management of asthmatic patient:**
  - Terminate dental therapy.
  - Position patient comfortably, usually sitting with arms thrown forward.
  - Administer bronchodilator by means of aerosol spray-epenephrine, isoproteronol or metaproteronol.
  - Administrate oxygen.
  - If episode continues, give epinephrine 1: 1000 i/m.
  - Aminophylline 250 mg by means of a very slow i/v infusion.
  - i/v hydrocortisone sodium succinate, 100-200 mg.
  - Summon medical assistance if episode is refractory to management.
  - Permit patient to recover fully and terminate therapy for the day.
  - Fluoride supplements should be given to patients taking β2 agonists.

- Oral hygine should be reinforced to reduce incidence of gingivitis and periodontitis.
- Avoid dental materials that can precipitate an attack.
- Schedule the patients in late morning.
- Care should be used in the positioning of suction tips as they may elicit a cough reflex.

PULMONARY EMBOLISM

- Main concern in the provision of dental care in the patient who is being managed with oral anticoagulants.

AIRWAY OBSTRUCTION

- Management of swallowed objects:
  - An object may enter the oropharynx when the patient is in supine or semisupine position. Position the chair in Trendlenberg position allowing gravity to turn the object to oral cavity which can then be retrieved by patient 'coughing it up' or magill forcep.
  - If not retrieved, radiographs (flat plate of abdomen or AP/lateral view of chest) are needed to localise the object.
  - If the object is determined to be in the tracheobronchial tree, it is most often located in the right bronchus. Retrieval from bronchus may involve the use of fibreoptic bronchoscope or thoracotomy.
- Recognition of airway obstruction:
  - Suprasternal retraction
  - Victim usually grabs at the throat.
- Non invasive procedures for airway obstruction:
  - Back blows.
  - Mineral thrusts, Chest thrust, Heimlich manoeuver.
  - Finger sweeps.
- Invasive procedures for obstructed airways
  - Tracheostomy
  - Cricothyrotomy

HYPERVENTILATION SYNDROME

Clinical manifestations

Body system	Clinical manifestations
CVS	Palpitations, Tachycardia, Precordial discomfort
Neurologic	Dizziness, Light headedness, Disturbance of consciousness or vision
	Numbness and tingling of the extremities
	Tetany (rare)
Respiratory	Shortness of breath, Chest pain, Xerostomia

GIT	Epigastric pain
Musculoskeletal	Muscle pains and cramps, Tremors, Stiffness, Tetany
Psychologic	Tension, Anxiety, Nightmares

Management

- Anxiety reduction
- Correction of respiratory alkalosis
  - Breath CO_2 enriched air
  - Diazepam or midazolam i/v (titrate) or i/m (10 mg diazepam or 5 mg midazolam)
  - Oral 10-15 mg diazepam
- Determine cause of anxiety and treat anxiety through psycho sedation

LUNG CANCER

- Dental treatment under LA should be uncomplicated.
- Conscious sedation should preferably be avoided.
- GA is a matter for specialist management .
- Muscle relaxants should not be given.
- Oral cancers may be associated with lung cancer and vice versa.
- Pigmentation of soft palate is a rare early oral manifestation.
- Metastasis to mandible occurs frequently.
- Most common pulmonary malignancies are squamous cell carcinoma, small cell carcinoma, adenocarcinomas and large cell carcinomas.

CYSTIC FIBROSIS

- Liver disease and diabetes may complicate treatment.
- L.A. is satisfactory.
- Conscious sedation is usually contraindicated.
- G.A is contraindicated if respiratory function is poor.
- Most patients have recurrent sinusitis and nasal polyps.
- Xerostomia is a common complaint.
- Salivary gland enlargement can occur due to high salivary sodium concentration.
- Pancreatin may cause oral ulcers if held in mouth.
- Tetracycline staining of teeth can occur.
- Enamel hypoplasia, delayed dental development and eruption and high caries prevalence is seen.

POST OPERATIVE RESPIRATORY COMPLICATIONS

- Segmental or lobar pulmonary collapse and infection.
- Mendelson's syndrome (aspiration of gastric contents into the lower respiratory tract causes pulmonary oedema)

GASTROINTESTINAL SYSTEM

OESOPHAGEAL DISORDERS

- Deglutition is initiated by sensory impulses from the oropharynx to the brainstern primarily through 7th, 9th, and 10th cranial nerves.
- The efferent function of swallowing is mediated by 9th, 10th and 12th cranial nerves.

Reflux oesophagitis (Gastro- oesophageal reflux disease)

- The gastric contents can have a pH as low as 1 and regurgitation, if chronic, can cause dental erosion. Erosion is typically, seen on palatal aspects of upper anteriors and premolars.
- Other oral manifestations include dysgeusia, burning sensation, dental sensitivity, pulpitis.
- Drugs used to treat GERD can cause Erythema multiforme (Ranitidine), Xerostomia (Proton pump inhibitors), Dysgeusia (Omeprazole).
- Such patients should be treated in semisupine position and premedicated with antacids.
- Any medication that may cause nausea should be avoided.
- Mild baking soda rinsing may reduce disgeusia.

Post cricoid web

- The association of post-cricoid dysphagia, upper oesophageal webs and iron deficiency anaemia is known as Plummer - Vinson syndrome or Paterson-Brown-Kelly syndrome or Sideropenia.
- This is a precancerous condition. Such patients are at a higher risk for hypopharyngeal, oesophageal and oral cancers.

Cancer of oesophagus

- Usually associated with oesophageal webs.
- Patients who have had oesophageal cancer have a greater chance of developing a second cancer in head and neck region.
- Rare patients have tylosis and oral leukoplakia.

STOMACH AND INSTESTINAL DISORDERS

Peptic ulcer

- Helicobacter pylorus is the most common contributory cause to peptic ulcers.
- H. pylori may be transmitted in saliva. There are conflicting findings as to whether dental plaque and dentures are an important reservoir for H. pylori and significant in transmission of the organisms.
- After resections, deficiencies of vitamin B12, folate or iron may cause ulcers, sore tongue or angular stomatitis.
- Persistent regurgitation of gastric acid as a result of pyloric stenosis can cause severe dental erosion (perimylolysis), typically of the palatal aspects of upper anterior teeth.
- Labial vascular anomalies may be associated with peptic ulcer disease
- Anaemia may also complicate treatment, particularly G.A.

- There may be an association with halitosis.
- Drugs like aspirin and other NSAID'S and corticosteroids are contraindicated as they can cause gastric irritation or promote bleeding.
- Oral adverse effects like xerostomia may result from proton pump inhibitor pirenzepine and sucralfate.
- Ranitidine can cause Erythema multiforme.
- Loss of taste from omeprazole.
- Antacids impede absorption of ciprofloxacin, erythromycin, metronidazole and tetracyclines.
- Cimetidine and omeprazole may delay clearance of lidocaine and benzodiazepins.
- Long appointments should be avoided to reduce stress.

Cancers of stomach

- Anaemia or obstructive jaundice may complicate dental treatment.
- Pernicious anaemia may preceed development of gastric cancer, when oral signs like glossitis, ulcers, and angular stomatitis can be early features.
- Usually, metastasis from a gastric carcinoma may be first detected in a lower cervical lymph node, usually on left side (Troisier's sign). Metastasis to jaws is rare.

Coeliac disease/Gluten-sensitive enteropathy, coeliac sprue, nontropical sprue.

- Most common genetic disease in Europe. This is a genetic hypersensitive or toxic reaction of the small intestine mucosa to the gliadin component of gluten (Protamine).
- Coeliac disease may be found in upto 5% of patients with recurrent aphthae and should be suspected if there are any other symptoms suggesting intestinal disease.
- Patients usually have anaemia and bleeding tendencies.

Crohn's disease (Regional enteritis or Ileitis)

- It is an inflammatory bowel disease, which appears to be caused by commensal bacteria in persons with a genetically determined dysregulation of mucosal T-Lymphocytes.
- Dental management may be complicated by any of the problems associated with malabsorption or by corticosteroids or other immunosuppressive treatment.
- NSAID's should be avoided.
- Antibiotics like amoxicillin and clindamycin should be avoided as it can aggravate diarrhoea.
- Oral lesions of Crohn's disease include:
  - Recurrant aphthae ulcers
  - Pyostomatitis vegetans
  - Facial or labial swelling
  - Mucosal tags or 'cobblestone' proliferation of the mucosa.
  - Anaemia
  - Angular stomatitis
  - Cheilitis granulomatosa and granulomatous changes of salivary gland ducts.
  - Melkersson-Rosenthal syndrome

- Oral lichenoid reactions
- Candidiasis
- High prevalence of caries and periodontitis.
- MPDS
- Atypical facial pain

- The findings of non-caseating granulomas beneath cobblestone proliferation of the oral mucosa is strongly suggestive of Crohn's disease.

CHRONIC PANCREATITIS

- Factors predisposing to or resulting from pancreatitis that might influence dental management includes:
  - Bleeding due to vitamin K malabsorption
  - Alcoholism
  - Diabetes mellitus
  - Hyperparathyroidism
  - Cystic fibrosis
  - Narcotic abuse due to severe pain.
- L.A. is satisfactory for pain relief. Conscious sedation may be given for control of anxiety
- Oral ulceration can result from holding pancreatic enzyme in the mouth.

ASSOCIATED SYNDROMES

ANOREXIA AND BULIMIA

- Anorexia involves individuals who intentially starve themselves when they are already underweight.
- Persons with bulimia nervosa consume large amount of food during "binge" episodes in which they feel out of control of their eating.
- Associated with dental erosions and parotid enlargements.

GARDNER'S SYNDROME

- Intestinal polyposis (premalignant lesion).
- Multiple impacted supernumerary teeth.

PLUMMER VINSON SYNDROME

- Lemon tinted pallor of mucosa, atrophic glossitis, angular cheilitis associated with iron deficiency anaemia.
- Eosophageal stricture.
- Spoon shaped finger nails.
- Splenomegaly.

PEUTZ JEGHER SYNDROME:

- Multiple intestinal polyposis of small intestine.
- Pigmentation of face, lips and oral cavity.
- Facial pigmentation fades later in life although the intraoral pigmentation persists.

COWDEN'S SYNDROME

- Facial trichilemmomas.
- Gastrointestinal polyps.
- Breast and thyroid neoplasms.
- Pebbly papilloma like lesions and multiple fibromas of oral cavity.
- Cutaneous marker of intestinal malignancy.

LIVER DISEASES

CONGENITAL HYPERBILIRUBINAEMIA

- Can lead to kernicterus or cause epilepsy or choreoathetosis.
- Associated with Gilbert's syndrome, Crigler-Najjar, Dubin Johnson and Rotor syndrome.
- Disorders associated with an early rise in serum levels of conjugated bilirubin (Mainly rhesus disease and biliary atresia) can cause dental hypoplasia and discoloration of the teeth.

ACQUIRED (PARENCHYMAL) LIVER DISEASE

- Impaired haemostasis. Patients can present serious bleeding problems if surgery is needed.
- CT and PT are indicated.
- If PT is prolonged, vitamin K1 10 mg parenterally (phytomenadione) should be given daily for several days preoperatively to improve haemostatic functions.
- If there is an inadequate response with vitamin K, a transfusion of fresh blood or plasma may be required.
- Repeated GI bleeding may cause anaemia.
- Anticoagulants can cause uncontrolled haemorrhage.
- Broad-spectrum antibiotics may further reduce vitamin K availability by destroying the gut flora.
- Drugs particularly barbiturates, liable to cause respiratory depression is especially dangerous.
- Drugs which, in varying degrees are hepatotoxic and should be avoided include tetracyclines, erythromycin estolate, chlorpromazine, azole antifungal, Co-amoxiclav, co-trimoxozole, metronidazole, aspirin, codeine, indomethacin, mefanamic acid, NSAIDs, opioids, paracetamol, MAO inhibitors, suxamethonium, lidocaine (given in low doses), halothane, thiopentone, diazepam, midazolam, phenothiazines, propofol, prednisone, anticoagulants, anticonvulsants, biguanides, diuretics, oral contraceptives.
- Antibiotics, which can be safely used in normal doses, include penicillins, cephalexin, cefazolin, imipenem.

- Analgesia is best achieved with paracetamol or codeine in lower than normal doses.
- Premedication with opioids must be avoided. Benzodiazepines are preferable to thiopentone for induction of G.A.
- L.A. is safe given in normal doses. Prilocaine or articaine are preferred to lidocaine.

MANIFESTATION OF LIVER DISEASES

Disorder	Main causes	Consequences	Clinical features
Impaired bilirubin metabolism	- Congenital hyperbilirubinaemia - Extrahepatic obstruction	Hyperbilirubinaemia	Jaundice
Impaired bilirubin excretion	Hepatocellular disease	- Hyperbilirubinaemia - Bilirubinuria	Jaundice Dark urine Pale stools
Impaired excretion of bile salts	- Extrahepatic obstructions - Hepatocellular disease	- Rise in serum alkaline phosphatase and 5' nucleotidase - Malabsorption of fat-soluble vitamins and fats - Prolonged PT	Pruritis Fatty stools Bleeding tendencies
Impaired liver cell metabolism	Hepatocellular disease	- Impaired clotting factor synthesis - Prolonged PT - Impaired albumin synthesis - Impaired drug metabolisms - Increase AST - Portal venous hypertension - Disorganized liver structure - Cirrhosis - Oesophageal bleeding	Bleeding tendencies Oedema Coma Neurological disorders Splenomegaly

VIRAL HEPATITIS

Causes of viral Hepatitis

1. Hepatitis A virus
2. Hepatitis B virus.
3. Delta agent (Hepatitis D)
4. Non A, Non B (Hepatitis C, G, E)
5. Transfusion transmitted virus
6. SEN – virus.
7. EBV
8. Herpes simplex
9. CMV
10. Coxsackie B-virus.
11. Yellow fever.

Clinical features and Biochemical changes

Stage	Clinical features	Serum bilirubin	AST	ALT	Alkaline Phosphatase
Prodrome	- Anorexia - Lassitude - Nausea - Abdominal pain.	N or ↑	↑	↑↑	N or ↑
Clinical Hepatitis	- As above plus - Jaundice - Pale stools - Dark Urine - Pruritis - Fever - Hepatomegaly	↑	↑	↑↑↑	N or ↑

HEPATITIS A (INFECTIOUS HEPATITIS)

- Spread is largely oro-faecal, but can also occur by close contact, sexual transmission.
- Diagnosis is confirmed by demonstrating serum antibodies to virus (HA-Ab).
- There appears to be no risk of transmission during dental treatment.

Comparative features of viral Hepatitis

	A	B	C	D	E	F
Type Of virus	Picornavirus (RNA)	Hepadna virus (DNA)	Flaviviridae (RNA)	Delta virus (RNA)	RNA	Flavavirus
Incubation period	2-6 week	2-6 months	2-22 weeks	3 weeks – 2 months	2-9 weeks	?
Main Route of transmission	Faecal oral	Parenteral	Parenteral	Parenteral	Faecal oral	Parenteral
Vaccine available	+	+	–	–	–	–
Severity	Mild	May be severe	Moderate	Severe	May be severe	No consequences are known
Complications	Rare Acute mortality 0.1%	- Chronic lever disease in 10-20% - Hepatoma - Polyarteritis nodosa - Chronic glo-merulo nephritis - Acute mortality 1-2%	- Many chronic liver disease >70% - Hepatoma	Can cause fulminant Hepatitis	Rare except in pregnancy	–

HEPATITIS B

- HBsAg (also known as Australian antigen, hepatitis associated antigen) is a non- infectious protein found transiently in those with acute hepatitis B and persist in the serum in carriers and in some who are non-infectious. HBs Ag develops 20-100 days after exposure, is detectable in serum for 1-120 days and then disappears. Presence of HBsAg beyond 13 weeks of the clinical illness often implies that a carrier state is developing.
- HBeAg indicates active disease and high infectivity. If HBeAg persists beyond about four weeks of the onset of symptoms, the patient will probably remain infectious and develop chronic liver disease.
- HBeAb usually indicates complete recovery and loss of infectivity, provided HBeAg is lost.
- HbcAg is found in liver biopsies in acute hepatitis B, but not in serum.
- Hepatitis B core antibody is a sensitive marker of viral replication indicating either current or recent infection.
- Drug of choice for treatment of Hepatitis B is lamivudine or interferon.
- Vaccination confers 90% protection against Hepatitis B and also protects indirectly against Hepatitis D.
- All the hepatotoxic drugs should be used with caution.
- There may be bleeding tendencies if platelet count is low or if PT is prolonged. Patients with a normal BT and PT can undergo routine dental treatment.
- Presence of HBsAg in saliva can be attributed to gingival exudate and may be a source of non-parenteral transmission.
- As little as 1×10^{-7} ml of HBsAg positive serum can transmit hepatitis B.

Serum markers of hepatitis B infection

	HbsAg	Anti-HBs	HBeAg	AntiHBe	HBcAg	Anti-HBc	DNA Polymerase
Late incubation	+	-	+	-	Liver only	-	++
Acute hepatitis	++	-	±	-	Liver only	++	+
Recovery (Immunity)	-	++	-	+	-	+	-
Asymptomatic carrier state	++	-	-	±	-	++	±
Chromic active Hepatitis	++	-	+	-	-	+	±

* HbeAg presence implies high infectivity.

HEPATITIS C

- Accounts for at least 90% post transfusion non -A, non-B hepatitis.
- About 15% of patients infected with HCV are co-infected with HGV. Co-infection with HBV is also common.
- There are associations of HCV in some populations with Sicca syndrome, lichen planus, lymphoma, cryoglobulinemia, and other extrahepatic manifestations.

- HCV is found in saliva.

HEPATITIS D

- HDV is an incomplete virus carried within the hepatitis B particle and will only replicate in the presence of HBsAg.

CHRONIC HEPATITIS

- Hepatotoxic agents, aspirin and paracetamol should be avoided.
- Other management problems include chronic liver disease, HBV or HCV carriage, and corticosteroids, complicating disorders such as other autoimmune diseases, diabetes, and Wilson's disease or alpha-1- antitrypsin deficiency.
- Sjogren's syndrome is relatively common and oral lichenoid lesions may develop.

DRUG INDUCED LIVER DISEASE

- The major problems in dentistry are those created by tetracyclines, erythromycin estolate, halothane and aspirin.
- Reye's syndrome- consists of liver damage with encephalopathy and abnormal accumulations of fat in liver and other organs, along with severe rise in intracranial pressure seen in children after ingestion of aspirin.

CIRRHOSIS

- Routine dental treatment can be carried out without any particular problem though alcoholism may influence treatment planning and procedures.
- Precautions that apply to other parenchymal disease should also be followed.
- Patients may become encephalopathic due to ammonia build up from incomplete detoxification of nitrogenous wastes.
- There may be induction of liver enzymes, leading to a need for increased dosages of certain medications.
- Patient with ascitis may not be able to fully recline in the dental chair.
- Surgery is hazardous, particularly in view of bleeding tendencies but also because of diabetes, anaemia, drug therapy, possible HCV or HBV infection, poor wound healing and a liability to peritonitis.
- Oral findings may be associated with vitamin deficiencies and anaemia.
- Antibiotic prophylaxis may be considered before invasive dental procedures. Amoxicillin orally 2-3 g, with metronidazole 1 h preoperatively or intravenous imipenem are recommended.
- There is an association between liver cirrhosis and oral carcinoma.
- Some patients have sialosis, or tooth erosion from gastric regurgitation.
- Liver transplantation patients who are on immunosupressive therapy should be monitored for systemic infection of oropharyngeal origin, oral viral infections and oral ulcers of unknown origin.

RENAL DISEASES

PROSTATIC CANCER

- Blood prostatic acid phosphatase levels and digital rectal examination are helpful for diagnosis.
- Metastasis frequently involve the jaws and are typically osteosclerotic.
- Cancer chemotherapy may cause mucositis and immunosuppresion.

RENAL FAILURE

- Main management problem include bleeding tendencies. Dental treatment should be best carried out day after dialysis, when there has been maximum benefit from the dialysis and the effect of the heparin has worn off.
- Should bleeding be prolonged, DDAVP (desmopressin) may provide hemostasis for upto 4 hours. If this fails, cryoprecipitate may be effective, has a peak effect of 4-12 hrs. and lasts upto 36 hrs. Conjugated estrogens may aid haemostasis, the effect takes 2-5 days to develop but persists for 30 days.
- Infections are poorly controlled by the patient with CRF, especially if immunosuppressed, and may spread locally as well as give rise to septicaemia.
- Infection may be difficult to recognize as signs of inflammation are masked.
- Haemodialysis predispose to blood borne viral infections such as viral hepatitis.
- Extra pulmonary tuberculosis is common.
- Odontogenic infections should be treated vigorously.
- **Drug modification in CRF patients**
  (a) Safe – No dosage change usually required:
    - Erythromycin
    - Cloxacillin
    - Azithromycin
    - Doxycycline
    - Flucloxacillin
    - Minocycline
    - Metronidazole
    - Rifampicin
    - Lidocaine
    - Paracetamol
    - Diazepam
  (b) Fairly safe – Dosage change only in severe renal failure:
    - Ampicillin
    - Amoxycillin
    - Benzylpenicillin

- Clindamycin
- Co – trimoxazole
- Ketoconazole
- Codeine

(c) Less safe – Dosage reduction indicated even in mild renal failure:
- Acyclovir
- Cephalosporins except cephalothin and cephaloridine which are contraindicated
- Ciprofloxacin
- Fluconazole
- Levofloxacin
- Ofloxacin
- Vancomycin
- NSAIDs and aspirin

(d) Avoided – Best avoided in any patient with renal failure:
- Aminoglycosides
- Gentamycin
- Sulfonamides
- Tetracycline
- Opioids

- Patients who should be considered for antimicrobial prophylaxis prior to extraction, scaling or periodontal surgery include –

(a) Those with polycystic kidneys

(b) Those receiving peritoneal dialysis

(c) Some on haemodialysis

(d) Those with prosthetic grafts or catheters

(e) Uraemia related chemical trauma to heart valves

(f) Those with transplants

An alternative is to give 400 mg teicoplanin i.v. during dialysis, which gives cover for at least a day.

- Aspirin and other NSAID's should be avoided since they aggravate GIT irritation and bleeding associated with CRF. Their excretion may also be delayed and they may be nephrotoxic.
- Even COX – 2 inhibitors may be nephrotoxic and should be avoided.
- Systemic fluorides shouldn't be given .
- Many patients are on antihypertensive therapy which may complicate management.
- Major surgical procedures may be complicated by hyperkalaemia as a result of tissue damage, acidaemia and blood transfusion.
- Dialysis is deferred postoperatively if possible since heparinization is required.
- Consideration must be given to the underlying diseases and complication such as hypertension, diabetes, SLE, amyloidosis or peptic ulceration.

- LA is safe unless there is severe bleeding tendency.
- CRF is invariably complicated by anaemia, which is a contraindication to GA if Hb is below 10g/dl.
- **Orofacial manifestations of chronic renal failure includes:**
  (a) Loss of lamina dura
  (b) Osteoporosis
  (c) Osteolytic area
  (d) Secondary hyperparathyroidism may lead to giant cell lesions
  (e) Abnormal bone repair after extraction with socket sclerosis
  (f) Xerostomia
  (g) Halitosis (uraemic)
  (h) Metallic taste
  (i) Insidious oral bleeding and purpura
  (j) Swelling of salivary glands
  (k) In children with CRF, jaw growth is usually retarded and tooth eruption may be delayed, malocclusion, enamel hypoplasia
  (l) Oral ulceration
  (m) Pallor of mucosa
  (n) Lower caries rate and less periodontal disease
  (o) Pulpal calcifications
  (p) Tooth erosion due to extensive vomiting
  (q) Gingival bleeding
- As renal failure develops, one of the early symptoms may be a bad taste and odor in the mouth, particularly in the morning. This is known as uremic factor or ammonical odor, is typical of any uremic patient and in caused by the high concentration of urea in the saliva and its subsequent breakdown to ammonia.
- An acute rise in BUN level may result in uremic stomatitis, which may appear as an erythemopultaceous form characterized by red mucosa covered with a thick exudate and a pseudomembrane or as an ulcerative form characterized by frank ulcerations with redness and a pultaceous coat, all intra oral changes are related to BUN levels > 150 mg/dl.
- Apart from serving as a potential site for infection, the arteriovenous site should never be jeopardized. The aim with the patent vascular access should be identified and noted on the patient's chart with instructions to avoid both intramuscular and intravenous infections. The blood flow through the arm should not be impeded by requiring the patient to assume a cramped position or by using that arm to measure blood pressure. When access site is located in a leg, the patient should avoid sitting for long periods.

NEPHROTIC SYNDROME

- Long term corticosteroid therapy is the main problem.
- Hypoproteinemia, hypoimmunoglobulinaemia treatment with corticosteroids and other factors such as electrocyte imbalance predispose to infections.

- Prophylactic antimicrobials are indicated for procedure likely to cause bacteremia.
- Cardiovascular and haematological disorders may complicate care.

HEMATOLOGY

POLYCYTHEMIA (VAQUEZ'S DISEASE, OSLER'S DISEASE)

- Ruddy cyanosis is seen on the face and extremities, owing to the presence of deoxygenated blood in cutaneous vessel.
- A purplish red discoloration of the oral mucosa.
- Gingiva are red and may bleed spontaneously.
- Petichae and ecchymosis are seen in patients with platelet abnormalities.
- Varicosities on the ventral tongue is exaggerated.
- Dental treatments present a risk because of the possibility of bleeding or thrombosis. Patients should have a complete blood count prior to treatment.
- To prevent complications, it is recommended that Hb be reduced below 16g/dl and the hematocrit to below 47%.
- Special emphasis should be given to local hemostasis.

IRON DEFICIENCY SYNDROME

- In addition to symptoms common to all anaemias, there is tendency of the nails to crack and split.
- Pallor of oral mucosa.
- Loss of normal keratinization and atrophy of oral epithelial cells.
- Tongue becomes smooth due to atrophy of the filliform and fungiform papillae.
- Glossodynia
- In long standing cases, esophageal strictures or webs can develop, resulting in dysphagia.
- Elective oral surgical or periodontal procedures should not be performed on patients with marked anaemia because of potential for increased bleeding and impaired wound healing.
- GA should not be a administered unless the Hb is at least 10g/dl.

PLUMMER – VINSON SYNDROME

- Characterized by dysphagia and microcytic hypochromic anaemia. A smooth and sore tongue, dry mouth, spoon-shaped nails and angular stomatitis are common features.
- Many patients with this syndrome are edentulous, having lost their teeth early in life.
- Complain of sore mouth and inability to wear dentures is common.
- It is potentially serious because pharyngeal and intraoral carcinoma are more common in these patients.

HAEMOLYTIC ANAEMIA

- In contrast to anaemia produced by bleeding or by factor deficiencies, the hemolytic anaemia produce jaundice caused by the hyperbilirubinemia secondary to erythrocyte destruction. This is best seen in sclera, but the skin, soft palate and tissues of the floor of mouth also becomes icteric as the serum bilirubin increases.

G6PD DEFICIENCY

- The severity of anaemia and its correction should be evaluated before major dental interventions; because the decline in Hb can reach 3-4 g/dl during hemolytic episodes.
- Drugs that may induce hemolysis such as – Dapsone, sulfasalazine, phenacetin should be avoided.
- Blood transfusions may be used prior to dental treatment in severe cases.

MEGALOBLASTIC ANAEMIA (VITAMIN B$_{12}$ DEFICIENCY / PERNICIOUS ANAEMIA / ADDISON'S ANAEMIA / BIEMER'S ANAEMIA)

- More frequently, due to impaired absorption of Vitamin B$_{12}$ due to failure of gastric mucosa to secrete intrinsic factor.
- Glossitis and Glossodynia are the classic oral symptoms. The tongue is *"beefy red"* and inflamed, with small erythematous areas on the tip and margins.
- The erythematous macular lesions also can involve the buccal and labial mucosa.
- Patients may complain of dysphagia and taste aberrations.
- Gradual atrophy of papillae of tongue occurs, which leads to bald tongue. Also known as *Hunters/ Moeller's glossitis.*
- *"Burning mouth"* can be due to neuropathy.
- Oral mucosa biopsy results from patients with pernicious anaemia show epithelial atrophy, enlarged basal cell nuclei, increased mitosis in basal epithelium, epithelial dysplasia and lymphocyte infiltrations.
- *"Howell-Jolly" bodies and "Cabot's rings"* are seen on histopathology.
- To diagnose pernicious anaemia, *"Schilling test"* is used.

FOLIC ACID DEFICIENCY ANAEMIA

- Oral manifestation may include angular cheilitis and with severe cases, ulcerative stomatitis and pharyngitis.

APLASTIC ANAEMIA

- There is pancytopenia due to bone marrow depression.
- *"Fanconi Syndrome"* – congenital and sometimes familial aplastic anemia associated with a variety of other congenital defects like bone, abnormalities microcephaly, hypogenitalism and a generalized olive brown pigmentation of skin.
- Presents as petichae, purpura, frank heamatomas, spontaneous gingival hemorrhage, ulcerative lesions, lack of resistance to infection.

- Tranexamic acid is given in a dosage of 20 mg/kg body weight QID, starting 24 hrs before oral procedures and continued for 3-4 days afterwards.
- Intramuscular injections and nerve block anesthesias are avoided. Intraligamentary anesthesia can be used safely.

SICKLE CELL ANEMIA

- Normal adult HbA is genetically altered to produce sickle Hb (HbS) by the substitution of valine for glutamine at the 6th position of the β globin chain.
- Patient is weak, dyspnoeic, has pain in joint, limbs and abdomen.
- Jaundice usually occurs.
- Pallor of oral mucosa.
- Delayed eruption and hypoplasia of dentition is seen.
- *"Ladder like"* effect is seen on IOPA between the roots of teeth. Lamina dura appears dense and distinct.
- In skull, diploe are thickened and trabeculae are coarse and tend to seen perpendicular to the inner and outer tables, giving a radiographic appearance of *"hair on end"* appearance.
- Patient are particularly prone to develop osteomyelitis, because of hypovascularity of bone marrow secondary to thrombosis.
- Osteoporosis is also a common finding.
- Elective dental procedures involving the soft tissues should not be performed in patients with poorly controlled disease unless absolutely necessary because of increased risk of complications secondary to chronic anaemia and delayed wound healing.
- GA should be used with caution.

THALASSEMIA (COOLEY'S ANAEMIA / MEDITERRANEAN DISEASE / ERYTHROBLASTIC ANAEMIA)

- Characterized by mongoloid features, flaring of maxillary arteries, depressed bridge of nose, unusual prominence of premaxilla, poor spacing of teeth, a marked open bite, prominent malar bones and a saddle nose (chipmunk facies).
- Pneumatization of the maxillary sinuses is delayed.
- Generalized rarefaction of alveolar bone, thinning of cortical bone, enlarged marrow spaces and coarse trabeculae.
- *"Hair-air-end" or "crew cut"* appearance is seen on skull radiographs.
- Intraoral radiographs show *"salt & pepper appearance"*.
- Cranial nerve palsies have also been described.
- Discoloration of teeth can occur due to increased iron deposits.
- Presence of *"safety pin" cells and "target cells"* on histological study.

GRANULOCYTOPENIA & AGRANULOCYTOSIS

- The most common oral sign is ulceration of oral mucosa. These ulcers differ from other oral ulcers in that they usually lack surrounding inflammation and are characterized by necrosis.

- Oral ulcers, advanced periodontal disease, pericoronitis and pulpal infections in patients with severe neutropenia should be considered potentially life threatening because they can lead to bacteremia and septicemia. Patient should be placed on the appropriate combination of parenteral broad-spectrum antibiotics. Topical application of antibacterial mouth sinus may also be helpful.

CYCLIC NEUTROPENIA

- Most common oral manifestation are oral mucosal ulcers and periodontal disease.
- Oral ulcers occurs with each new bout of neutropenia and resemble the large deep scaring ulcers seen in major aphthous stomatitis.
- A series of 3 TLC and DLC per week for 4-6 weeks is necessary to rule out this disease.
- Routine treatment should be confined to the periods when the absolute neutrophil count is above 2000/mm^3.

CHEDIAK- HIGASHI SYNDROME

- Gingival and periodontal disease are common findings in patients and leads to early loss of teeth.

CHRONIC IDIOPATHIC NEUTROPENIA

- Severe rapidly advancing periodontal disease.
- Gingiva appears intensely red with granulomatous margins.
- Recurrent oral ulcers which correspond to decreased neutrophil counts.

LEUKEMIA

- Dental treatment should be carried out after consultation with physician.
- Elective surgeries should be deferred until a remission phase.
- Main dental management problems are:
  - Bleeding tendencies.
  - Susceptibility to infection.
  - Patient may be kept in isolation, where strict asepsis is indicated.
  - Antimicrobial cover is needed for any surgery.
  - Anaemia.
  - Hepatitis B or C and HIV infection.
  - Corticosteroid treatment.
  - Disseminated intravascular coagulopathy.
  - Complication of bone marrow transplantation.
  - Interaction between methotrexate and nitrous oxide.
  - Regional LA injections may be contraindicated if there is a severe hemorrhage tendency.
  - Anaemia may be a contraindication to GA.
  - Nitrous oxide, which interferes with Vitamin B$_{12}$ and folate metabolism is possibly contraindicated if the patient is being treated with methotrexate.

- Penicillin is the antibiotic of choice. Should not be given i.m., as it may lead to hematoma formation.
- Socket should not be packet, as it predisposes to infection.
- Aspirin and other NSAIDS can aggravate bleeding.
- Other oral findings include tonsillar swelling, paraesthesia, extrusion of teeth, painful swellings over the mandible and parotid.
- Bone changes include destruction of crypts of developing teeth, thinning or disappearance of lamina dura, loss of alveolar crestal bone, bone destructions near the apices of mandibular posterior teeth. These bony changes are reversible with chemotherapy.
- Many of the cytotoxic drugs can precipitate mucositis.
- Pulmonary fibrosis can result from busulphan.
- Interferon-α can disturb taste and cause xerostomia.
- Oral infection includes candidiasis, histoplasmosis, aspergillosis, mucormycosis, herpes zoster, herpes labialis etc.
- Leukemic infiltrates may cause oral signs and symptoms because of involvement of 5th and 7th cranial nerves.
- Craniofacial deformities and dental anomalies are common in children receiving chemotherapy. The most common anomalies include dental agenesis, arrested root development, microdontia, enamel dysplasia.

LYMPHOMAS

- The main problem from lymphomas may influence oral health care are:
  - Anemia
  - Corticosteroid tendencies
  - Bleeding tendencies
  - Impaired respiratory function
  - Acute leukemia
  - Lung or cardiac disease (due to mediastinal irradiation)
  - Oral manifestations
  - Painless cervical lymphadenopathy
  - Oral infection
  - Mucositis or oral ulceration caused by cytotoxic drugs
  - Xerostomia
  - LA regional blocks should be avoided if there is any hemorrhagic tendency
  - NHL is one of the most common types of non-epithelial tumor of salivary gland in adults
  - Involvement of Waldeyer's ring in more common in NHL than in Hodgkin's disease
  - Lymphoma in oral cavity are frequently seen in HIV infection

MULTIPLE MYELOMA

- Dental treatment may be complicated by
  - Anaemia
  - Infections
  - Bleeding tendencies
  - Renal failure
  - Corticosteroid therapy
- Skull radiographs show punched out radiolucencies in 70% cases.
- Small, punched out oesteolytic lesions involving the posterior mandible are typical. They are seen less frequently, but can be the first sign.
- Amyloid deposits in oral safe tissues with macroglossia.
- Root resorption, loosening of teeth, mental anesthesia and rarely, pathological fractures are often possible effects.
- Melphalan can cause severe mucositis. Bisphosphanates may cause osteonecrosis.
- Biochemical findings:
  - Hypergammaglobulinemia
  - Bence Jones proteinemia
  - Monoclonal IgG
  - Plasma cell proliferation
  - Uraemia
  - Hypercalcaemia
  - Hyperuriaemia (after treatment)
- Haematological findings.
  - Normocytic anaemia
  - Leukemia
  - Thrombocytopenia.
  - ESR increased.

POSTOPERATIVE BLEEDING

- Plasminogen and plasminogen activator are present in the oral environment under physiological conditions. Thus after surgery, fibrinolysis is triggered.
- Prolonged bleeding after dental extraction is one of the most common signs of hemorrhagic disease and may amount to a hemorrhagic emergency.
- The precise site or origin of bleeding must be discovered by cleaning the mouth with swabs and applying pressure. Suturing of socket is done under LA. Consider any underlying systemic cause, if the bleeding still persists.

Features of bleeding disorders

Platelet defects	Purpura	Coagulation defect
1. Gender affected	Females more than males	Males
2. Family history	Rarely	Usually positive
3. Nature of bleeding	Immediate after trauma Short-lived	Delayed Persistent
4. Effect when locally applied pressure removed	May stop bleeding	Bleeding recurs
5. Spontaneous bleeding from skin, mucosa or gingiva	Common	Uncommon
6. Bleeding from minor superficial injuries	Common	Uncommon
7. Deep hemorrhages or haemarthrosis	Common	Rare
8. Bleeding time	Prolonged	Normal
9. Torniquet test (Hess)	Positive	Negative
10. Platelet count	Often low	Normal
11. Clotting function	Normal	Abnormal

Typical findings in platelet disorders

Disorder	Bleeding time	Platelet count	Clot retraction	Platelet aggregation
Thrombocytopenia	↑	↓	↓	N
Thrombasthenia	↑	N	↓	↓
Storage pool deficiency	↑	N	N	Nor↓
Aspirin or Von-Willebrand's disease	↑	N	N	↓
Thrombocythaemia	↑	↑	Nor↓	Nor↓

Laboratory findings in clotting disorders

	PT	APTT	TT	FL	FDL
Hemophilia A,B; Von- Willebrand disease, Deficiency of factor XII, XII	N	↑	N	N	N
Warfarin or coumarin therapy, obstructive jaundice, Vitamin K, factor V or X deficiency	↑	↑	N	N	N
Heparin therapy, DIC	Nor↑	↑	N	N	N
Parenchymal liver disease	↑	↑	↑	↓	↑
Factor VII deficiency	↑	N	N	N	N

OSLER – RENDU – WEBER SYNDROME (HEREDITARY HEMORRHAGIC TELANGIECTASIA)

- Autosomal dominant condition characterized by telangiectasia on skin and mucosa, IgA deficiency and rarely Von Willebrand's disease.
- Telangiectases may be seen in any part of mouth and may be conspicuous on lips .
- Bleeding from oral surgery is unlikely to be troublesome.
- Rarely, brain abscess or other infections have followed oral procedures that cause bacteraemias but there is no need for antibacterial prophylaxis.
- Regional LA should be avoided because of risk of deep bleeding.
- GA, nasal intubation is best avoided and close postoperative observation is advisable.

ANGINA BULLOSA HAEMORRHAGICA / LOCALIZED ORAL PURPURA

- There are blood blisters often on palate of old patients may be seen in pharynx also.
- It can be due to platelet disorder amyloidosis, leukemia, infectious mononucleosis, HIV or rubella, trauma, corticosteroid inhalers, bleeding into subepithelial blisters such as in mucous membrane pemphigoid.

IDIOPATHIC THROMBOCYTOPENIC PURPURA

- Submucous purpura may be conspicous and sometimes seen as *"Black current jelly"* blood blisters.
- Haemorrhage is rarely severe.
- Regional LA injections can be given if the platelet levels are above 30×10^9/lt.
- Haemostasis after dentoalveolar surgery is usually adequate if platelet levels are above 50×10^9/Lt.
- Major surgery requires platelet levels above 75×10^9/Lt.
- Platelet rich concentrate (PRC) is the best source of platelets.
- Need for platelet transfusions can be induced by local haemostatic measures and use of desmopressin or tranexamic acid or topical administration of platelet concentrates and oxidized regenerated cellulose, collagen etc.
- Spleenectomy may predispose to infections.
- Over the long term, corticosteroids can cause well-recognized problem.
- Drugs such as aspirin and other NSAIDS should be avoided.

Drugs that may impair platelets or their functions

- Alcohol
- Antibiotics – Amoxycillin, ampicillin, azithromycin, carbenicillin, cephalosporin, gentamycin, penicillin G, rifampicin, sulfonamides, trimethoprim.
- Analgesics- Aspirin, NSAIDS, clopidogril.
- Cytotoxic drugs
- G.A. agent – Halothane

- Psychoactive drugs- Antihistamines, diazepam, ticyclic antidepressants chlorpromazine, haloperidol, valproate.
- Diuretics- Acetazolamide, chlorothiazide, furosemide.
- Antidiabetics- Chlorpropamide, tolbutamide.
- Cardiovascular drugs - Digitoxin, quinine, heparin, methyldopa.

HAEMOPHILIA A

- Teeth erupt and exfoliate without problems and non-invasive dental care in safe.
- Caries must be minimized or avoided. The use of fluorides, fissure sealants, dietary advice and dental check ups from early age are crucial.
- Difficulties in management of haemophiliacs may include:
  - Dental neglect necessitating frequent dental extractions.
  - Trauma, surgery and subsequent hemorrhage.
  - Factor VIII inhibition.
  - Hazards of anaesthesia, nasal intubation and i.m. injections.
  - Risk of hepatitis and liver disease.
  - HIV infection.
  - Aggravation of bleeding by drugs.
  - Anxiety
  - Drug dependence as result of chronic pain.
  - LA regional blocks, lingual infiltration or injections in floor of mouth must not be used in absence of factor VIII replacement because of risk of haemorrhage hazarding the airway. Rarely, even submucosal LA infiltration have caused widespread heamatomas.
  - Intraligamentary or intraosseous LA are safer.
  - i.m. injections of drugs should be avoided.
  - Non surgical dental treatment can usually be carried out under antifibrinolytic cover (usually tranexamic acid).

Conservative treatment

- Of primary dentition can be carried out without LA.
- Papillary or intraligamentary infiltration are preferred.
- Alternative techniques such as electronic dental anesthesia can be used.
- Care should be taken to prevent soft tissue injury by use of matrix bands, rubber dam, dry cotton rolls, high-speed vacuum aspiration, saliva ejectors.
- Avoid instrumentation beyond the apex while doing endodontic treatment.
- Intracanal injections of LA solution containing epinephrine may be helpful.

Periodontal surgery

Necessitates LA and factor VIII replacement to a level between 50-75%. Scaling should be carried out under antifibrinolytic cover.

Orthodontics

- There is no contraindicated to movement of teeth.
- Care should be taken to avoid sharp edges of appliances, wire etc.

Extraction and minor surgery

- Factor VIII level of between 50-75% is required.
- All necessary treatment should be carried out in one operation .
- Local measures for hemostasis should be taken .
- Minimal trauma during surgery.
- Non-traumatic needle should be used for suturing and number of sutures minimized. Vicryl sutures are preferred, catgut is best avoided. Suturing carries with it the risk of postoperative bleeding and cause blood to track down towards the mediastinum with danger to airway.
- Packing of sockets is unnecessary if replacement therapy has been adequate but a little oxidized cellulose soaked in tranexamic acid placed into the base of sockets may be used.
- Care should be taken to avoid hematoma formulation postoperatively.
- Infection also appears to induce fibrinolysis, so antimicrobials such as oral penicillin V 250 mg or amoxicillin 500 mg QID for 7 days.
- After trauma to head and neck, factor VIII should be given to achieve a level of 100% because of risk of bleeding into cranial cavity or fascial spaces of neck. If there are lacerations, that need suturing, a minimum level of factor VIII of 50% is required at the time with further cover for 3 days.

HEMOPHILIA B

- Factor IX replacement is needed before surgery but desmopressin is not used.
- All other precautions are similar to Hemophilia A.

VON WILLEBRAND'S DISEASE

- Desmopressin given as a nasal spray is used in type I Von Willbrand's disease, but contraindicated in Type 2 B and 3, which require clotting factor replacement.
- Intermediate purity factor VIII, cryoprecipitate and fresh frozen plasma are effective, though pure factor VIII may be ineffective.
- Aspirin and NSAIDS should be avoided.

ENDOCRINE SYSTEM

DIABETES MELLITUS

- DM in the term given to chronic hyperglycemia at a level sufficient to cause micro vascular complications and is a leading causes of death and disability.
- 3 types of DM

Type I – Insulin dependent

- Juvenile onset
- 5 – 10% of all diabetes
- Due to insulin deficiency
- In upto 90% cases, islet cell antibodies are formed
- HLA DR 3.4 in 95% case

Type II – Non insulin dependent

- Maturity onset
- 90 – 95% of all diabetes
- Due to insulin resistance
- Often associated with family history

Type III – Gestational diabetes

- Develops only during pregnancy
- Usually occurs in 2nd or 3rd trimester.
- Usually disappears after delivery

- The fasting plasma glucose is the preferred test. Diabetes is confirmed when

    (a) FBS is > 7.0 mmol / Lt

    (b) RBS is > 11.0 mmol / Lt

    (c) Blood glucose is > 11.1 mmol / Lt

       2 hr. after GTT giving 75 g glucose

    A diagnosis of DM is made when any one of the above three tests is positive with a second test positive on a different day.

- Predicaments is the term given when there is either:

    (a) Impaired fasting glucose

    (b) Impaired glucose tolerance test

- Long term assessment of glucose control can be made by estimation of the blood level of glycosylated Hemoglobin (HbAlc or HbAl), normal adult Hb that binds glucose, remains in circulation for the life of the erythrocyte and therefore acts as a cumulative index of diabetes control over the preceding 3 months. In general HbAlc of 4.5% is ideal. A value > 6.1% should prompt a change in regimen.

- Fructosamine is an alternative assay of long-term diabetes control.

- The main hazard during health care is hypoglycemia. Dental disease and treatment in particular may disrupt the normal pattern of food intake and interfere with diabetes control. It is best to give oral glucose just before the appointment. This will also minimize the risk of stress induced hypoglycemia.

- Autonomic neuropathy in diabetes can causes orthostatic hypotension; supine patient should be slowly raised upright in the dental chair and helped out of it.

- Aspirin and levofloxacin can enhance the effect of oral hypoglycemic agents. So, should be avoided.

- Orofacial infections should be treated vigorously to prevent ketosis.

- Diabetes controlled by diet alone can frequently tolerate minor oral surgical procedures, such as extraction under L.A. A brief GA can also be given without special precautions apart from monitoring the urine sugar before operation and on recovery. For major surgery, patient should be admitted to hospital preoperatively for assessment and possible stabilization with insulin.

- Patient controlled by oral hypoglycemic may tolerate minor oral surgical procedures under L.A., provided that normal meals are nor interrupted. Well controlled patient can safely have short simple procedures carried out under GA, but blood glucose levels should be monitored postoperatively, 2 hrly.

- If diabetes control is poor, if the patient is on large doses of drugs or if more major surgery is planned, a suggested regimen is as follows –

    (a) Preoperative assessment and stabilization.

    (b) Chlorpropamide should be stopped at least 3 days or preferably a week preoperatively because of its prolonged action and changed to tolbutamide or glibenclamide. It is better to give soluble insulin.

    (c) Metformin must be stopped at least 2 days preoperatively because of the risk of lactic acidosis.

    (d) Before of the surgery, infusion of 10% glucose (500 ml) containing 10 mmol KCl and insulin 5 units should be given.

    (e) Blood glucose is monitored regularly and thin regimen is contimed at 100 ml/hr until normal food can be taken orally. The infusion is then stopped and the oral hypoglycemics restated.

- In a well controlled diabetic on insulin, provided that normal diet is taken and the procedure carried out within 2 hr. of breakfast, the procedure can be carried out with no change in insulin regimen.

- In a well controlled diabetes, who requires surgical procedures, the following procedure is followed –

    (a) Preoperatively, the patient should be put on soluble insulin and stabilized.

    (b) Surgery should be done in early morning hours.

    (c) Blood should be taken for glucose estimation and an intravenous infusion set up giving glucose 10 g, soluble insulin 2 units and potassium 2 mmol/h should be given until normal oral feeding is resumed.

    (d) Blood glucose should be monitored at 2-4 hrly intervals until the patient is feeding normally.

- Generally anesthesia may be complicated in diabetes especially by –

    (a) Hypoglycemia

    (b) Chronic renal failure

    (c) Ischaemic heart disease

    (d) Autonomic neuropathy

- Oral manifestations in diabetes –

    (a) Periodontal disease

    (b) Severe dentoalveolar abscesses with fascial space involvement

    (c) Initially, tooth development appears to be accelerated but after the age of 10 years, is retarded.

(d) Xerostomia may result from dehydration and occasionally there is swelling of the salivary glands, due to autonomic neuropathy

(e) Glossitis, alterations in filliform papillae or burning mouth sensation in the absence of physical change may be possible.

(f) Lichenoid reactions due to oral hypoglycogenics.

(g) Grinspan syndrome.

(h) Chlorpropamide may cause facial flushing.

(i) Oral candidiasis and angular stomatitis.

(j) Mucormycosis

(k) Temporary lingual and labial paraesthesias may follow the removal of mandibular 3rd molar.

(l) Circumoral paraesthesia.

CUSHING'S DISEASE

- The most obvious features of cushing's disease are – central obesity affecting particularly the face (moon face), interscapular region (buffalo hump) and trunk with relative spacing of the limbs.
- Other features include hypertension, diabetes mellitus, osteoporosis, muscle weakness, thinning of skin, purpura, hirsuitism, acne, oligomenorrhoea, infection and psychoses.
- Cushing's disease is conformed by raised plasma control levels, low-dose overnight dexamethasone suspension test to measure plasma cortisol.
- Dental management complication may include –
  - Need for corticosteroid cover
  - Hypertension
  - Cardiovascular disease
  - Diabetes mellitus
  - Psychosis
  - Vertebral collapse
  - Myopathy
  - MEN I syndrome
- LA is preferred for pain control. Conscious sedation can be given, preferably with nitrous oxide and oxygen. G.A. must be carried out in hospital.

HYPERALDOSTERONISM

- In the untreated patients, hypertension and muscle weakness are the main complication.
- If bilateral adrenalectomy has been done, the patient is at risk for collapse during dental treatment and requires corticosteroid cover.
- LA is used for pain control. Conscious sedation may be helpful, especially if there is hypertension. GA should be carried out in hospital. Competitive muscle relaxants may be dangerous as they can cause profound paralysis.

PRIMARY HYPOADRENOCORTICISM (ADDISON'S DISEASE)

- The risk of precipitating hypertensive collapse is such that corticosteroid must be given preoperatively.
- Conscious sedation should generally be avoided unless the patient has had corticosteroid cover.
- G.A. is best given by expert.
- Brown or black pigmentation of mucosa is seen in 75% of the patients. Hyperpigmetation affects particularly areas, normally pigmented or exposed to trauma e.g. buccal mucosa at the occlusal line or the tongue.
- Acute adrenal insufficiency should be managed as follows:
    (a) Lay the patient flat with legs raised
    (b) Give 200 mg hydrocortisone i/v.
    (c) Summon medical assistance.
    (d) Take blood for glucose and electrolyte estimation.
    (e) Give glucose if there is hypoglycemia (25 g orally or i/v).
    (f) Put up an i/v infusion of normal saline or glucose saline. Give 1 lt over 2 hours together with 200 mg hydrocortisone succinate, repeating this at 4-6 hrly intervals as required and monitor the B.P.
    (g) Determine and deal with the underlying cause when the BP has been stabilized. Control of pain and infection are particularly important and steroid supplementation must be continued for at least 3 days after the B.P. has returned to normal.
- Systemic steroid therapy - Adrenocortical function may be suppressed if –
    (a) Patient is currently on daily systemic corticosteroid at doses above 7.5 mg prednisolone.
    (b) Corticosteroids have been taken regularly during previous 30 days.
    (c) Corticosteroid have been taken for more than 1 month during the past year.
- BP must be carefully watched during surgery and especially during recovery and steroid supplementation given immediately if the BP starts to fall.
- Dentoalveolar or maxillofacial surgery may result is stress and a control response, but most other forms of dental treatment cause little response .
- Minor operations under LA must be covered by giving the usual oral steroid dose in morning and giving oral steroids 2–4 hr pre and postoperatively (20-50 mg hydrocortisone or 20 mg prednisolone or 4 mg dexamethasone).
- Cover for major surgery can be provided by giving at least 25– 50 mg hydrocortisone sodium succinate i/m or i/v and then 6- hrly for a further 24 – 72 hr.
- Drugs, especially sedatives and GA are a hazard and it is extremely important to avoid hypoxia, hypotension or hemorrhage.
- Aspirin and other NSAIDS can increase the use of peptic ulceration.
- Osteoporosis induces the danger of fractions when handling the patient
- Susceptibility to infections like herpes simplex, chicken pox, varicella zoster, candidiasis and bacterial infections increases.

- Wound healing is impaired.
- Long-term profound immunosuppression may lead to the appearance of hairy leukoplakia, Kaposi's sarcoma, lymphomas, lip cancer or oral keratosis.
- Topical steroid for use in mouth are unlikely it have any systemic effect but predispose to oral candidiasis.

PHEOCHROMOCYTOMA

- LA is generally safe and epinephrine in modest amount is unlikely to have any significant adverse effects.
- Conscious sedation may be desirable to control anxiety and endogenous epinephrine production.
- Neutraleptic analgesia using a combination such as droperidol, fantanyl and midazolam may be the most satisfactory choice.
- Elective dental treatment should be deferred until after surgical treatment of pheochromocytoma as acute hypertension and dysrhythmias are likely to occur.
- If emergency treatment is required, BP should be controlled first.
- Patient who have had adrenal surgery, require steroid cover before dental surgery.
- Pheochromocytoma is occasionally associated with oral mucosal neuromas (MEN III Syndrome).

DIABETES INSIPIDUS

- LA is the most satisfactory mean of pain control. Conscious sedation may be needed to control anxiety.
- Dentistry is usually uncomplicated by this disorder except for presence of xerostomia.
- Transient diabetes insipidus can be a complication of head injury.
- Syndrome of in appropriate ADH (SIADH) secretion may be caused by –
  (a) Maxillofacial or head injury
  (b) Intracranial lesions
  (c) G.A.
  (d) Elective maxillofacial surgery
  (e) Pain
  (f) Fits
  (g) Smoking
  (h) Drugs like carbamazepine chlorpropamide, vinca alkaloids

ANTERIOR PITUITAY HYPOFUNCTION

Patients are at risk of adrenal crises and hypo pituitary coma.

GROWTH HORMONE EXCESS

- Dental management may be complicated by –
  (a) Blindness
  (b) Diabetes mellitus

- (c) Hypertension
- (d) Cardiomyopathy dysrhythmias
- (e) Hypopituitarism
- (f) Kyphosis
- Glottis opening may be narrowed and the cords mobility reduced. Goitre may further embarrass the airway.
- May be associated with MEN syndrome.
- Mandibular enlargement leads to class III malocclusion with spacing of teeth and thickening of soft tissues.
- The paranasal air sinuses are enlarged and skull thickened.
- Sialosis may develop.
- Sella turcica is enlarged on skull radiographs.

HYPERTHYROIDISM

- Patients with untreated hyperthyroid can be difficult to deal with, as a result of heightened anxiety and irritability.

  LA is the main means of pain control. The risk from epinephrine exacerbating sympathetic over activity is considerable.
- Benzodiazepins may potentiate antithyroid drugs and therefore nitrous oxide should be preferred.
- Providin iodine and similar compounds are best avoided.
- Carbimazole occasionally causes agranulocytosis, which may cause oral and oropharyngeal ulceration.

HYPOTHYROIDISM

- The main danger is of precipitating myxoedema coma by use of sedatives (diazepam or midazolam), opioid analgesics or tranquillizers.
- L.A. is satisfactory for pain control. Conscious sedation may be carried out with nitrous oxide and oxygen.
- GA may be complicated because of possible ischaemic heart disease and danger of coma. If unavoidable, GA should be delayed if possible until thyroxin has been started.
- May be associated with anemia, hypoadrenocorticism, hypotension, diminished cardiac output, bradycardia, Sjogren's syndrome.
- Congenital hypothyroidism may be associated with enlarged tongue.
- Delayed dental development and delayed eruption is usually present.

HYPOPARATHYROIDISM

- L.A. is satisfactory. Conscious sedation can be given preferably after replacement therapy
- Dental management may be complicated by –
- (a) Tetany
- (b) Seizures

(c) Psychiatric problem

(d) Learning disability

(e) Other endocrinopathies

(f) Dysrhythmias

- There may be facial paraesthesia and facial twitching caused by tetany (Chvostek's sign).
- Idiopathic hypoparathyroidism may feature enamel hypoplasia, shortened roots with osteodentin formation, delayed eruption and sometimes-chronic mucocutaneous candidiasis.

HYPERPARATHYROIDISM

- LA is the main means of pain control especially if there are hypertension and dysrhythmias.
- GA may be complicated because of cardiovascular complications and sensitivity to muscle relaxants.
- Dental treatment may be complicated by –
  (a) Renal disease
  (b) Peptic ulceration
  (c) Bone fragility
  (d) MEN syndrome
  (e) Hepatitis B or C
- Dental change include –
  (a) Loss of lamina dura
  (b) Generalized bone rarefaction
  (c) Giant cell lesions (Brown tumors)

MULTIPLE ENDOCRINE NEOPLASIAS

MEN I (Werner's Syndrome)

- Adenoma of pituitary, adrenals
- Hyperplasia of parathyroid

MEN II (II a / Sipple syndrome)

- Medullary cell carcinoma of thyroid
- Pheochromocytoma in 33% cases
- Dermal neuroma

MEN III (II b / Schmidt syndrome)

- Medullary cell carcinoma in 80 – 100% cases
- Pheochromocytoma in 70% cases
- Hyperplasia of parathyroid
- Oral mucosal neuromas
- Marfanoid skeletal anomalies
- Visual disturbances

INFECTIONS

SYPHILIS (LUES)

Congenital (prenatal) syphilis

(a) Frontal bossing

(b) Hypoplastic maxilla

(c) Saddle nose

(d) High arched palate

(e) Higoumenaki's sign

(f) Hutchinson's triad

(g) Saber shins or anterior tibial bowing

(h) Rhinitis and chronic nasal discharge with maculopapular eruptions

(i) Postrhagadic scarring

Primary syphilis

(a) Occurs mostly on genitals

(b) Chancre is the typical lesion

(c) Painless unless superinfected

(d) Lymph nodes are enlarged, rubbery, non tender

(e) Highly infectious

(f) Oral sites include lip, oral mucosa, lateral surface of tongue, soft palate, tonsillar area, pharyngeal lesion and gingiva

Secondary (Metastatic) syphilis

(a) Incubation period is 3 – 6 weeks after primary lesion

(b) Oral lesion are mucosal patches- occurs as multiple, painless, grayish white plaque covered ulcers

(c) Highly infectious

(d) Snail track ulcers

(e) Condyloma latum

(f) Split papule at angle of mouth

Tertiary (Late) syphilis

(a) Non infectious

(b) Occurs several years later

(c) Chronic granulomatous lesion "gumma" are formed, mostly involving tongue and palate

(d) Interstitial glossitis

(e) Tabes dorsalis

(f) General paresis

(g) Positive Romberg's sign

(h) Tabetic crisis

(i) Charcot's joint

(j) Argyll Robertson pupil

(k) Cardiovascular involvement

Radiographic features

(a) Bone involvement usually occurs in tertiary stage and in some cases in secondary stages

(b) Ill defined radiolucent areas or periostitis

Diagnosis

(a) Dark field examination

(b) Biopsy

(c) Serological test – Treponemal antigen test is confirmatory test. Non treponemal tests (VDRL, RPR) are of value in assessing efficiency of therapy

YAWS

- Also called framboesia or buba
- Caused by treponema pertenue
- Primary lesion are papules or ulcers
- Secondary lesions are found in warm, moist areas such as axilla, groin, mouth
- Bone and cartilage are involved
- Tertiary lesions are characterized by gummatous nodular ulcerative lesions
- Saddle nose defect is seen

GONORRHEA

- Oral lesions consists of multiple, painful and round elevated gray white eroded spots with or without pseudomembrane formation.
- Acute gingivitis.
- Tongue may be red, dry, ulcerated or become glazed and swollen with painful erosion.
- TMJ may be affected due to gonococcal arthritis.

LEPROSY

- Oral lesions are macules, well defined hypopigmented, anhydrotic and hyperesthetic or anestheti.
- Peripheral nerves such as facial and trigeminal nerves are frequently involved leading to facial paralysis, difficulty in phonation and mastication.
- Rhino maxillary changes include atrophy of anterior nasal spine, atrophy and recession of maxillary alveolar process, nasal collapse (saddle nose) and a specific chronic osteomyelitis.
- Small tumor like masses called lepromas develop on tongue, lips or hard palate.
- Gingival hyperplasia with loosening of teeth.
- Circumferential hypoplasia of enamel and cementum.

TUBERCULOSIS

- Miliary T.B – dissemination of microorganism by blood stream or lymphatics.
- Scrofula – tuberculous lymphadenitis.
- Lupus vulgaris – primary TB of skin.
- Tongue is the most common oral site.
- Tuberculous ulcers are irregular lesions with ragged undermined edges, minimum induration and yellow granular base. Surrounding mucosa is inflamed and edematous.
- Sentinal tubercle – Tiny single or multiple nodules surrounding the ulcer.
- Tubercle involvement of the periapical tissue and tooth pocket occurs.
- Tuberculous gingivitis- diffuse hyperemic or nodular papillary proliferation.
- Osteomyelitis of jaw bones and destructive involvement of TMJ.
- Chest radiograph in-patient with secondary TB may show fibronodular change. Most often in upper lobe, ill defined opacities, cavitations.

ACTINOMYCOSIS

- It may be localized to oral tissue or may involve salivary glands, bone or skin of the face and neck.
- It produces swelling and induration of tissue, may develop into one or more abscesses which tend to collapse upon the skin surface, liberating pus which contains typical sulfur granules.
- Periapical granulomas and osteomyelitis.
- Painful nodules on tongue which eventually ulcerates.
- Ray fungus appearance on histopathology.
- Penicillin is the antibiotic of choice.

SCARLET FEVER

- Caused by β - haemolytic streptococci which produce erythrogenic toxin.
- Usually seen in children.
- "Stomatitis scarlatina" – mucosa is fiery red, congested, particularly palate.
- "Strawberry tongue" is early stage.
- "Raspberry tongue" – when coating is lost.

DIPHTHERIA

- Involves upper respiratory tract.
- A pseudomembrane, grayish thick, fibrinous exudate overlying necrotic, ulcerated areas of mucosa, tonsils, pharynx and larynx. Bleeding surface if stripped away.
- Nasal regurgitation of liquids during drinking.
- "Bull neck" – swelling of neck.
- Temporary paralysis of soft palate.
- Complication can be myocarditis, polyneuritis, nephritis.

SARCOIDOSIS

- Multisystem granulomatous disease.
- There is depression of delayed type of hypersensitivity.
- Oral lesions may resemble "fever blisters" or diffuse bone destructions.
- Histopathology is same as tuberculosis except that caseation necrosis and AFB are absent.
- Kveim-Siltzback test is diagnostic.

UVEOPAROTID FEVER (HEERFORDT'S SYNDROME)

- Firm painless, bilateral parotid enlargement and occasionally submaxilla and lacrimal glands also. Eye lesions are seen.
- Unilateral / bilateral facial nerve paralysis.

TETANUS

- Incubation period – 14 days.
- Cranial nerve palsy of 7th nerve occurs in cephalic form.
- Pain and stiffness in jaw, neck muscles with muscle rigidity, producing trismus and dysphagia.
- Rigidity of facial muscles may occur producing the typical risus sardonicus.
- Sometimes, entire body may be affected leading to opisthotonus.

RHINOSCLEROMA

- Proliferating nasal masses "HEBRA NOSE"
- Oral proliferative granulomas
- Anaesthesia of soft palate and enlargement of uvula

GRANULOMA INGUINALE

- Oral lesions occurs secondary to genital lesions.
- Presence of Donovan bodies in tissue from lesions.
- 3 types of oral lesions are seen ulcerative exuberant and cicatricial.
- Fibrous scars on cheek or lip may restrict oral opening.

FUNGAL INFECTIONS

GILCHRIST'S DISEASE: (NORTH AMERICAN BLASTOMYCOSIS)

- Granulomatous infection.
- Resembles squamous cell carcinoma.
- Abscess formation is usually all prominent.

LUTZ DISEASE (SOUTH AMERICAN BLASTOMYCOSIS)

- Organism may enter the body through periodontal tissues and subsequently reaches lymph nodes.

- Oral ulcers
- Periapical granulomas

HISTOPLASMOSIS (DARLING'S DISEASE)

- Sore throat, painful chewing, hoarseness, difficulty in swallowing.
- Nodular, ulcerative or vegetative oral lesions.
- Ulcerated base covered with preudomembranous phagocytes cells.
- Chiefly affects Reticuloendothelial system.

MUCORMYCOSIS (PHCOMYCOSIS)

- Ulceration of palate, due to necrosis and invasion of palatal vessels.
- Early manifestation is reddish black nasal turbinate and septum with nasal discharge.
- Apparent predilection for blood vessels.
- May be associated with diabetes, cellulitis, opthalmoplegia and meningioenphalitis.

CANDIDIASIS

- Thrush - acute pseudomembranous form
- Antibiotic sore mouth – Acute atrophic candidiasis
- Denture sore mouth – Chronic atrophic candidiasis
- Chronic hyperplastic candidiasis – Leukoplakia type
- Id Reaction of skin is seen with oral lesions
- Stained with PAS or methanamine silver

VIRAL INFECTIONS

HERPES SIMPLEX INFECTION

- Oral lesions are usually caused by HSV I.
- Herpetic whitlow – primary lesion of fingers.
- Generalized acute marginal gingivitis is seen in primary lesions, with oral ulcers.
- Intramuscular inclusions called lipschultz bodies are present. Scrapings from fresh vesicles show multinucleated giant cells, ballooning degeneration and syncitium.
- Recurrent lesions are usually seen on lips, gingiva, palate and alveolar region.

MEASLES (RUBEOLA)

- Occurs in endemic form, mainly in children.
- Incubation period 8 – 10 days.
- Skin lesion begin on face, in hair line behind the ears.
- Oral lesions are Koplik's spots that usually occur on buccal mucosa. Bluish white specks, surrounded by a bright red margin.

- Palatal and pharyngeal petichae, ulceration and congestion is seen.
- Oral lesion precede 2-3 days before cutaneous lesions.
- Complications – Encephalitis, otitis media, noma, Hodgkin's lymphoma.

VARICELLA ZOSTER INFECTION

- Lesions occur in successive crops. So many vesicles in different stages of formation or resorption are seen.
- Oral lesions involved buccal mucosa, tongue, gingiva, palate, pharynx, forms small eroded ulcers with red margins, closely resembling aphthous lesion.

HERPES ZOSTER (SHINGLES/ ZONA)

- Unilateral vesicles on an erythematous base appears in clusters, chiefly along the course of nerve and give picture of a single dermatome involvement.
- Most commonly involved nerves are C_3, T_5, L_1, L_2 and Ist division of trigeminal nerve.
- If Hutchinson's sign is present then the probability of ocular involvement is more.
- Most common sequel is postherpetic neuralgia.
- James Ramsay Hunt Syndrome – Zoster infection of geniculate ganglion with involvement of external ear and oral mucosa. Presents as facial paralysis.

HERPANGINA

- Occurs in epidemic, unlike HSV.
- Clinical manifestation are generally wider than HSV.
- Lesions occur in pharynx and posterior portions of oral mucosa.
- Acute gingivitis is absent.
- Lesions are smaller than HSV.

RUBELLA (GERMAN MEASLES)

- Koplik's spots do not occur.
- Oral mucosa is not inflamed .
- Infection during 1st trimester of pregnancy can lead to congenital defects such as blindness, deafness, cardiovascular abnormalities or miscarriage.

CONDYLOMA ACUMINATUM

- Small multiple nodules which coalesce and form papillomatous, bulbous masses scattered over tongue, buccal mucosa, palate and gingiva.
- Intranuclear viral inclusions may be seen in the lesional epithelial cells.

MUMPS (EPIDEMIC PAROTITIS)

- Unilateral, or bilateral swelling of salivary glands, usually parotid, rubbery or elastic, elevates the ear.

- Common complications are orchitis (most common), pancreatitis, deafness, mastitis, meningioencephalitis.
- Serum amylase and lipase are often elevated.

REITER'S SYNDROME

- Typical tetrad of manifestations
  - (a) Urethritis
  - (b) Arthritis
  - (c) Conjunctivitis
  - (d) Mucocutaneous lesions

25 | History of Radiology

- **William Morgan** (1785) – Unknown to him, he was the first man to produced X-rays during an experiment.
- **Wilhelm Hittorf** (1870) – Discovered cathode rays. His work was subsequently verified by Goldstein (1879).
- **William Crookes** (1880's) – Worked on fluorescence. Unknowingly generated X-rays.
- **Philip Lenard** – "Lenard Rays" – Cathode rays which cause air to glow in front of window of discharge tube.
  - Also proposed "Inverse square Law"
- **Wilhelm Konrad Roentgen** – Prof. at Wurzberg Bavaria (1895), Discovered X-rays.
- First property of X-rays to be discovered –
  - Fluorescence
  - Penetration
- First medical radiograph – Mrs. Roentgen's hand
- First industrial Radiograph – Roentgen's shotgun
- **Prof Wilhelm Koenig and Dr. Otto Walkhoff** – first dental radiograph.
- **Frank Harrison** – First reported radiation hazards
- **William J. Morton** – First dental radiograph on a skull (VS)
- **Edmund Kells** (1880) – first intraoral radiograph. Gave paralleling technique
- **Coolidge W.D** (1913) – Developed Hot cathode tube.
- **William Rollins** (1895) – First dental X-ray apparatus.
- **Rollins** – Father of Radiation protection
- **Weston A. price** (1904) – Gave bissecting angle technique.
- **Raper** (1909) – Introduced bitewing technique

- **Gordon Fitzgerald** (1940's) – Designed a long-cone for dental X-ray Machine
- **S.S White Co.** (1964) – first panoramic Machine
- First dental X- ray film was an emulsion made on glass plate enclosed in black paper.
- Later flexible celluloid base was used.
- Eastman Kodak co. – first prepacked intraoral film.

26   Radiation Physics

- **Ionization** – Production of ions.
- **Excitation** – The process of raising an electron to a higher level. Excitation of biological material is an important cause of biological damage caused by radiation.
- **Binding energy** – Electrons are maintained in their orbits by the electrostatic force of attraction, between the positive nucleus and the negative electrons. This is known as binding energy. It is measured in eV (electron volts).

1 KeV = 1000 eV.

- Ionization is usually followed by emission of X-rays while excitation is followed by emission of visible or UV rays.
- **Radiation** – Defined as the emission and propagation of energy through space or a substance in the form of waves or particles.
- **Ionizing radiation** – Defined as radiation that is capable of ionizing the atoms. It is of 2 types.
  - (a) **Particulate radiation** – these are tiny particles of matter that possess mass and travel in straight lines and at high speeds. e.g. Electrons (Beta particles, Cathode rays), Alpha particles, Protons, Neutrons.
  - (b) **Electromagnetic radiation** – propagation of wave like energy through space or matter.

    Electromagnetic spectrum

Electric waves	– 10^{15} Å wavelength
Hertz waves	– $10^{16} - 10^{13}$ Å
Radio waves	– $10^{13} - 10^{8}$ Å
X-rays	– $0.1 - 1$ Å
UV rays	– 10^{-6} cm
Visible light	– 10^{-5} cm
Infra red rays	– 10^{-2} cm

- Electromagnetic radiations follow **dualistic theory** –

  (a) Wave theory- These radiations propagate as waves.

$$\nu = hc / \lambda$$

299

Where ν = frequency of waves

h = Planck's constant $(6.61 \times 10^{-34}$ J/sec)

c = speed of light

λ = wavelength.

(b) Quantum theory – According to this concept, electromagnetic radiations are discrete bundles of energy called photons or quanta.

$$E = h\nu$$

Where   E = photon energy in eV.

- $E = hc / \lambda$ (combining the wave and quantum theory)
- **Properties of electromagnetic rays** –

(a) Travel in straight line.

(b) Have no mass or weight.

(c) No electrical charge.

(d) Travel at speed of light $(3 \times 10^8$ m/sec)

(e) Give off an electric field at right angle to the path of propagation and a magnetic field at right angle to both propagation and electric field.

(f) Transfer energy as quanta.

(g) Undergo attenuation, absorption and scattering.

(h) Obey inverse square law.

$$I = 1 / d^2$$

Where   I = Intensity of beam

d = distance from source

- **Uses of various electromagnetic rays in dentistry**.

Radio waves - Short wave diathermy

- Treatment of sinusitis

- Cancer therapy.

- Reduce postoperative swelling and trismus arising from traumatic procedures.

- In Magnetic resonance imaging

Infra red rays - Thermography

- Surgical diathermy

- Altering properties of various dental materials.

- Tooth vitality testing.

Visible light - Dental photography

- Operative field illumination.

UV light - Disclose plaque on unclean surfaces by fluorescence.

- Photo polymerization of compositor

- PUVA therapy for autoimmune disorders.

X-rays 1-2 Å **(Grenz or super soft X- rays)** -Treatment of superficial lesions

1-0.5 Å **(soft X- rays)** - contact therapy

0.5 – 0.1 Å **(Medium X-rays)-** Diagnostic or superficial therapy.

0.1 Å **(hard X-rays)** - Deep x ray therapy, Fluoroscopic examination Radiography, Monitoring film badges

Gamma rays - Treatment of tumors e.g., Radon needles or seeds that are implanted at the tumor site.

PROPERTIES OF X-RAYS

- X-rays are electromagnetic rays that possess all the properties of electromagnetic rays-
    (a) Travel in a straight line, in a wave like motion.
    (b) Travel with speed of light.
    (c) Produce electric and magnetic field perpendicular to the path of propagation.
    (d) Invisible to eyes.
    (e) Cannot be focused by a lens.
    (f) Cannot be reflected, refracted or deflected by an electric and magnetic field.
    (g) Show property of interference, diffraction and polarization.
    (h) Donnot require a medium for propagation.
    (i) Obey inverse square law.
- X-rays are produced by collision of electrons with tungsten atoms. The collision which occurs are of 2 types, giving 2 types of spectra –
    a) **Continuous / General / Bramstrahlung / Braking radiations -** The incoming electron penetrate the outer electron shell and passes close to the nucleus. The speed of the electron is dramatically slowed down and energy is emitted as continuous spectrum.
    b) **Characteristic spectrum / Line spectrum -** The incoming electron displaces an inner shell electron to an outer shell (excitation) or displaces it from the atom (ionization). When the electron jumps back to the original shell, X-ray, photons with characteristic spectrum is emitted.
- **Attenuation** – Reduction in intensity of radiation as it passes through the matter. It depends upon thickness, density of object and photon energy.
- **Absorption** – Degree of absorption of X-ray depends upon density of matter.
- **Penetration** property helps in diagnosing various lesions and radiotherapy.
- **Coherent / Elastic/ Unmodified/Classical/ Thompson and Rayleigh Scattering** – Deflection of X-rays photons occur, without losing energy. This process occur more in higher atomic number materials and with low energy radiations. In radiology, effect of coherent scattering is negligible. It results in production of fog.
- **Photoelectric effect** – It is the process of interaction of the incident photon and the bound electron leading to emission of characteristic radiation. It constitutes 30 % of photons absorbed from dental X-ray beam. These radiations are of little diagnostic value.
- **Compton / Inelastic/ Modified/ Incoherent scattering** - Interaction of photons with free or loosely bound outer shell electrons. The photon handover some of its energy to the electron and itself continues in a new direction, but with reduced energy. Accounts for 62% interactions in dentistry.

- **Annihilation radiation** – When a photon having excess energy passes close to the nucleus of an atom, the photon may completely disappear and replaced by a positive and negative electron. The positive ion is very unstable and combines with another electron to produce annihilation radiation (i.e. Changing back into energy equivalent to their masses).
- **Phosphorescence** – "After-glow". In this phenomenon, a material continues to emit light for a period of time after the X-ray absorption has taken place.
- **Fluorescence** – Here, the emission of light is instantaneous, following X-ray irradiation. This property is used in intensifying screens and mass miniature Radiography.
- **Thermo luminescence** – Emission of visible radiations during or after irradiation of X – rays, but only if heated to a few 100°C. This phenomenon is used in comparative dosimetry and TLD badges.
- Various devices which work on the principle of ionization are –
  - (a) Ionization chamber
  - (b) Thimble chamber
  - (c) Condenser chamber
  - (d) Geiger Muller counter
  - (e) Scintillating counter.
- **Diagnostic properties of X-rays**
  - (a) Travel in straight line
  - (b) Penetration
  - (c) Absorption
  - (d) Ionization
  - (e) Fluorescence
  - (f) Photographic effect
  - (g) Biological effects.
- **Bragg ionization curve** – relative ionization of material is more as the distance from the source increases.

PRODUCTION OF X-RAYS

- X-rays are produced by the sudden deceleration or stoppage of a rapidly moving stream of electrons at a metal target in a high vacuum tube.
- **Parts of dental X-rays machine**
  1. *Control panel* - On and off switch
                     - An exposure button
                     - Control devices to regulate X-ray beam
  2. *Extension head*
  3. *Tube head* – contains X-ray tube
- **Component of tube head**
  1. *Metal housing* – It is filled with oil. It protects the X-ray tube and grounds the high voltage component. Also adds to filtration.

2. *Insulating oil* – It prevent overheating of tube and adds to filtration.

3. *Tube head seal* – Made up of aluminum or leaded glass. Seal the oil in tube head and acts as a filter to x-ray beam.

4. *X-rays tube* – generates X-rays

5. *Aluminum disks* – placed in path of X-ray beam, filters the beam (added filtration).

   – Inherent filtration is provided by metal housing and insulating oil. It is 0.5-1mm of Aluminum

   – Added filtration added in 0.5mm increments.

   – Total filtration = Inherent + added.

   At or below 70 kvp – 1.5mm of aluminum

   Above 70 kvp – 2.5mm

6. *Collimator* – Made up of lead. Used to restrict the size and shape of X-ray beam. Thus, reduce patient exposure. It can be fixed or adjustable and may have a round, rectangular opening.

7. *Position Indicating Device (PID)* – "Cone" It can be conical, rectangular or round. Usually lined by lead, to prevent scattering of radiation. Available in 2 lengths- short (8 inches) and long (16 inches). Rectangular PID reduces patient exposure the most.

- **Component of x ray Tube**

   1. *Glass housing* – Leaded glass vacuum tube, which prevent escape of X-rays. It is provided with a window that permits exit of X-rays towards the PID. Also used for earthing.

   2. *Cathode* – Made up of 2 components.
      - Filament
      - Focussing cup.

      Filament – Made up of Tungsten wire.
      - Source of electrons.
      - Approximately 0.2 cm×1cm in size.
      - Produce electrons by a process called "Thermionic emission".
      - A milliampere control adjusts the voltage across the filament and in turn the flow of heating current through it. Thus, regulates the current.

      Focusing cup – Made up of Molybdenum
      - Houses the filament.
      - Focuses the electrons emitted by filament on the focal spot.

   3. *Anode* (Positive electrode)
      - Consists of wafer thin Tungsten target embedded in a copper stem.
      - Tungsten acts as ideal target material due to –
         – High atomic member
         – High melting point (3380^0C)
         – Low vapour pressure.
         – High specific heat

- Copper stem dissipates the heat through conduction and a radiation device is attached to copper stem, which dissipates heat, by radiation.
- *Two type of anodes* –Stationary/ fixed and Rotating anode.
  - Rotating anode helps to dissipate heat. These are used in extra oral or cephalometric machines.
- Target is inclined at an angle of 20° to the central ray of electron to cause effective focal spot be smaller in size (1×1 mm) in contrast to actual focal size (1×3 mm). This is known as **"Line focus principle"**.
- Angle of 20° is called as **"the angle of truncation"**.
- Sharpness of image increases by reducing the effective focal spot size.
- **HEEL EFFECT**- Due to relatively low intensity of X-ray beam on anode side of the central ray, heel effect is seen. So, after a certain degree of inclination of anode, there is no further increase in sharpness of image. Heel effect is not seen in dentistry due to small size of film.
- Dental X-ray tube acts as a *self - rectifier* as it changes AC to DC while producing x rays.
- **Circuits used in production of X-rays**
  1. *Filament circuit*   – Low voltage (3-5V)
     - Regulates flow of current to filament.
     - Controlled by mA setting in control panel.
  2. *High voltage circuit*   – Uses 65,000 – 1,00,000 V.
     - Controlled by KVp setting in control panel.
     - Accelerates electrons.
- **Transformers**
  1. *Step Down transformer* - Reduces voltage from the incoming 110-220 line voltage to 3-4 V as required for filament circuit. Have more coils in primary coil.
  2. *Step up transformer*- Increase voltage from the incoming 110-220 line voltage to 65000-100000 V as required by high voltage circuit.
  3. *Auto transformer*-This serves as a voltage compensator that corrects the minor fluctuations in the current.
- **Timer**– A timer completes the circuit with the high voltage transformer.
  - Controls the time for which high voltage is applied to the tube.
- **Tube rating** – It refers to the maximum safe intervals (seconds) the tube may be energized at a given range of voltage (KVp) and the tube current (mA) values.
- **Duty cycle** – Refers to how frequently successive exposures can be made. The heat build up at the anode is calculated as

$$\text{Heat unit (HU)} = \text{KVp} \times \text{mA} \times \text{Sec (watt sec)}$$

- Less than 1% of energy of electrons is converted to X-rays at anode 99% is lost as heat.

- **Types of X-rays produced** –
  1. Bremsstrahlung / Braking / General Radiation
     - 70% of X-rays are produced in this matter.
     - Consists of X-rays of many different energies and wavelengths.
  2. Characteristics Radiation –
     - Accounts for a very small part of X-rays produced in dental X-ray machine.
     - Occurs only at 70 KVP and above.
- **Half value Layer** – The thickness of absorbing material (usually aluminium) necessary to reduce the X-ray intensity to one half of its original value.
- KVp – P stands for peak, not potential.

FACTORS CONTROLLING X-RAY BEAM

- **Exposure time** – Determines Quantity
  - When exposure time is doubled, the number of photons generated doubles, but range of energies is unchanged.
- **Tube voltage** – Determines Quality.
  - Increases number of photons generated
  - Increases mean energy of photon.
  - Increases maximum energy of photons.
  - Increase penetration power of rays (Rays with greater voltage are called hard rays)
- **Tube current** – Determines Quantity.
  - Although the exposure time varies inversely to KVp, no definite relationship exists between the two.
- **Quantity Q = mA × Sec.**
- Theoretically, there is a linear relationship between milliampere and tube output. Thus, doubling the tube current should double the number of photons produced.
- **Filtration** – Reduces the intensity of beam, yet increases the mean energy (i.e. hardens the beam).
- **Inherent filtration = 0.5-2.0 mm of aluminium**
  - It is due to a) Glass wall of tube; (b) Insulating oil; (c) Barrier material
  Total filtration – 0.5 mm of aluminium below 50 KVp
  - 1.5 mm of aluminium between 50-70 KVp
  - 2.5 mm of aluminium for all higher KVp
- **Materials used for filtration** depend upon the energy of beam used-
  30-120 KVp – Aluminium
  100-250 KVp- Copper
  200-600 KVp- Tin
  600 KVp- 2 MV- Lead
  >2 MV- None

- **Thoreus Filter** – 0.4 mm Tin + 0.25 mm copper + 1.0 mm aluminium.
- **Collimation** – Reduces size of x-ray beam and thus volume of irradiated tissues. This reduces patient exposure and increases film quality.
- **Types of collimators**- Diaphragm, tubular, rectangular, slit, light.
- **Inverse square law** -Intensity is the number of photons per cross sectional area per unit time.
  - Intensity is inversely proportional to the square of the distance from the source.
  - $I_1/I_2 = (D_2)^2/(D_1)^2$
  - A practical formula to adjust exposure factors is

Original mAs / New mAs = (Original source film distance)^2/ (New source film distance)^2

27 Radiation Biology

- *Deterministic Effects*- In that the severity of response is proportional to the dose.
- *Stochastic effects* – Those for which the probability of occurrence of a change, rather than its severity, is dose dependent.
- *Direct effect* – When the energy of a photon or secondary electrons ionizes biological macromolecules, the effect is called direct.
- *Indirect effects* – When the photon ionizes water molecules and the resulting free ions form free radicals that in turn produce biological effects.

RADIATION EFFECTS AT CELLULAR LEVEL

- *Nucleus*
  - Breaking of one or both DNA strands.
  - Cross -linking of DNA strands within the helix, to other DNA strands or to proteins.
  - Change or loss of a base.
  - Disruption of hydrogen bonds between DNA strands.
  - Chromatid aberration – when irradiation occurs in G_2 or mid and late S phase.
  - Chromosome aberration – When irradiation occurs in G_1 or early S phase.
- *Proteins* – denaturation
- *Mitochondria* – Swelling, increased permeability and disorganization of the internal cristae.

CLASSIFICATION OF CELLS BASED ON THEIR RADIO SENSITIVITY

- *Vegetative intermitotic cells*
  - Most radiosensitive.
  - Divide regularly.
  - Have long mitotic future.
  - Do not undergo differentiation between mitosis.
    e.g. Early precursor cells such as those of spermatogenic or erythroblastic series.
  - Basal cells of oral mucosa.

- *Differentiating intermitotic cells*
    - Somewhat less radiosensitive.
    - Divide less often
    - Undergo some differentiation between divisions.
        - e.g. – Inner enamel epithelium cells
            - Cells of hematopoietic series
            - Spermatocytes, oocytes
- *Multipotential connective tissue cells*
    - Intermediate radio sensitivity
    - Divide irregularly.
    - Limited differentiation.
        - e.g. – Vascular endothelial cells.
            - Fibroblast
            - Mesenchymal cells.
- *Reverting post mitotic cells*
    - Generally radio resistant.
    - Divide infrequently.
    - Specialized function.
        - e.g. – acinal and ductal cells of salivary glands.
            - Pancreatic cells
            - Parenchymal cells of liver, kidney and thyroid.
- *Fixed post mitotic cells*
    - Most resistant
    - Highly differentiated
    - Incapable of mitosis
        - e.g. – Neurons
            - Striated muscle cells.
            - Squamous epithelial cells that are differentiated.
            - Erythrocytes.

RADIO SENSITIVITY OF VARIOUS ORGANS

- *High*
    - Lymphoid organs.
    - Bone marrow.
    - Testes
    - Intestines
    - Mucous membranes.
- *Intermediate*
    - Fine vasculature.
    - Growing cartilage and bones.
    - Salivary glands

- - Lungs, kidney, Liver.
- **Low**   – Optic lens.
  - Mature erythrocytes.
  - Muscle cells
  - Neurons.

Radiation effect on oral Tissues

- **Oral mucosa** – Mucositis initially.
  - Desquamation of epithelium
  - Fibrosis and atrophy after 2 months.
  - Ulceration.
- **Taste buds**   – Loss of taste acuity within 2-3 weeks.
- **Salivary glands**

  - Progressive loss of salivary secretion. Complete xerostomia occurs at 60 Gy. Parotid parenchyma is more commonly affected.
  - Decreased pH of saliva.
  - Viscous saliva with decreased buffering capacity.
  - Acute inflammation of acini followed by progressive fibrosis, adiposis, loss of fine vasculature and concomitant parenchymal degeneration.

- **Teeth**   – Before calcification – destruction of tooth bud.
  - After calcification – Malformation.
  - General growth arrest.
  - Premature eruption.
  - Adult teeth are resistant. Pulp may show long-term fibro atrophy.
  - Hard tissues solubility does not increase.

Radiation caries

Occurs due to exposure of salivary glands which results in xerostomia and changes in saliva. Irradiation of teeth by itself does not influence the course of radiation caries. They are of 3 types –

- Superficial lesion attacking buccal, occlusal, incisal and palatal surfaces.
- Involving cementum and dentin in cervical region.
- Dark pigmentation of the entire crown.
- **Bone**   – Damage to vasculature of periosteum.
  - Destruction of osteoblasts.
  - Replacement of normal marrow by bone marrow.
  - Marrow becomes hypovascular, hypoxic and hypo cellular.
  - Endosteum atrophy.
  - Reduction of mineralization and necrosis (Osteoradio necrosis)

EFFECTS OF WHOLE BODY IRRADIATION

- **Acute radiation syndrome**

  1-2 Gy   – Prodromal symptoms (characteristic of GIT disturbances)

  2-4 Gy   – Mild haemopoietic symptoms.

  4-7 Gy   – Severe haemopoietic symptoms.

  7-15 Gy – Gastrointestinal symptoms.

  50 Gy – Cardiovascular and CNS symptoms.

- **Radiation effects on embryo**

  - Most sensitive period for inducing developmental abnormalities is during the period of organogenesis (18 – 45 days).
  - Irradiations after 50 days of gestation cause general growth retardation and increased risk of childhood cancer.

- **Other late somatic effects**

  (a) Carcinogenesis especially of colon, leukemia, stomach and lungs.

  (b) Growth retardation in children.

  (c) Mental retardation.

  (d) Cataracts.

- **Gene mutations**

  Doubling dose – Amount of radiation, a population requires, to produce in the next generation, as many additional mutations as arise spontaneously (2 SV in humans).

28 Radiation Protection

- **ALARA** (As low as reasonably achievable) – Based upon the principle that there is a possibility of some stochastic effect, no matter how small the dose is.
- An average person is exposed to an additional 0.76 to 1.01 mSv per year from other source like global fall out, occupational exposure, treatment and diagnostic radiation procedures and other miscellaneous causes.
- **Natural or Background exposure**

  External – Cosmic (non terrestrial) – 0.27 mSv

  – Terrestrial – 0.28 mSv

  (National average in India – 13 mSv per year.)

  Internal – From radionuclides, approximately 0.40 mSv.
- *Artificial* – Medical X-rays – 0.39 mSv

  – Nuclear Medicine – 0.14 mSv

  – Consumer products – 0.10 mSv

  – Other – < 0.01 mSv
- **Radiation Quantities and Units**

Quantity	SI unit	Traditional Unit	Conversion
Exposure	Air kerma	Roentgen (R)	1Gy = 100 rad
Absorbed dose	Gray (Gy)	Rad	1Gy = 100 rad1 rad = 0.01 Gy = 1c Gy
Equivalent dose	Sievert (Sv)	Rem	1 Sv = 100 Rem1rem = 0.01Sv = 1c Sv
Radioactivity	Becquerel (Bq)	Curie (Ci)	1Bq = 2.7×10^{-11}Ci1Ci = 3.7×10^{10}Bq
Effective dose	Sievert (Sv)	–	–

- **Dose** – Amount of radiation at a given point or the amount of energy absorbed per unit mass at the site of interest.
- **Exposure** – Measure of radiation quantity, the capacity of the radiation to ionize air.
- **1Gy = 1 Joule/kg.**

- **Absorbed dose** – Energy absorbed by any type of ionizing radiation per unit mass of any type of matter.

  Absorbed dose = Ed/m

  Where Ed = energy imparted by an ionizing radiation to the matter in a volume of element.

  m = Mass of matter.

- **Equivalent dose (H_T)** – Used to compare the biologic effects of different types of radiation to a tissue or organ.

  $H_T = \sum W_R \times D_T$

  Where D_T = Sum of products of absorbed dose averaged over a tissue.

  W_R = radiation weighing factor.

- **Effective dose (E)** – Used to estimate the risk in humans.

$$E = \sum H_T \times W_T$$

- **Quality factor (QF)** – Relates all radiation to biologic systems in terms of its biological effects relative to standard exposure of X-rays.

- In diagnostic radiology **1R = 1r = 1 rem.**

- **Relative Biological effectiveness (RBE)** – Its application is only in laboratory investigation. It is the unit of measuring radioactivity of substance.

- **Maximum permissible dose (MPD)** – It is the equivalent that a person shall be allowed to recieve in a stated period of time.

  - Average weekly exposure for either patient or operator = 0.001 Sv.

  - A maximum of 13 week exposure or maximum exposure = 0.05 Sv.

  - For general public, the maximum permissible dose is limited to 1/10th or 0.005 Sv/yr.

- **Operator Accumulated dose (OAD)-** also called MAD (Maximum accumulated dose)

  This is equal to 5 (N- 18)

  Where N = Age of the patient.

- A full mouth radiographic examinations produce gonadal dose of –

  - Males - < 1 mSv

  - Female – 0.02 mSv

- Mean skin exposure per single dental film in intraoral radiography.

  - 360 mR for periapical

  - 325 mR for bitewing

- Tolerance dose of different organs.

  - Skin – 60 Gy / 5 weeks

  - Epiphysis – 5Gy / 3weeks

  - Brain, liver, kidney, lungs – 40 Gy / 3weeks

  - Eyes – 50 Gy / 3 weeks

  - Gonads – 4 Gy / single dose

    - Males – 0.003Gy

    - Females – 0.005Gy

- **1 Roentgen** = 2.095×10^9 ion pairs (1 ESU)
- **MPD (whole body)** = 100mR per week (5 R/ year)
- Recommended limit of whole body exposure to ionizing radiations for first 30 years of life, excluding background radiation is 10 R.
- Exposure from 1 IOPA radiograph – 100-600MR
- From complete intraoral examination – 5 R (0.0005 R of this dose would expose male genetic cells)
- Daily whole body exposure from natural background = 0.0004 R.
- Sources of radiation in dental radiology.
    - Primary beam
    - Scattered or secondary radiation that originates from irradiated tissues.
    - Leakage or stray radiation from X-ray tube housing.
    - Scattered radiation from filters and cones.
    - Scattered radiation from other objects.
- **Position distance Rule** – Operator should stand at least 6 feet away from the source of radiation or the operator should be at an angle of $90° – 135°$ with respect to direction of the central ray.
- **Methods to reduce patient exposure**
    - Use of high speed films.
    - Use of screen films.
    - Use of intensifying screens.
    - Longer focal spot film distance.
    - Use of collimators – The recommended beam size is not more than 2 ¾ inches in diameter at patient's face, when the source film distance is 18 cm or more.
    - Filtration.
    - Use of high KVp.
    - Use of position indicating device.
    - Film holding devices.
    - Use of protective barriers.
    - Use of adequate timer.
- Thickness of lead apron should be $1/4^{th}$ mm of lead.
- Walls made of 3" of concrete; 16" of steel or 1mm or lead suffice to protect adjacent rooms.
- Barium plaster or Barium concrete provides good alternative to lead.
- **Radiation monitoring devices.**

    Electrical   –   Ionization chamber
                    –   Thimble chamber
                    –   Proportional chamber
                    –   Geiger counter

    Chemical   –   Film
                    –   Chemical dosimeter.

Light   –   Scintillation counter.

            –   Gerenkov counter

Thermolumuniscence dosimeter (TLD)

Heat   –   Calorimeter.

- **Personal monitoring devices.**
  - Pocket dosimeter
  - Film Badge
  - TLD
  - Electronic dosimeter.

29 | Ideal Radiograph

- **5 rules for accurate image formation:**
    - X- Rays should arise from as small a focal spot as conditions would allow.
    - The source-object distance should be as great as possible.
    - The film should be as close as possible to the object being radiographed.
    - The central ray should be as nearly perpendicular to the film as possible.
    - As far as possible, the long axis of the object should be parallel to the film.
- **Density** – Overall "blackness" or "darkness" of a dental radiograph.
    - Density α mAs
    - Higher the mAs – greater the density.
    - Density α $(KVp)^2$
    - As KVP increases – wavelength decreases, penetration increases, exposure increases, increases density.
    - As a thumb rule, an increase in 10 KVP doubles the output of the machine.
    - Density α 1/Source-film distance.
    - Increase in thickness and density of object -density decreases.
    - Filtration of beam decreases density.
    - High-speed film – Increased density.
    - Use of grids – decreases density.
    - Use of screen – Increase density.
- **Optical Density = $\log I_0 / I_t$**
    Where I_0 = Intensity of incident light (from a view box)
        I_t = Intensity of light transmitted through the film.
        D = 0 – 100% light is transmitted
        D = 1 – 10% light is transmitted
        D = 2 – 1% light is transmitted

Useful range of film densities – 0.3-2.0

- **Contrast** – Difference in densities.
  - Contrast is primarily a function of KV_p.
  - As KVP increases-Energy of Xrays increases, penetration of tissues increases; Contrast decreases i.e. a long scale contrast is obtained.
  - Double emulsion – decrease contrast
  - Increased developing – Increase contrast.
  - Only Elon in developing solution – Indistinct contrast.
  - Only hydroquinone – High contrast.
  - Combination of elon & hydroquinone – Better contrast.
  - Film fog – Poor contrast.
  - Increased thickness and density of object – Increase contrast.
  - Increased exposure time – Increase contrast.
- When contrast is changed, density is altered. However, when density is altered there is no obvious change in contrast.
- Caries diagnosis needs – high contrast, Low gray scale.
- Periodontal disease – Low contrast, High gray scale
- 30-40% mineral loss or 13% cortical bone loss should be present for radiographic evidence.
- Low KVP is most advantageous for early / small carious lesions.
- **Characteristic curve/ H and D curve/ Hurler and Driffield curve-** A graphic plot of relationship between film density and exposure.

Sharpness (Detail, Definition, Resolution)

- Smaller the effective focal spot – more is the sharpness.
- 0.8 to 1.5 mm is the ideal focal spot size.
- Actual image – Umbra.
- Fuzzy area at edges – Penumbra.
- Criss crossing of rays which produces penumbra – Undercutting.
- To avoid magnification –
  - Object film distance –Small
  - Source object distance - Large
- $Ug = F \times d/D$
  - Ug = Penumbra size
  - F = focal spot size
  - d = Object- film distance
  - D = Source-object distance.
- Large the grain size – faster the film – less sharp is the image.
- Intensifying screen produce unsharpness due to screen mottle or quantum mottle.
- Fogging causes unsharpness.

Distortion

- Distortion of image can occur due to
    - wrong alignment
    - Wrong angulations
    - Bending of film.

Magnification

- Large source object distance - Less magnification
- Small Object film distance - Less magnification
- **Percentage Magnification =**

(Source-Film distance/ Source-Film distance – Object-Film distance) – Object-Film distance × 100 %

NOTES

30   X-rays Films

- **Composition**
  - *Emulsion*
    - Silver halide grains – Sensitive to X-rays and visible light.
    - Vehicle matrix – Gelatinous or non-gelatinous.
    - Silver halide – Mainly AgBr (0.7 – 0.75 mm) crystals. Few AgI and sulfur compounds.
    - Ultraspeed film is composed of globular crystals (1 mm size)
  - *Base*
    - Cellulose triacetate.
    - Polyester polyethylene terephthalate.
- *Direct action films – (non-screen film or wrapped or packet film).*
  - Sensitive to X ray photon.
  - Excellent image quality and details.
  - All intra oral films.
- *Indirect action / Screen films*
  - Used with intensifying screen
  - Require short exposure
  - Low radiation dose to patient
  - Inferior image quality.
  - Extra oral films
- Different emulsions are sensitive to different colors of light emitted by different types of intensifying screens.
  - Standard AgBr – Blue light sensitive
  - Orthochromatic – Green light sensitive
  - Panchromatic – Red light sensitive
- Purpose of lead foil in film packet is to shield the film from secondary radiation and reduce patient explosure.

- If the film is placed in mouth with lead foil towards tube – *"Tyre-track" pattern or "Herring-bone" pattern* is obtained.
- *IOPA films*.
    - 0 – for children (22 × 35 mm).
    - 1 – Anteriors (24 × 40 mm).
    - 2 – Standard film for adults (31× 41 mm)
- *Bite wing films*
    - Size 2 – Adults
        - 1– children
- *Occlusal films* – 3 times the size of number 2 film (57 × 76 mm)
- *Speed of film* depends upon size of emulsion crystals.
    - A (slow speed)   – single emulsion
    - B (Medium speed) – Double emulsion
                                         – Requires half the exposure time as compared to A films.
    - C (High speed)   – Requires ½ the exposure time as compared to B films.
    - D, E, F speeds are also available.
- Single emulsion film has increased sharpness.

31 Faulty Radiographs

Light radiographs

- Processing errors
  - Underdevelopment (temperature too low, short time, thermometer inaccurate)
  - Depleted developer
  - Contaminated / diluted developer
  - Excessive fixation.
- Under exposure
  - Insufficient mA, KVp, time.
  - Film source distance too great
  - Film packet reversed in mouth.
  - Dark radiographs

Dark radiographs

- Processing errors
  - Over development.
  - Concentration of developer too high
  - Inadequate fixation
  - Accidental exposure to light
  - Improper safe light
- Overexposure
  - Excessive mA, KVp and time
  - Film source distance too short
  - Fogging.

Insufficient contrast

- Under development
- Excessive KVp
- Scattered radiation
- Under exposure
- Excessive film fog
- Failure to use intensifying screen in extra oral radiography.

Excessive contrast

- Overexposure
- Over development
- Insufficient KVp

Film fog

- Improper safe light
- Light leakage
- Over development
- Contaminated solution
- Damaged film during storage

Dark spots on lines

- Fingerprint contamination
- Black paper wrapping sticking to film
- Film in contact with tank or another film during fixation
- Film contaminated with developer before processing
- Excessive bending of film
- Static electricity
- Excessive roller pressure
- Dirty rollers

Light spots

- Film contaminated with fixer before processing
- Film in contact with tank or other film during developing
- Excessive bending of film
- Bubbles of air sticking to film during developing.

Yellow or brown stains

- Depleted developer
- Insufficient fixation
- Insufficient washing
- Contaminated solution

Herring-bone pattern

- Film kept reversed in mouth during exposure.

Unsharpness

- Large focal spot.
- Decreased source film distance
- Increased object film distance
- Movement of patient or tube
- Coarse grained screens
- Bad contact between film and screen.

32 Normal Anatomical Structures on Intraoral Radiographs

RADIOLUCENT

Maxilla

Maxillary sinus

Nasal cavity

Incisive foramen

Mid palatal suture

Mandible

Mental foramen

Mental fossa

Sub mandibular fossa

Nutrient canals

RADIOPAQUE

Maxilla

Coronoid process of mandible

Zygoma

Hamular notch

Anterior nasal spine

Nasal septum

Mandible

External oblique ridge

Mylohyoid ridge

Genial tubercles

- **Coronoid process** is seen in IOPA of maxillary 3rd molar when mouth is wide open.
- **Y- Line of Ennis** – Junction of floor of nasal fossa and anterolateral wall of maxillary sinus. Seen in maxillary canine premolar region.

NOTES

33 Processing

- **Latent image** – When an X-ray film is exposed to X-rays, the photosensitive silver halide crystals in the film emulsion interact with photons, and get chemically changed. These chemically changed crystals constitute latent image.
- Metallic silver is deposited at latent sites, which reacts with developer to form visible image.
- **Developer contains**
  1. *Reducing agents*
     - Hydroquinone
     - Mentol / Elon – Bring out details
     - Less sensitive to temperature
     - When used together, hydroquinone and elon produce adequate details and contrast at 68° F or 20°C.
     - Metal phenidone – Activator for hydroquinone.
     - Used in automatic processing.
  2. *Preservative*
     - Sodium sulphite
     - Prevents oxidation of developer.
  3. *Activator*
     - Potassium carbonate / sodium carbonate.
     - Maintains alkalinity with sodium carbonate give higher contrast.
  4. *Restrainer*
     - Potassium bromide or benzotriazole.
     - Prevents excessive fogging.
     - Increase contrast.
  5. *Hardener*
     - Gluteraldehyde used in automatic processors to prevent emulsion from softening and damage.

6. *Fungicide*
7. *Buffer*
8. *Solvent* – Water
   – In automatic processor sulphate compounds are added to the developer to minimize the swelling of emulsion.

- Function of developer is to reduce the exposed silver halide crystals into metallic silver and create dark or black areas on radiograph.

- Film is washed after developing to remove any remaining develops for 30 seconds. This slows down developing, removes alkali activator, which may neutralize acidic fixer.

- **Fixer contains**
  1. *Clearing agent* – Ammonium thiosulphate or sodium thiosulphate (hypo)
     – Remove silver bromide (undeveloped)
  2. *Preservative* – Sodium sulfite
     – Prevents oxidation of hypo.
     – Prevents any carried over developer from staining the film.
  3. *Acidifier* – Acetic acid (pH – 4 to 4.5)
     – Promote diffusion of hypo into emulsion.
     – Neutralizes any carried over developer.
  4. *Hardener* – Aluminium chloride or aluminium sulphate or potassium alum.
     – Hardens the softened gelatin to prevent mechanical damage.
  5. *Solvent* – Water

- Film should be fixed for at least twice the developing time.
- Lights should not be switched on until the film has been in fixer for 30 seconds.
- After fixing, film is washed in water for 20 minutes.
- Areas of unexposed silver halide crystals that have been removed during processing and have no metallic property.
- A safe light uses a GBX- 2 filter and 15-watt bulbs, in red spectrum of visible light, which is placed at least 4 feet above the whole surface in darkroom.
- Film handling under a safe; light should be restricted to 5 minutes.
- *Different methods of processing-*
  1. Manual
     (a) Time temperature method
     (b) Visual
     (c) Rapid processing
  2. Automatic method
  3. Monobath method
  4. Day light method
  5. Digitized processing
  6. Self-developing films.

34 | Intra Oral Radiology

- **Basic Principals of shadow casting.**
  1. Focal spot should be as small as possible.
  2. Focal spot – object distance should be as long as possible.
  3. Object – film distance should be as small as possible.
  4. The long axis of the object and the film planes should be parallel.
  5. X ray beam should strike the object and film planes at right angles.
  6. There should be no movement of the tube, film or patient during exposure.
- Smaller the focal spot – sharper the image.
- Larger the focal spot – greater the amount of penumbra – greater the unsharpness.
- Longer the target film distance – less is the magnification.
- Less the object film distance – less the magnification.
- If central ray is not perpendicular to tooth – shortening occurs.
- **Advantages of long cone / Paralleling Technique**
  1. Dimensionally accurate
  2. Simple
  3. Can be easily duplicated.
  4. Decreased secondary radiation.
- **Advantages of Bissecting angle Technique**
  1. No film holder is required.
  2. Positioning of film is more comfortable for the patient.
  3. Exposure time decreased.
  4. More effective when the palate is shallow.
- **Angulations for Bissecting angle Technique**

Teeth	Maxillary	Mandibular
Incisors,	+40°	–20°
Canines,	+45°	–25°

Premolars,	+30°	–15°
Molars	+20°	–0 to (–10)°

- Excessive vertical angulations – foreshortening.
- Decreased vertical angulations – elongation.
- Correct finger placement in bissecting angle technique is near the crown gingival junction.
- **Le Masters technique:** - A cotton roll is fastened to the front side of film to rest on palatal surface of molars to make the film parallel to molars and vertical angulation is decreased. This prevents superimposition of zygomatic process on molar roots.
- *Bite Wing Technique* is indicated for
  1. Inter proximal caries.
  2. To monitor progression of dental caries.
  3. Detection of secondary caries.
  4. To evaluate bone loss.
  5. To detect calculus in inter proximal areas.
- IOPA is used to detect proximal caries in anterior teeth.
- Bitewing is also known as Raper's view.
- **Occlusal view** – Used to
  1. Locate retained roots of extracted teeth.
  2. Locate supernumerary, unerupted or impacted teeth.
  3. Locate foreign bodies.
  4. Locate sialoliths.
  5. Evaluate extent of lesions.
  6. Evaluate boundaries of maxillary sinus
  7. Evaluate fractures.
  8. Cleft palate.
- Maxillary cross sectional view is also called "Bird- eye" view.
- Angulations for occlusal view
  1. Maxillary cross- sectional   +65°
  2. Maxillary topographic (anterior)   +65°
  3. Maxillary topographic (lateral)   +60°
  4. Mandibular topographic (anterior)   –55°
  5. Mandibular topographic (lateral)   –90°
  6. Mandibular cross sectional   –90°
- **Methods used to localize objects**
  1. Buccal object Rule / Tube shift technique/ Clark's Rule / SLOB Rule.
  2. Right angle Technique (Miller's Technique)

Extra Oral Radiology

- **Drawbacks**
    1. More magnification due to greater Source-Film distance.
    2. Loss of details due to use of intensifying screen.
    3. Reduced contrast because of production of more secondary radiation.
- **Canthomeatal line**
    1. Imaginary line drawn from outer canthus of eye to the tragus of ear.
    2. Used as radiological base line.

RADIOGRAPHY OF PARA NASAL SINUSES

1. **Granger Projection (PA – occipito frontal view)**
    - Central ray is perpendicular to the film.
    - Used to view para nasal sinuses.
2. **Cadwell Projection (Inclined PA view, occipito frontal projection)**
    - Central ray angled at 23° to canthomeatal line and enters 3 cm above external occipital protuberance.
    - Used to view para nasal sinuses.

RADIOGRAPH FOR MAXILLARY SINUSES

1. **Standard occipitomental Projection (0° OM)** – central ray perpendicular to the film.
    - To see facial skeleton
    - Maxillary antra.
    - Middle third fractures
    - Coronoid fractures.
2. **30° Occipetomental Projection**
    - Central ray angled at 30° to horizontal centered through orbit.
    - Middle third fractures
    - Coronoid process fractures.

3. PA Waters
- Only chin touches the cassette.
- Maxillary, frontal and ethmoidal sinuses are primarily seen.
- Sphenoidal sinus is seen if the patient keeps the mouth open.
- Orbits, frontozygomatic suture, nasal cavity, coronoid process of mandible, zygomatic arch are also seen.

4. Bregma Menton view
- Canthomeatal line is parallel to the cassette and central ray projected through vertex.
- Demonstrates walls of maxillary sinus (especially posterior areas), orbits, zygomatic arches and nasal septum.

RADIOGRAPHY OF MANDIBLE

1. PA Mandible – Used to see
- Posterior third of body of mandible.
- Angles
- Rami
- Lower condylar necks
- Mesiolateral expansion of body and ramus.
- Mandibular hypoplasia or hyperplasia.

2. Rotated PA mandible
- To investigate parotid gland and ramus of mandible, submasseteric infection.

3. Lateral oblique
- To evaluate impacted teeth, fractures and lesions located in the body of mandible and ramus.

RADIOGRAPHY OF BASE OF SKULL

1. Submento vertex projection- Used to study – Destructive / expansile lesions affecting palate, pterygoid region, base of skull, sphenoidal sinus.

2. Jug Handle view - A modification of submento vertex by reducing the exposure time to approximately 1/3rd the normal time for SMV view. Used to visualize zygomatic arches.

RADIOGRAPHY OF TMJ

1. Transcranial

(a) Lindblom Technique – Point of entry of central ray is ½ inch behind and 2 inches above the auditory meatus.

(b) Grewcock approach – Central ray enters through a point 2 inches above the external auditory meatus.

(c) Gill's approach – Central ray enters ½ inch anterior and 2 inches above the external auditory meatus.
- Helps to evaluate arthritic changes on articular surface and the bony relationship of joint.

2. **Transpharyngeal / Infracranial / Mc Queen Dell / Parma Technique** – To view superior and lateral aspect of condylar head and neck.

3. **Transorbital / Zimmer projection** –
   - To visualize articular surface and the articular eminence.
   - To evaluate mediolateral displacement of condylar fractures.

4. **Reverse Towne's**
   - To view condylar neck and head fractures, intracapsular fractures of TMJ, articular surfaces, condylar hypoplasia or hyperplasia.

RADIOGRAPHY FOR SKULL

1. **Lateral cephalogram**
   - To evaluate facial growth and development trauma, diseases and developmental anomalies.
   - Film source distance is 5 feet.

2. **True lateral**
   - To evaluate skull and facial bones for evidence of trauma, disease or developmental abnormality.
   - Nasopharyngeal tissue, Para nasal sinuses and palate are also seen.
   - Pathologies of sella turcica can be seen.

3. **PA cephalogram**
   - To evaluate skull vault and facial bones.
   - Frontal sinuses
   - Conditions affecting cranium (Paget's disease, Multiple myeloma, hyper parathyroidism), intracranial calcifications.

4. **Towne's projection**
   - To observe the occipital area of skull.
   - Neck of condyle can also be viewed.

RADIOGRAPHIC VIEWS ADVISED FOR FRACTURES OF VARIOUS SITES

1. **Angle of mandible**
   - OPG
   - Lateral oblique

2. **Condyle**
   - OPG
   - Lateral oblique
   - Reverse town's
   - Transorbital

3. **Body of mandible**
   - OPG
   - Lateral oblique
   - PA mandible
   - Lower occlusal for symphysis
   - IOPA of involved tooth.

4. **Ramus**
   - OPG
   - Lateral oblique
   - PA mandible

5. **Coronoid process**
   - OPG
   - Lateral oblique
   - Standard occipitomental

6. **Dento Alveolar fractures**
   - IOPA
   - Occlusal (true and topographic)

7. **Le fort I**
   - Standard occipitomental
   - True lateral

8. **Le fort II**
   - Standard occipitomental
   - 30° Occipitomental
   - True Lateral

9. **Le fort III**
   - Standard occipitomental
   - 30° Occipitomental
   - True lateral
   - Coronal / 3D CT scan

10. **Zygomatic complex**
    - Standard occipitomental
    - 30° Occipitomental
    - Submentovertex
    - Jug handle

11. **Naso-ethmoidal complex**
    - True lateral
    - Standard occipitomental
    - 30° Occipitomental
    - Soft tissue lateral view of nose
    - PA cadwell
    - CT scan

12. **Orbit**
    - Standard Occipitomental
    - True lateral
    - PA cadwell
    - CT scan

13. **Maxillary sinus**
    - IOPA
    - OPG
    - PA water's
    - Topographic occlusal
    - True lateral
    - CT scan

14. **Sphenoidal sinus and ethmoidal sinus** – Standard Occipitomental
    - True lateral
    - Submento vertex
    - Tomography
    - CT
15. **Frontal sinus**   – Standard Occipitomental
    - PA skull
    - True lateral
    - CT scan.
16. **Recommended views for salivary glands**
    Parotid   – OPG
    - Lateral oblique
    - Rotated AP view
    - PA view (rotated)
    - Cheek blow out view
    - Intraoral view of cheek

    Submandibular   – OPG
    - Lateral oblique
    - Lower true occlusal
    - Lower posterior topographic occlusal
    - True lateral skull

NOTES

- **Curative therapy** – Here the intention is to eradicate the disease permanently in the treated area.
- **Palliative therapy** – Here the aim is to achieve temporary improvement in the patient's condition in circumstances where the experience has shown that cure is rarely possible.
- **Transcutaneous Irradiation** – Irradiation from sources at a distance from the body (X-ray, teletherapy with radium 226, cobalt – 60 or cesium - 137)
- **Local Irradiation (Brachytherapy)** – Irradiation from source in direct contact with tumor.
  - (a) Surface irradiation with applicators loaded with radioactive material.
  - (b) Intracavity irradiation.
  - (c) Interstitial irradiation using removable needles.
  - (d) Direct radiotherapy to epithelial lesion by means of cones.
- **Internal or systemic irradiation** – Irradiation by radioactive sources administered intravenous or parenterally.
- **Fractionation of Radiotherapy** – Clinical effect of fractioned radiotherapy are influenced by ability to –

Repair sublethal damage.

Reoxygenation of the tumor.

Repopulation of tumor and normal tissues between fractions.

Redistribution of cells into a more sensitive phase in cell cycle treatment.

- **Types of fractionation** –
  1. Conventional – Daily doses of 180-200 cGy and 5 fractions per week.
  2. Hyper fractionation – 2 or more fractions per day of reduced dose (115-120 cGy). It increases total dose without increasing late reactions.
  3. Accelerated – Decrease overall duration of treatment.
  4. Accelerated hyper fractionation – 2 or more fractions per day of normal dose per fraction reduce treatment time without risk of late complications.
  5. Concomitant (Boost technique) – Treatment given once daily for 1st three weeks and then twice daily.

6. Hypo fractionation – Useful in selective case.

7. Split course therapy – Small course with a rest period in between.

- **Tumor Lethal Dose** – Dose of radiation that produces complete or permanent regression of tumors. It is advisable to go upto 90% level, even in curative therapy.

- **Relative biological efficiency (RBE)** – Ionization produced by a radiation along the track differs with the type of energy of the radiation. These differences are expressed as RBE.

- **Therapeutic ratio = normal tissue tolerance/tumor lethal dose.**
  - In case of radiosensitive tumors, the ratio is high.
  - In case of radioresistant tumors, this ratio is low.

- **Methods of increasing therapeutic ratio:**
  - Use of hyperbaric oxygen.
  - Radiosensitizers like metronidazole
  - Radioprotective agents.
  - Hyperthermia

- **Advantage of supervoltage radiation:**
  - Increased penetration
  - Skin sparing effect
  - Differential absorption in bone
  - Sharply defined beam

37 Digital Imaging

- Three Methods to obtain a digital Image
  1. **Direct digital imaging** – Here a sensor is placed in the mouth and exposed. The sensor captures the image and transmits to a computer monitor.
  2. **Indirect digital Imaging** – An X-ray film is digitized using a CCD cameras which scans the image, digitizes and converts the image to display it on computer screen.
  3. **Storage phosphor imaging** – Wireless digital system. Here, a reusable imaging plate coated with phosphors is exposed and a high-speed scanner is used to convert information to electronic files.
- A pixel is the digital equivalent of a silver halide crystal in conventional radiography.
- Production of digital image requires a process called analog to digital conversion.
- *Advantages of digital radiography*

  Superior gray scale resolution

  Easy reproducibility

  Reduced exposure

  Increased speed

  Lower equipment and film cost.

  Increased efficiency.

  Enhancement of diagnostic image.

  Excellent quality.

  Image processing, enlargement and reconstruction for specific diagnostic purpose is possible.

  Effective patient education.
- **Digital subtraction radiography** –
  - Radiographs are digitized and subtraction of the gray levels between the two images in then performed. Any change that has occurred between the two radiographs shows up as light or dark areas.
  - Assess subtle changes in bone.

NOTES

38 Specialized Imaging

- *Relative exposure from various examinations*
  IOPA – 1
  Bitewing – 10
  Full mouth IOPA – 14-17
  Panoramic – 1-2
  CT/head – 25-800
  Skull – 30.

TOMOGRAPHY

It is the process by which an image layer of the body is produced, while the images of the structures above and below that layer are made invisible by blurring.

- **Three types –**
  (a) Conventional Tomography
  (b) Computed Tomography
  (c) Emission Tomography

CONVENTIONAL TOMOGRAPHY

- In tomography, the film and tube move in opposite directions, in a synchronized manner.
- Object closest to the film are seen more sharply and object away from film appear blurred.
- Thickness of the image layer depends on the angle of rotation or the amount of movement of the tube. If the path of X ray tube is short, and the angle is small, the image layer is relatively thick.
- Used to examine sinuses, facial bones, mandible, TMJ and for dental implants.

COMPUTED TOMOGRAPHY

- **CT scan** – Produce sectional images but the radiographic film is replaced by very sensitive crystal or gas detector. The tomographic layer is not contaminated by blurred structures from adjacent anatomy.

- Image consists of a matrix of individual points called **pixels**. Each pixel represents a calculation of actual attenuation of X-ray beam by material within the body. These CT numbers are also known as **"Hounsfield Unit".** This helps to detect minute differences in tissue alterations.
- HU for air –1000

  Water – 0

  Muscle – 35-70

  Trabecular bone – 150-900

  Cortical bone – 900-1800

  Dentine – 1600-2400

  Enamel – 2500-3000
- **Voxels** – The CT image is recorded and displayed as a matrix of individual blocks called "Voxels".

CONE-BEAM CT

- Uses a round or rectangular cone - shaped X-ray beam centered on a 2-D X-ray sensor to scan a 360° rotation about patient's head.
- Scan time ranges from 17 seconds to more than a minute.
- Rasolution power is 4 times that of CT Scan.
- Radiation dose is 3-20% that of a conventional CT.

SCANOGRAPHY

- Uses a narrowly collimated, fan shaped beam of radiation to scan the area of interest, sequentially projecting image data relative to this area onto a moving film.
- Produces images with a higher contrast and greater detail.
- Useful for assessment of periodontal disease and detection of periapical lesions.

MAGNETIC RESONANCE IMAGING (MRI)

- Works on nuclear magnetic resonance to produce signal that can be used to construct an image.
- Uses non-ionizing radiations from the radio frequency band of the EMS.
- T_1 **weighed image**
  - Short repetition time between RF pulses and a short signal recovery time.
  - Intense MR signal is obtained.
  - Used to visualize normal anatomical structures.
- T_2 **weighted images**
  - Long repetition time and long signal recovery time.
  - High intensity signal and dark image is produced.
  - Used to see inflammatory or pathologic changes.

RADIONUCLIDE IMAGING / FUNCTIONAL IMAGING

- Assess physiologic changes that are a direct result of biochemical alteration.
- Here, the patient is the source of radiation.

- Gamma cameras are used to detect the signal.
- Various radioisotopes used are 99m Tc- pertechnetate (for thyroid, salivary glands, bone marrow, bone scans and brain scans); I – 131(for thyroid, liver, cardiovascular blood pool scans); 67-Ga (for abscess scans, infections, osteomyelitis, tumors etc.)
- Initial changes that are not seen on radiographs can be detected.
- Poor resolution of images leads to minimum information about the anatomy.
- High radiation exposure to the patient.
- Images are not usually disease specific.

SPECT (single photon emission computed tomography)

- When photons (gamma rays) are emitted from the patient and detected by a gamma camera rotating around the patient and the distribution of radioactivity is displayed as a cross sectional image, enabling the exact anatomic site of the source of the emissions to be determined.

PET (POSITRON EMISSION TOMOGRAPHY)

- Annihiliation radiation emitted by 2 positrons is detected simultaneously by oppsosite radiation detectors that are arranged in a ring around the patient. Exact site of origin of each signal is recorded and cross sectional image is displayed as a PET scan.
- Radioisotopes used are ^{11}C, ^{18}F, ^{15}O, ^{13}N (alone or incorporated into diverse and biologically important compounds like glucose, amino acids and ammonia).
- Used to study tissue perfusion, substrate metabolism, cell receptors, neurotransmitters, drug pharmacokinetics.

PET-CT

- Co- localization technique to determine a lesion's exact anatomic position.

ULTRA SOUND

- As sound waves pass through any material, it encounters **"acoustic impedance"**. The greater the difference in acoustic impedance of the tissue, greater is the sound reflected. This reflected sound is picked up by transducer, converted into electric impulses and finally displayed on screen.
- USG uses vibratory frequency in range of 1-20 MHz.
- USG signals are produced and detected by certain type of crystals (like quartz, piezoelectric crystals). These crystals change their shape when subjected to an electric voltage.
- USG is used to differentiate between solid and cystic lesions, examine salivary glands, lymph nodes and neck masses.
- Shows good differentiation between soft tissues.

XERORADIOGRAPHY

Provides benefits like enhanced edge effect, high contrast, good details, wide latitude and choice of positive and negative images. Caries and periodontal diseases are better appreciated.

ARTHROGRAPHY

- Supplies information on soft tissue state of TMJ.
- Helps to differentiate disk derangement from bony pathologies and other non-bony problems like capsulitis, myofascitis and MPDS.
- Contraindicated in patients with hypersensitivity to iodine and in acute joint infections.

NOTES

39 Question on Radiology

1. **Cross sectional occlusal radiograph is used for:** [AIPGEE 2008]
    1. Sialoliths in Warthin's duct
    2. Determination of root position
    3. Determination of position of impacted canine
    4. Detection of antroliths

Ans. **1**

2. **If an object is placed lingually & viewed with the tube moved mesially then the object will be seen:** [AIPGEE 2008]
    A. Mesially
    B. Distally
    C. Lingually
    D. Buccally

Ans. **1**

(Use SLOB Rule-Object located on the lingual side shifts to the same side as the movement of the tube)

3. **Acceptable percentage of magnification on a cephalogram is:** [AIPGEE 2008]
    1. 1-2 %
    2. 10-13 %
    3. 6-7 %
    4. 14-16 %

Ans. **2**

4. **Percentage of demineralization required to be seen upon a radiograph is:** [AIPGEE 2008]
    1. 30 %
    2. 20 %
    3. 40 %
    4. 10 %

Ans. 1

5. **The actual size of a lesion as compared to that on a radiograph is:** [AIPGEE 2008]
   1. Smaller
   2. Deeper
   3. Same
   4. Depends upon the angulation

Ans. 2

Because of the fact that at least 30% demineralization of the area is necessary to be visible on the radiograph.

6. **Advantage of paralleling technique is:** [AIPGEE 2008]
   1. Object can be placed far away
   2. Object can be placed parallel to the tooth
   3. Distortion of image is decreased
   4. Decreased patient exposure

Ans. 3

Advantages of long cone / Paralleling Technique
- Dimensionally accurate
- Simple
- Can be easily duplicated.
- Decreased secondary radiation.

7. **True regarding intensifying screens:** [AIPGEE 2008]
   1. Decreases exposure time
   2. Increases clarity
   3. Prevent backscatter radiation
   4. Increased patient exposure

Ans. 1

There is loss of clarity of image and patient radiation dose is reduced.

8. **The distance between the film & the source in cephalometric radiology is:** [AIPGEE 2008]
   1. 4 feet
   2. 6 feet
   3. 7 feet
   4. 5 feet

Ans. 4

9. **A pear shaped radiolucency present between the maxillary lateral incisor & canine is most likely to be:** [AIPGEE 2008]
   1. Globulomaxillary cyst

2. Nasopalatine cyst
3. Dentigerous cyst
4. Periapical cyst

Ans. `1`

Nasopalatine cyst- Heart shaped radiolucent area

Dentigerous cyst- Perocoronal radiolucency

10. **The three features of a radiograph are:** [AIPGEE 2008]
    1. Definition, density & detail
    2. Definition, density & distortion
    3. Definition, contrast, detail
    4. Definition, distortion & detail

Ans. `3`

11. **Incipient carious lesions can be detected by:** (AIPGEE 2008)
    1. Air drying & exploring with probe
    2. Radiograph
    3. Ultrasound
    4. Digital subtraction radiography

Ans. `1`

For a lesion to appear on radiograph, 30% demineralization is necessary.

Ultrasound may be helpful when there is discontinuity of the enamel surface.

Digital subtraction radiography is helpful to monitor the progression of the lesion.

12. **Name the lesion, which is not a radiolucent lesion of the jaws -** [AIPG 2005]
    1. Ameloblastoma.
    2. Cherubism.
    3. Focal periapical osteopetrosis.
    4. Odontogenic.

Ans. `3`

Other three lesions are radiolucent.

13. **Reduced salivary flow following irradiation is dose dependent. At what dose does the flow reach essentially zero?** [AIPG 2005]
    1. 4000 rads.
    2. 5000 rads.
    3. 6000 rads.
    4. 7000 rads.

Ans. `3`

The extent of xerostomia following radiotherapy is dose dependent and reaches essentially gets at 60 Gy. pH value decreased 1 value below the normal. Compensatory hypertrophy of the residual salivary glands can also be seen.

14. **In radionuclide imaging the most useful radiopharmaceutical for skeletal imaging is -** [AIPG 2005]

    1. Gallium 67 (^{67}Ga).
    2. Technetium-sulphur-colloid (^{99m}Tc-Sc).
    3. Technetium (^{99m}Tc).
    4. Technetium –99m linked to methylene diphosphonate (^{99m}Tc-MDP).

Ans. **4**

Ga- 67 is used for infections, inflammation, sarcoidosis and lymphoma.

^{99m}Tc-Sc is used for thyroid, renal, lung, myocardial imaging and bone metastasis

^{99m}Tc-MDP can detect bone diseases even in early stage.

15. **In which one of the following conditions the sialography is contraindicated?** [AIPG 2005]
    1. Ductal calculus.
    2. Chronic parotitis.
    3. Acute parotitis.
    4. Recurrent sialadenitis.

Ans. **3**

Sialography is contraindicated in case of allergy to contract media and acute infections as it may flare up the symptoms due to retrograde flow of contrast media.

16. **The technique employed in radiotherapy to counteract the effect of tumour motion due to breathing is known as -** [AIPG 2005]
    1. Arc technique.
    2. Modulation.
    3. Gating.
    4. Shunting.

Ans. **3**

17. **Gamma camera in nuclear medicine is used for -** [AIPG 2005]
    1. Organ imaging.
    2. Measuring the radioactivity.
    3. Monitoring the surface contamination.
    4. RIA.

Ans. **2**

Rectilinear and anger or gamma scintillation camera record the gamma emissions from patients injected with appropriate tracers. These are used in scintigraphy, SPECT and PET.

18. **Which of the following is used to show the base of the skull, sphenoid sinus, position and orientation of the condyles and fractures of the zygomatic arch?** [AIPG 2005]

    1. The TMJ surgery.
    2. Submentovertex projection.
    3. Reverse-Towne projection.
    4. The facial profile survey.

Ans. **2**

Reverse Towne's is used to see mediolateral displacement of condylar fractures.

Facial profile survey is helpful for orthodontic study.

TMJ surveys are mainly used to see arthritic changes for TMJ.

19. **Which survey has the purpose of examining fractures of the condylar neck of the mandible?** [AIPG 2005]

    1. Lateral jaw projection.
    2. Lateral skull projection.
    3. Waters projection.
    4. Reverse-Towne's view.

Ans. **4**

Lateral jaw projection is meant for fractures of body and ramus of mandible.

Water's projection for paranasal sinuses, infraorbital, supraorbital margins & frontozygomatic fractures.

20. **In cephalometrics, the frankfort plane is constructed -** [AIPG 2005]

    1. Horizontally from nasion through portion.
    2. Horizontally from nasion to the superior aspect of external auditory meatus.
    3. Vertically from orbitale through the maxillary canine.
    4. Horizontally from orbitale to the superior aspect of the external auditory meatus.

Ans. **4**

Frankfurt plane is an imaginary plane extending from lower most point on infraorbital rim to superior most point of external acoustic meatus.

21. **Which of the following is the most penetration beam?** [AIPG 2004]

    1. Electron beam
    2. 8 MV photons
    3 18 MV photons
    4. Proton beam

Ans. **3**

Higher the energy, more is the penetration power.

22. **The principle reason for placing an aluminium filter in the primary beam of radiation is to?**

    [AIPG 2003]

    1. Reduce exposure time
    2. Decrease development time of the films
    3. Reduce radiation to the skin of the patient
    4. Obtain greater definition of the images of teeth.

Ans. **3**

Use of filters removes the scattered radiation, which does not have any diagnostic value. Thus, patient exposure is reduced.

23. **Periapical cementifying fibroepulis is similar to a granuloma in that the former:**

    [AIPG 2002]

    1. Radiolucent initially and the tooth is vital
    2. Radiopaque initially and the tooth is vital
    3. Occurs in males only
    4. Occurs in the mandible.

Ans. **1**

In later stages, it appears as radiopaque, but the tooth is still vital.

24. **All the following have similar radiographic features except:**   [AIPG 2002]
    1. Ameloblastoma
    2. Lateral periodontal cyst
    3. Complex odontoma
    4. Radicular cyst.

Ans. **1**

Ameloblastoma is usually multilocular. Other 3 are unilocular

25. **Radiographic irregularities associated with the roots of mandibular central incisor can be:**

    [AIPG 2002]

    1. Root caries
    2. Sublingual calculus
    3. Hyperplastic cementum
    4. Cementoma

Ans. **2**

Most common radiopaque structure seen between the roots of mandibular incisors is calculus.

26. **The lamina dura is the radiographic image of:**   [AIPG 2002]
    1. Periodontal ligament space
    2. Alveolar bone proper
    3. Cortical bone
    4. Cancellous bone.

Ans. `2`

Due to presence of higher calcium content in the shadow.

27. **Most penetrating radiation is:** [AIPG 2002]

    1. Alpha rays
    2. Beta rays
    3. Gamma rays
    4. Cathode rays

Ans. `3`

Due to shorter wavelength and negligible mass.

28. **X-ray of the mandible shows the mandibular foramen in:** [AIPG 2002]

    1. Anterior region
    2. Ramus region
    3. Maxillary anterior region
    4. Maxillary sinus region.

Ans. `2`

It is a radiolucency seen in the middle of ramus.

29. **Which of the following conditions cannot be assessed by a cephalogram?** [AIPG 2001]

    1. Mandibular lateral asymmetry
    2. Vertical facial discrepancy
    3. Increase posterior height
    4. Decreased anterior height

Ans. `1`

For lateral symmetry, PA view is needed.

30. **In a patient of operated cleft lip and palate with anterior cross-bite cephalogram will show:**
    [AIPG 2001]

    1. Maxillary retrusion
    2. Mandibular protrusion
    3. Maxillary protrusion
    4. 1 and 2

Ans. `1`

Due to cleft palate, maxilla is hypoplasia. So skeletal class II malocclusion is there.

31. **In paralleling technique the X-ray film is held parallel to the teeth. To accomplish this the film needs to be positioned away from the teeth within the oral cavity resulting in distortion. To overcome this:** [AIPG 2000]

    1. Increase the KVP
    2. Decrease the KVP

    3.   Increase the target film distance

    4.   Decrease the target film distance.

Ans.   **3**

To reduce geometric distortion caused by placing the film away from the teeth, source-object distance is increased. The use of long source-object distance reduces the apparent size of focal spot. This leads to increased deformation and decreased magnification. This is why, paralleling technique is also known as long cone technique.

32. "Brachytherapy" is: **[AIPG 2000]**

    1.   Irradiation of tissues from a distance

    2.   Irradiation of tissues from a distance of 3 cm

    3.   Irradiation of tissues by implants within the tissues

    4.   Irradiation of tissues by radiopharmaceuticals.

Ans.   **3**

Radioactive cobalt and caesium implants are placed in the tumor mass to provide radiotherapeutic effect. Irradiation from distance is called teletherapy.

33. X-ray of a permanent Ist molar with early acute pulpal abscess will show: **[AIPG 2000]**

    1.   Furcation involvement

    2.   Little change from normal

    3.   Widening of PDL

    4.   Narrowing of PDL.

Ans.   **2**

34. X-ray to view the superior compartment of TMJ is: **[AIPG 2000]**

    1.   Transpharyngeal

    2.   Transcranial

    3.   Orthopantomograph

    4.   Transorbital.

Ans.   **2**

Transcranial view gives a clear picture of glenoid fossa and joint space. Transpharyngeal shows the medial and superior surface of condyle clearly. OPG gives lateral view of condyle. Transorbital shows mediolateral displacement of fractured segments.

35. Intensifying screens are used with extraoral radiography to: **[AIPG 2000]**

    1.   Increase the KVP

    2.   Increase the exposure time

    3.   Decrease the fixing time

    4.   Decrease the patient exposure.

Ans.   **4**

Intensifying screens are based upon the property of florescence. Once they are exposed to X-ray, they emit visible light, which further helps in image formation. Thus, total radiation dose to the patient is reduced. But, there is loss of sharpness and details of the image.

36. **The skin of a patient 2 days after radiotherapy will show:** [AIPG 99]
    1. Erythema
    2. Depigmentation
    3. Radiation induced carcinomas
    4. No change

Ans. **1**

Depigmentation and carcinomas occur due to chronic radiation exposure.

37. **Radiodensity can be increased by:** [AIPG 99]
    1. Decreasing mA
    2. Decreasing kVp
    3. Decreasing the target film distance
    4. Increasing the object-film distance

Ans. **3**

Increasing mA, increasing KVP and decreasing object film distance, can increase radiodensity.

38. **Cephalometric growth changes in a patient can be evaluated by superimposing on the:**
    [AIPG 99]
    1. FHP
    2. S-N plane
    3. Mandibular plane
    4. Facial plane

Ans. **2**

Because S-N plane remains constant through out life.

39. **Bitewing radiographs are used for:** [AIPG 99]
    1. Periapical lesions
    2. Proximal caries
    3. Reducing patient radiation exposure
    4. Reducing fog

Ans. **2**

Bitewing are used for proximal carries and interdental bone loss.

40. **Sialogram of a salivary gland will resemble:** [AIPG 99]
    1. Leafy tree
    2. Leafless tree
    3. Sialdenitis
    4. Sialolithiasis

Ans. 2

41. Oblique posterior mandibular occlusal view is done for: [AIPG 98]
1. Fractures of the angle of the mandible
2. Submandibular duct calculi
3. Symphyseal fracture
4. None of the above

Ans. 2

This view gives better visualization of any calcification in proximal part of wharton's duct in the floor of mouth.

Best view for angle of mandible fracture is lateral oblique or PA mandible and for symphyseal fracture, it is mandibular anterior occlusal view.

42. Moth eaten appearance is seen in: [AIPG 97]
1. Sclerosing osteomyelitis
2. Garre's osteomyelitis
3. Osteoradionecrosis
4. Fibrous dysplasia

Ans. 1

In Garre's osteomyelitis, onion peel appearance in seen due to periosteal reaction. Osteoradionecrosis appears as an ill-defined radiolucency. In fibrous dysplasia, initial stage is marked by well-delineated radiolucency, which is replaced by opacity in later stages.

43. Ideal distance between patient and X-ray source for taking cephalogram is: [AIPG 97]
1. Four feet
2. Five feet
3. Six feet
4. Nine feet

Ans. 2

The object tube distance is fixed for cephalogram for the purpose of standardization and growth evaluation.

44. Ideal position for the dentist to stand while taking radiographs is: [AIPG 97]
1. Behind the head of the patient
2. At an angle of 90-135 degrees and six feet away from patient
3. In 11'O clock position
4. At an angle of 180 degrees and ten feet away from patient

Ans. 2

Because the scattered radiation is minimum at an angle of 90°-135° and six feet distance from the patient.

45. **A patient requires tooth extractions from an area that has been subjected to radiation therapy. Which of the following represents the great danger to this patient?** [AIPG 97]

1. Alveolar osteitis
2. Osteoradionecrosis
3. Prolonged healing
4. Fracture of the mandible

Ans. **2**

Due to hypocellular, hypovascular and hypoxic bone, there are chances of osteoradionecrosis, if the tooth is extracted within 6 months to one year after radiotherapy.

46. **In radiobiology, the "latent period" represent the period of time between:** [AIPG 97]

1. Cell rest and cell mitosis
2. The first and last dose in radiation therapy
3. Film exposure and image development
4. Radiation exposure and onset of symptoms

Ans. **4**

This is the period when the patient doesn't show any symptoms.

47. **In radiographic study of impacted teeth:** [AIPG 96]

1. Bite wing X-rays are of no use
2. Occlusal view is useless
3. Bite wing X-rays are indispensable
4. All of the above

Ans. **1**

Bitewing X-rays are used for diagnosis of proximal caries and interdental bone loss. They do not reveal the periapical region. Occlusal view helps in localization of the impacted teeth.

48. **Most radiosensitive tissue is:** [AIPG 96]

1. Cartilage
2. Bone
3. Bone marrow
4. Nails

Ans. **3**

Rapidly dividing cells are most radiosensitive. Bones are cartilage have intermediate sensitivity. Nails are dead tissue, so radioresistant.

49. **Best X-ray view for TMJ is:** [AIPG 96]

1. Lateral skull
2. Lateral oblique
3. Transpharyngeal
4. Panoromic

Ans. ■3

In transpharyngeal, TMJ can be viewed with minimal superimposition by other osseous structures.

50. Which radiograph would give the best view of fracture of zygomatic bone? [AIPG 1995]

1. PNS view
2. Submentovertex
3. Lateral oblique mandible
4. Transpharyngeal view

Ans. ■2

Submentovertex view - indications

- Destructive / expansive lesions affecting the palate, pterygoid region or base of skull
- Investigation of sphenoidal sinus
- Zygomatic arches.

51. To restrict X-ray beam which of the following is done: [AIPG 94]

1. Collimation of beam
2. Increase KVP
3. Decrease target object distance
4. Use a grid

Ans. ■1

Collimation prevents the scattering of the incident rays, thus reducing the amount of low energy photons and patient exposure.

52. Filters of which metal is used to remove long wavelength X-rays from the primary beam: [AIPG 94]

1. Platinum
2. Aluminium
3. Copper
4. Lead

Ans. ■2

53. Which of the following have the largest wavelength? [AIPG 94]

1. Cosmic waves
2. Radio waves
3. Infrared waves
4. Visible waves

Ans. ■2

Radio waves – 3×10^5 cm to 1.0 cm.

Infra red rays – 10^{-2} cm to 10^{-5} cm

Visible light – 7×10^{-5} cm to 4×10^{-5} cm.

UV rays – 10^{-5}cm to 10^{-6} cm

X and γ rays – 10Å – 0.001Å

54. Grid is used in radiography to: [AIPG 94]

1. Reduce KVP
2. Reduce exposure time
3. Reduce fogging
4. Increase contrast

Ans. 4

A grid is composed of a large number of long parallel strips of lead held apart and parallel to each other by an X-ray transparent interspace material. They remove 80-90% of the scattered radiation, thus improving the contrast.

55. Radiolucent area in relation to 11,21: [AIPG 93]

1. Mesiodens
2. Median maxillary anterior alveolar cleft
3. Globulomaxillary cyst
4. Nasopalatine cyst

Ans. 4

Most common site of nasopalatine cyst in apical to 11, 21. It appears as a heart shaped radiolucency. Globulomaxillary cyst is seen as tear drop shaped radiolucency in lateral incisor canine region.

56. Osteoradionecrosis results from: [AIPG 93]

1. Infection, trauma, radiation
2. Radiation, trauma, infection
3. Trauma, radiation, infection
4. Infection, radiation, trauma

Ans. 2

This is the most appropriate sequence in the pathogenesis of osteoradionecrosis. Due to radiation therapy, there is hypoxia of bone. Trauma to the region leads to impaired healing and superimposed infection which causes osteoradionecrosis.

57. In an OPG of 25-year-old asymptomatic patient, a radiolucent area below 35 was seen, it could be: [AIPG 93]

1. Mental foramen
2. Periapical cyst
3. Periapical granuloma
4. None of the above

Ans. 1

Mental foramen is the anatomical landmark located at the apex of mandibular premolar, which is mostly mistaken for periapical radiolucency.

58. All of the following have same radiographic features except: [AIPG 93]

1. Periodontal odontoma
2. Dentigenous cyst
3. Ameloblastoma
4. Keratocyst

Ans. **1**

All the other three may have a cystic appearance, associated with an impacted tooth or can be multilocular with soap-bubble radiolucency. Periodontal odontoma is radiopaque.

59. All of the following show opacity in X-ray except: [AIPG 93]

1. Ameloblastic fibroma
2. Ameloblastic odontoma
3. Cementoblastoma
4. Ameloblastic fibrodontoma

Ans. **1**

All others show a radiopaque shadow at least at some stage of development.

60. Of the following, the best radiographic examination of the maxillary sinus is performed with: [AIPG 91]

1. A panorex
2. Periapical view
3. A Waters view
4. A cephalometric view

Ans. **3**

Panorex is used for general survey of teeth, periapical view is used to visualize floor of the maxillary sinus. Cephalometric view reveals the floor and posterior wall of maxillary sinus.

61. The most anterior point on bony chin is: [AIPG 91]

1. Gonion
2. Menton
3. Gnathion
4. Pogonion

Ans. **4**

Gonion – Bisector drawn from the point of intersection of mandibular and ramal plane at the angle of mandible.

Menton – Most inferior point on bony chain

Gnathion - Most anteroinferior point on bony chin.

62. Frankfurt horizontal plane is obtained by joining: [AIPG 91]

1. Nasion and sella
2. Porion and Nasion

3. Porion and Orbitale

4. Porion and sella

Ans. **3**

Frankfurt horizontal plane is obtained by joining inferior most point on bony orbit (Orbitale) and superior most point on external auditory meatus (Porion).

63. **Ground glass appearance in X-rays may suggest the patient is suffering with:** [AIPG 1990]

1. Hyperparathyroidism

2. Fibrous dysplasia

3. Paget's disease

4. None of the above

Ans. **1**

It may also be seen in monoostotic fibrous dysplasia but, almost always seen in hyperparathyroidism. In Paget's disease cotton wool appearance with hypercementosis and loss of lamina dura is seen.

64. **Which of the following is a unilateral landmark on a cephalogram?** [AIPG 1990]

1. Orbitale

2. Porion

3. Basion

4. Gonion

Ans. **3**

Basion is the midpoint on anterior margin of foramen magnum.

1, 2, and 4 are bilateral.

65. **Hand and Wrist X-rays predict:** [AIPG 1990]

1. Timing of growth

2. Direction of growth

3. Amount of growth

4. All of the above

Ans. **1**

Specific and definite schedule of appearance and ossification of bones of hand and wrist are evaluated.

66. **Periosteal bone formation occurs in all except:** [AIPG 1990]

1. Paget's disease

2. Garre's osteomyelitis

3. Ewing's sarcoma

4. Osteocarcinoma

Ans. **1**

Other 3 shows onion peel appearance due to periosteal bone formation.

67. **"Y" shaped line of Ennis is found radiographically on:** [AIPG 1990]

1. Incisors
2. Canines
3. Premolars
4. Molars

Ans. **3**

It is formed by intersection of floor of nasal cavity and anterior wall of maxillary sinus.

68. **Which of the following can usually be identified by radiographic means alone?**

[AIPG 1989]

1. Cementoma
2. Apical cyst
3. Mental foramen
4. Chronic apical periodontitis

Ans. **3**

Mental foramen: is an anatomic landmark not observed clinically. Located only by radiographs in the lower first and second premolar apical regions.

69. **Which of the following is most sensitive to radiation?** [AIPG 1989]

1. Nerves
2. Female breast
3. Thyroid
4. Skin

Ans. **2**

Nerves, thyroid & skin have reverting & fixed post mitotic cells, which are the most radioresistant.

70. **The speed with which electrons travel from the filament of the cathode to the target of the anode depends upon the:** [AIPG 1989]

1. Size of the electron cloud
2. Voltage in the filament
3. Angle between the filament and the target
4. Potential difference between the two electrodes.

Ans. **4**

Size of electron cloud – the milliampere controls the quantity of electrons. The filament emits, which in effect controls the tube current & fine adjustment of voltage across the filament.

Angle between the filament & target angled at 20 degrees with respect to the central rays of x-ray beam.

- The sharpness increases as focal spot decreases in size
- The use of an anode with the target angulated such that the effective focal spot is smaller than the actual focal spot size is refer to as line focus principle.

71. Coronoid process of the mandible is best viewed on: [AIPG 1989]

    1. Water's view

    2. Towne's view

    3. PA view

    4. Submentovertex view

Ans. **1**

PA view

- Skull, frontal and ethmoid sinus, nasal fossa and orbits.

Water view – Occipitomental projection

- Maxillary, frontal & ethmoid sinuses, orbit, frontozygomatic suture, nasal cavity, coronoid process between maxilla & zygomatic arch.

Towne's view

- Subcondylar areas

Submentovertex view: Base or full axial projection

- Base of skull, position and orientation of condyles, the sphenoid sinus, curvature of mandible, lateral wall of maxillary sinus

- Displacement of fractured zygomatic such, medial and lateral pterygoid plates & foramina of base of skull.

72. The usual radiographic appearance of osteosarcoma is: [AIPG 1989]

    1. Radiolucent with regular borders

    2. Soap-bubble appearance

    3. Sun-burst appearance

    4. Cotton-wool appearance

Ans. **3**

Sunburst or 'sun ray' appearance

- Osteosarcoma

- Central hemangioma

- Ewing's sarcoma

Soap bubble appearance

- Ameloblastoma

- Aneurysmal bone cyst

- Odontogenic myxoma

- Osteoclastoma

Cotton wool appearance

- Paget's diseases

- Chronic diffuse sclerosing osteomyelitis

NOTES

40   Miscellaneous

RADIOLOGICAL FEATURES

- **Ball-in-Hand Appearance**
  - Benign salivary gland tumors.
- **Balloon –like appearance**
  - Follicular cyst
  - Aneurysmal bone cyst
- **Candlestick appearance**
  - Pyknodysostosis
  - Progressive systemic sclerosis
- **Chalk – like appearance**
  - Osteopetrosis
  - Hyperparathyroidism
  - Pyknodysostosis
- **Drumstick appearance** - osteochondroma
- **Cherry – Blossom pattern**
  - Sjogren's syndrome
  - Mikulicz's disease
- **Cotton wool appearance**
  - Paget's disease
  - Chronic sclerosing diffuse osteomyelitis
- **Codman's triangle**
  - Osteosarcoma
  - Osteochondroma
  - Ewing's sarcoma.

- **Crew cut or Hair-on-end appearance**
  - Thalassemia
  - Sickle cell anaemia
- **Driven snow appearance** – CEOT or pindborg tumor
- **Copper – Beaten appearance of skull** – Craniosynostosis
- **Filling defect** – Salivary gland tumor
- **Floating tooth appearance**
  - Squamous cell carcinoma
  - Malignant Lymphoma
  - Burkitt's lymphoma
  - Eosinophillic granuloma
- **Ground glass appearance**
  - Monostotic fibrous dysplasia
  - Ossifying fibroma
  - Osteosarcoma
  - Hyperparathyroidism
- **Honey – comb appearance (soap-bubble appearance / Tennis racket appearance)**
  - Ameloblastoma
  - Central hemangioma
  - Odontogenic myxoma
  - Giant cell lesion
  - Odontogenic keratocyst
  - Pindborg tumor
  - Aneurysmal bone cyst.
- **Moth-eaten appearance (worm-eaten)**
  - Squamous cell CA
  - Malignant Lymphoma
  - Chronic osteomyelitis
  - Histiocytosis –X
  - Degeneration of condyle
  - Eosinophillic granuloma
- **Mottled appearance**
  - Fibrous dysplasia
  - Ossifying fibroma
- **Onion-peel appearance**
  - Ewing's sarcoma
  - Garre's osteomyelitis
  - Osteosarcoma

- **Ghost appearance** – Regional odontodysplasia
- **Permeated type**
  - Carcinoma of gingiva
  - Squamous cell carcinoma of maxilla
  - Malignant Lymphoma
- **Pear-shaped appearance**
  - Globulomaxillary cyst
  - Radicular cyst
- **Pencil – line appearance**
  - Ameloblastoma
  - Traumatic bone cyst
  - CEOC (Gorlin cyst)
- **Pressure -type appearance** – Squamous cell carcinoma of gingiva.
- **Punched - out Radiolucency.**
  - Multiple Myeloma
  - Hand -schuller Christian disease.
- **Sand -like appearance**
  - Adeno ameloblastoma
  - CEOC
  - CEOT
- **Salt and pepper appearance**
  - Hyperparathyroidism
  - Traumatic bone cyst
  - Aneurysmal bone cyst
  - Giant cell lesion
- **Orange-peel appearance** – Fibrous dysplasia
- **Heart shaped radiolucency** – Nasopalatine cyst
- **Scalloping appearance**
  - Dentigerous cyst
  - Traumatic bone cyst
  - Aneurysmal bone cyst
  - Giant cell tumor
- **Spiked root**
  - Malignant histiocytoma
  - Burkitt's Lymphoma.
- **Sunburst appearance**
  - Osteosarcoma
  - Central Hemangioma

- Ewing's sarcoma.
- **Hanging-drop sign** – Blow out orbital fracture.
- **Step-Ladder effect** – Sickle cell anaemia
- **Tram like appearance**
  - In CSF rhinorrhoea (on face)
  - Sturge-Weber syndrome (on skull radiograph)
  - Inferior alveolar canal
- **Salt and pepper effect on MRI** – Sjogren's Syndrome
- **Snow -storm / Branchless fruit-laden appearance / Punctate sialectasis**
  - Sjogren's syndrome
- **Leafless tree appearance** – Normal sialogram
- *PDL widening*
  - Osteosarcoma.
  - Scleroderma.
  - Acro sclerosis.
- *Loss of lamina dura*
  - Periapical infections
  - Fibrous dysplasia
  - Paget's disease
  - Osteoporosis
  - Hyperparathyroidism
  - Leukaemia
  - Cushing syndrome
  - Hypophosphatasia
  - Osteomalacia
  - Multiple myeloma

LABORATORY TESTS

- *Schillers test* – Carcinoma of cervix.
- *Dick's test* – Scarlet fever.
- *VDRL* – Syphilis (non-specific test)
- *FTA-Antibodies* – syphilis (Specific)
- *Frei's test* – Lymphogranuloma venerum.
- *Gordons Biological test* – Hodgkin's disease
- *Schilling's test* – Vitamin B_{12} deficiency.
- *Schick test / Elek's test* – Diphtheria.
- *Tzank test* – Pemphigus

- Herpes simplex
- Herpes zoster
- *Kveim- Siltzbach's test* – Sarcoidosis
- *Paul-Bunnel test/ Monospot test* – Infectious mononucleosis
- *Schimmer's test* – Sjogren's syndrome.
- *Weil-Felix test* – Rickettsial infection
  - Lymphogranuloma venerum.
- *Argyll Robertson pupil* – Neurosyphilis.
- *Rothera test* – Ketone bodies in urine.
- *Rose Waller test* – Rheumatoid arthritis.
- *Figlu excretion test* – Folic acid absorption.
- *ELISA* – HIV / AIDS (non specific).
- *Western Blot* – Detects proteins (specific for AIDS).
- *Southern Blot* – for DNA assay.
- *Northern Blot* – RNA assay.
- *Auspitz sign* – Psoriasis.
- *Mantoux or Hee's test* – T.B.
- *NBT (nitro blue tetrazoline) test* – Neutrophil functioning.
- *Coomb's test* – Erytheroblastosis fetalis.
- *Paget's test* – for small swellings.
- *Patch test* – for allergy.
- *Lupus band test*- SLE
- *RAST (radioallergosorbent test)* – Specific allergy sensitivity testing based on circulating levels of IgE.
- *Rumpel Leede / Torniquet test* – Capillary fragility
  - Scurvy
- *Lacrimal gland function tests* – Schimer test
  - BUT (Break up time)
  - Rose Bengal dye.

MOST COMMON SITES AND LESIONS

- Fordyces granules – Buccal mucosa.
- Static bone cyst – Between mandibular canal and inferior border of mandible.
- Talon cusp – Lateral incisor.
- Supernumerary tooth – Mesiodens.
- Tumor of oral mucosa – Squamous cell carcinoma
- Dens in dente – Permanent maxillary lateral incisor.

- Dens evaginatus – Premolar.
- Globulomaxillary cyst – Between maxillary lateral incisor and canine.
- Nasoalveolar cyst – Between maxillary central incisors.
- Epstein pearls – Along the median palatine raphae.
- Bohn's nodules – Scattered over hard palate near junction of hard and soft palate.
- Branchial cleft cyst – Lateral aspect of neck
- Thyroglossal duct cyst – Midline of neck.
- Basal cell carcinoma – middle third of face
- Tumor of parotid – Pleomorphic adenoma
- Primordial cyst – Retained, erupted deciduous teeth.
- Dentiguous cyst – Third molar region.
- Enameloma – Near furcation of root.
- Pindborg's tumor – Unerupted or impacted tooth.
- Compound composite odontoma – Anterior maxilla.
- Complex composite odontoma – posterior mandible.
- Viral infection – Herpes simplex.
- Ameloblastoma – Mandibular molar / ramus area.
- Adenomatoid odontogenic tumor – Maxillary canine region.
- Keratoacanthoma – Lips
- Granular cell myoblastoma - tongue
- Leukoplakia – Buccal mucosa.
- Erythema multiforme – Lips
- Mucocele – lower lip
- Necrotizing sialometaplasia- Hard palate
- Papilloma – Tongue.
- Taurodontism – Permanent / deciduous molar.
- Most rapid metastasis – Burkitt's lymphoma.
- Ankylosis of primary tooth / submerged tooth – Deciduous mandibular second molar.
- Anomalous tooth – third molars.
- Anomalous succesional tooth – Maxillary lateral incisor.
- Arch most commonly affected by caries – Maxillary.
- Benign oral cancer – fibroma.
- Bifid mandibular canal – Neuro fibromatosis.
- Missing permanent tooth – 3rd molars.
- Missing deciduous tooth – Upper lateral incisor
- Natal and neonatal tooth – Decidous mandibular central incisor.
- Cleft – Unilateral complete cleft lip.
- Greatest variation in onset of mineralization – Mandibular second premolar.

- Tooth affected by caries – Mandibular first molar.
- Odontogenic tumor – Compound odontoma.
- Odontogenic cyst – Radicular cyst.

AUTOIMMUNE DISORDERS

- Recurrent aphthos ulcers
- Behcet's disease
- Pemphigus
- Pemphigoid
- Dermatitis herpetiformis
- Sjogren's syndrome
- Mikulicz disease
- Pernicious anaemia
- Purpura
- SLE
- Scleroderma
- Rheumatoid arthritis
- Myasthenia gravis
- Dermatomyositis
- Oral submucous fibrosis

ORAL HAMARTOMAS

- Dens invaginatus
- Dens evaginatus
- Talon's cusp
- Enameloma
- Dentinoma
- Odontoma
- Gigantiform cementoma
- Dental lamina cyst
- Pigmented cellular nevus
- Hemangioma
- Lymphangioma
- Glomus tumor
- Torus
- Neurofibromatosis

TONGUE

- Atrophic or interstitial glossitis – Syphilis
- Beefy red – Niacin deficiency
- Magenta – Riboflavin, B_2 deficiency.
- Strawberry/ Raspberry – Scarlet fever.
- Hairy – Filliform papillae hypertrophy.
- Hunter's / Moeller's glossitis – Pernicious anaemia
- Bald tongue of Sandwith – Pellagra.
- Ageusia – Complete loss of all taste stimuli.
- Hypogeusia – Impairment of taste sense.
- Dysgeusia / parageusia – A distortion or perversion in perception of taste.
- Phantogeusia or gustatory hallucination – Perception of a taste in the absence of any recognized taste stimulus.
- Cocogeusia – Bad taste.
- Torquegeusia – Twisted taste.
- Hypergeusia – Increased sensitivity for all taste stimuli, some or single stimulus.
- Gustatory agnosia – Loss of ability to classify, contrast or identify a taste stimulus verbally.
- Glossodynia – Painful tongue.
- Glossopyrosis – Burning tongue.
- Glossoplegia – Paralysis of tongue.
- Trefoil tongue (clover leaf pattern) – due to genetic ability
- Gorlin's sign (hyperextensibility) – Ehler Danlos syndrome
- Baked tongue – Typhoid fever
- Parrot tongue- chronic low grade fever

TUBERCULOSIS

- Scrofula – T.B of lymph nodes.
- Lupus vulgaris – Skin.
- Phithiasis – Lungs.
- Pott's disease / Cervical caries – Spine.
- Miliary T.B- Hematogenous spread.
- Cold abscess
- Cori's abscess
- Collar stud abscess

HALITOSIS

- Poor oral hygiene
- Periodontal pockets.
- Pericoronal infection.
- Decayed teeth.
- ANUG- fetid odour
- Diabetes- acetone odour
- Oral cancer.
- Rhinitis
- Pharyngitis
- Sinusitis.
- Tonsillitis
- Xerostomia
- Diseases of lungs (gangrene, T.B, abscess)
- Uraemia – urinous odour
- Kidney dysfunction - urinous odour
- Digestive dysfunction – sour odour
- Gangrene/ necrotic lesion – strench odour
- After use of GA – fruity odour
- Chronic liver dysfunction – mousy odour
- Internal haemorrhage – bloody odour

OSTEOPOROSIS

- Hyperthyroidism
- Old age
- Diabetes
- Renal acidosis
- Rickets
- Leukaemia
- Histiocytosis
- Cyclic neutropenia.
- Acromegaly.
- Multiple myeloma
- Cushing's syndrome.
- Sickle cell anaemia.
- Thalassaemia.

- Osteogenesis imperfecta
- Hypovitaminosis C.

OROFACIAL PAIN

- *Allodynia* – Pair to a stimulus that doesn't usually causes pain.
- *Hyperalgesia* – Increase response to a stimulus of pain.
- *Hyperaesthesia* – Increased response to a stimulus which is not painful.
- *Hyperpathia* – Increased reaction to stimulus of pain at an increased threshold.
- *Causalgia* – Syndrome of burning pain, allodynia and hyperpathia after a traumatic nerve lesion.
- *Neuropathy* – Disturbance of function or pathologic change of a nerve.
- *Neuralgia* – Pain in the distribution of a nerve.
- *Paraesthesia* – abnormal sensation.
- *Dysesthesia* – Unpleasant abnormal sensation.
- *Anaesthesia Dolorosa* – Paradoxic pain in a region of sensory loss following an injury to a cranial nerve or nerve root.

SPECIFIC CELLS ON HISTOPATHOLOGICAL EXAMINATION

- *Ghost cells* – CEOT
    - Odontomas
    - Ameloblastic fibro odontoma
    - Craniopharyngioma
- *Reed Sternberg cells (Dorothy Reed cells)* – Hodgkin's lymphoma.
- *Lacunar cells* – Nodular sclerosing type of Hodgkin's disease.
- *Heart failure cells* – Hemosiderin laden phagocytes in lungs.
- *Langhans giant cells* – T.B, Leprosy.
- *Safety pin cells* – Thalassemia.
- *Tzank cells* – Pemphigus, Herpes zoster, Acute herpetic stomatitis
- *Hyaline cells* – Pleomorphic adenoma.
- *Nevus cells* – Pigmented mole.
- *Anitschkow cells* – Recurrent aphthous, Iron deficiency anaemia, Sickle cell anaemia, Megaloblastic anaemia, Children receiving chemotherapy.
- *LE cells* – SLE (occasionally DLE)
- *Warthen-Frenkeldey giant cells* – Measles
- *Clear cells* - Lateral periodontal cysts, Gingival cysts of adults, Mucoepidermoid carcinoma, Acinic cell carcinoma.
- *Target cells* – Thalassemia.
- *Pericyte of Zimmerman* – Glomus tumor.

- *Ribbon cells / Roquet cells* – Rhabdomyosarcoma.
- *Angulate cell* – Myoblastoma.
- *Downey cells* – Kissing disease
- *Dilapidated brick wall effect-* familial benign chronic pemphigus
- *Benign dyskeratotic cells (corps, Ronds and grains)* – Dyskeratosis follicularis.
- *Tobacco cells or cells in cells-* hereditary benign intraepithelial dyskeratosis
- *Giant cells* – fibrous dysplasia, Cherubism, Hyperparathyroidism, Central giant cell granuloma, Osteoclastoma, Eosinophilic granuloma, Peripheral giant cell granuloma, Herpes zoster, Sarcoidosis, Wegener's granulomatosis, Osteosarcoma.

SPECIFIC FEATURES

- *Carpet tack extension* – Erythema multiforme.
- *Crush man's spirals* – sputum of asthmatics.
- *Cytoid bodies / Civette bodies* – lichen planus
- *Asteroid bodies* – Spirotrichosis
- *Denovan bodies* – Granuloma inguinale.
- *Guarnier bodies* – small pox
- *Haberden's nodes* – Osteoarthritis.
- *Handerson-paterson / Molluscum bodies* – Molluscum contagiosum
- *Hinge bodies* – Thalassemia
- *Verrucay / Hyaline bodies* – Neurolemmoma, B-type schwannoma.
- *Russel body* – Chronic inflammation, Periapical granuloma, Multiple myeloma.
- *Rushton bodies* – Radicular cyst, Inflammatory cyst
- *Pseudo rhagades* – Ectodermal dysplasia
- *Negri body* – Rabies.
- *Saddle nose* – Syphilis
- *Reily bodies* – Hurler's syndrome.
- *Lipschutz bodies* – Primary herpetic stomatitis.
- *Ballooning degeneration* - Primary herpetic stomatitis
- *Domle bodies* – Chediak Higashi syndrome.
- *Herba nose* – Rhinoscleroma.
- *Herald's spot* – Pityriasis rosea.
- *Iris / bull eye / target lesions* – Erythema multiforme.
- *Mallory bodies* – Cirrhosis of liver.
- *Intern's thrush* – food debris on mucosa
- *Cabot's rings* – Pernicious anaemia.
- *Leisgang rings* – Pindborg tumor

- *Munro's abscess* – Geographic tongue, Psoriasis, Psoriasiform lesions.
- *"Jigsaw puzzle" of bone* – Paget's disease
- *"Honey-comb" / "Swiss-cheese" pattern* – Adenoid cystic carcinoma.
- *"Picket fence" / "Tomb stone" appearance* -Odontogenic keratocyst, Primordial cyst.
- *"Starry-sky"* – Burket's lymphoma.
- *"Cart wheel" / "Checker board" appearance* – Multiple myeloma.
- *"Chinese-Character" appearance* – Monostotic fibrous dysplasia, Central ossifying fibroma.
- *Mosaic bone pattern* – Paget's disease, Chronic diffuse sclerosing Osteomyelitis.
- *Polyclonal staining* – Inflammatory cells
- *Monoclonal staining* – Malignant cells.
- *Hutchinson's teeth* – Congenital syphilis (notched incisors)
- *Fournier's molar / Mulberry molars / Moon's molars* – Hypoplasia of molars in congenital syphilis
- *Ghost teeth* – Regional odontodysplasia
- *Turner's teeth* – Hypoplasia due to trauma or infection of primary teeth.
- *Pink teeth* – Internal resorption.
- *Shell teeth* – Dentinogenesis Imperfecta.
- *Rootless teeth* – Dentin dysplasia
- *Chloasma or Melasma* – Pigmentation of oral mucosa in pregnancy
- *Micro cyst formation*
  Acinic cell carcinoma
  Mucoepidermoid carcinoma
  Neurilemmoma
  Squamous odontogenic tumor.
- *Perineural spread*
  Mucoepidermoid carcinoma
  Kerato acanthoma
  Adenoid cystic carcinoma.
- *Nikolsky's sign*
  Pemphigus
  Chronic desquamative gingivitis
  Hallay-Hallay disease
  Epidermolysis bullosa.
- *Café-au-lait spots*
  Neurofibroma.
  Polyostotic fibrous dysplasia
  Peutz Jegher's syndrome
  Hypothyroidism

- *Blue sclera*
  Fetal rickets.
  Osteogenesis imperfecta.
  Marfan syndrome
  Ehler Danlos syndrome
  Osteopetrosis
  Infants.
- *Angle face* – Cherubism
- *Mask like face* – Scleroderma, Bell's palsy
- *Grotesgue / simian appearance* – Paget's disease
- *Petrified man* – Myositis ossificans (generalized)
- *Rubberman* – Ehler Danlos syndrome
- *Moon face / dusky plethoric appearance/ buffalo hump / Match stick appearance / Lemon appearance* – Cushing syndrome.
- *Parrot beak like nose* – Craniofacial dysostosis, Congenital syphilis
- *Bird like facies* – Ankylosis, Mandibulo facial dysostosis, Pierre Robin syndrome.
- *Claw hand* – Scleroderma, Leprosy, Hurlers syndrome.
- *Hypomobility of joints* – Achondroplasia.
- *Hypermobility of joints* – Marfan syndrome, Osteogenesis imperfecta, Down's syndrome
- *Peripheral neuritis with "Wristdrop" or " foot drop"* – Lead poisoning, Hypochromic anaemia, Encephalitis
- *Lock jaw* – Tetanus
- *Lump jaw* – Actinomycosis
- *Phossy jaw* – Phosphorus poisoning
- *African jaw* – Burkitt's lymphoma.
- *Aschoff nodules*-Rheumatic fever.
- *Bitot's spots* – Vitamin A deficiency in children.
- *Pink spot* – Internal resorption
- *Koplik's spots* – Measles
- *Roth spot* – SABE
- *Adie's pupil* – A benign condition in which one pupil is dilated and reacts only very slowly to light and convergence.
- *Palmer planter hyperkeratosis*- Gorlin Goltz syndrome, Papillon lefevre syndrome , Follicularis keratosis
- *Cytoplasmic inclusions* – Pox virus, Rabies, Molluscum contagiosum
- *Nuclear inclusions* – Herpes virus, Polio virus
- *Both nuclear + cytoplasmic inclusions* – CMV, Measles
- *Cobblestone appearance*- Keratosis follicularis, Crohn's disease

- *Overripe strawberry appearance-* Palatal papillary hyperplasia
- *Burtonian line* – Plumbism
- *Neonatal line* – Enamel hypoplasia at birth.
- *Incremental lines of retzius* – Enamel
- *Incremental lines of von Ebner* – Dentin
- *Incremental lines of salter* – Cementum
- *Reversal line* – Hypercementosis, Paget's disease, Benign cementoblastoma.
- *Mesenteric lines* – Brown pigmented dental plaque on enamel margins.
- *Skin pigmentation*
  Sprue – Brown
  Aplastic anaemia – Olive brown.
  Neurofibromatsis – Café –au-lait spots (Coast of California appearance)
  Albright's syndrome - Café –au-lait spots (Coast of Maine appearance)
- *Bence Jones proteins-* Multiple Myeloma, Leukaemia, Polycythemia.
- *Telangiectasia*
  Scleroderma.
  CREST syndrome.
  Sarcoid disease.
  Lupus erythematosis.
- *Solutions for Cryotherapy*
  CO_2 snow (-78°C).
  Liquid N_2 (-180°C).
- *Sclerosing solution* - Sodium morrhuate or psyllate, sodium tetra decyl sulfate.
- *Periosteal Bone formation*
  Garre's osteomyelitis.
  Infantile cortical hyperostosis.
  Hypervitaminosis A.
  Syphilis.
  Leukaemia.
  Ewing's sarcoma.
  Metastatic neuroblastoma.
  Fracture callus.
- *Macroglossia*
  Down's syndrome.
  Amyloidosis.
  Hurler's syndrome.
  Hyalonosis cutis.
  Lymphangioma.

Hemangioma.

Acromegaly.

Congenital hypothyroidism or cretinism.

- *Immuno fluorescent studies*
  (a) Granular pattern – Pemphigus
  (b) Irregular – Lichen planus, LE
  (c) Patchy, linear – Pemphigoid, Erythema multiforme

CRITERIA FOR DIAGNOSIS OF DYSPLASIA

- Increased abnormal mitosis.
- Individual cell keratinization.
- Epithelial pearls within spinous layer.
- Alteration in nuclear cytoplasmic ratio.
- Loss of polarity and disorientation of cells.
- Hyperchromatism of cells.
- Large, prominent nucleoli.
- Dyskaryosis or nucleus atypism.
- Poikilokaryocytosis or division of nuclei without division of cytoplasm.
- Basilar hyperplasia.

TNM CLASSIFICATION OF MALIGNANT TUMORS IN ORAL CAVITY

T – Primary tumor

T_{IS}– CA in situ.

T_1 – Tumor 2 cm or less in greatest diameter

T_2 – Tumor greater than 2 cm but less than 4 cm in greatest diameter.

T_3 – Tumor greater than 4 cm in greatest diameter but less than 6 cm.

T_4 – Tumor greater than 6 cm in greatest diameter.

N – regional lymph nodes.

N_0 – No clinically palpable cervical lymph nodes or palpable nodes but metastasis not suspected.

N_1 – Clinically palpable ipsilateral cervical node(s), none of them > 3 cm in largest diameter.

N_2 – Ipsilateral LN involvement > 3cm or multiple ipsilateral nodes

N_2a – Single ipsilateral nodes > 3 cm and<6 cm

N_2b – Multiple ipsilateral nodes < 6cm

N_2c – bilateral or contralateral nodes < 6cm

N_3 – Lymph nodes > 6 cm

M (Distant metastasis)

M_0 – No metastasis

M_1 – Distant metastasis

Clinical staging of CA

Stage I   - $T_1N_0M_0$

Stage II   - $T_2 N_0M_0$

Stage III - $T_3 N_0M_0$

            $T_1N_1M_0$

            $T_2 N_1M_0$

            $T_3 N_1M_0$

Stage IV - $T_1N_2M_0$ $T_1N_3M_0$

            $T_2 N_2M_0$ $T_2 N_3M_0$

            $T_3 N_2M_0$ $T_3 N_3M_0$

            or any T and N category with M_1

Premalignant Lesions

An altered tissue in which malignancy is known to occur more commonly than the normal counterpart. Eg. Leukoplakia, Erythroplakia, CA in situ, smoker's palate.

Premalignant condition

Generalized condition to which there is increased tendency of malignant transformation.

E.g. Syphilis

      Plummer Vinson syndrome

      Oral submucous fibrosis

      Fibrous dysplasia

      Dyskeratosis congenita

      Gorlin-Goltz syndrome

      Actinic keratosis

TEETH

Delayed eruption of teeth

- Cleidocranial dysostosis
- Polyostotic fibrous dysplasia
- Rickets
- Cretinism
- Hypothyroidism
- Hypoparathyroidism
- Hemifacial atrophy

Premature exfoliation of primary teeth

- Hypophosphatasia
- Hyperthyroidism
- Hand Schuller Christian disease
- Facial hemihypertrophy
- Cherubism
- Acrodynia
- Cyclic neuropenia
- Down's syndrome
- Litter siewe disease

Pink teeth

- Mercury poisoning
- Cobalt poisoning
- Asphyxia
- Barbiturate poisoning

Malformed teeth

1. Local infection and trauma
2. Radiotherapy
3. Congenital syphilis
4. Down syndrome
5. Ectodermal dysplasia
6. Rickets

STAINS USED FOR ORAL LESIONS

1. Candida albicans – Wright's stain, PAS stain
2. Inflammatory cells – Polyclonal staining
3. Neoplastic cells – Monoclonal staining
4. Amyloid

   Iodine

   Congo red

   PAS

   Metachromatic

   Thioflavin S

   Thioflavin T
5. Herpes simplex – Papanicoleau stain

6. Glycogen – Mucarmin stain
7. Fat – Sudan red
8. Reilly bodies – Alcian blue.
9. Collagen – Masson's trichome stain, Von – griesen stain

RESULTS OF ASPIRATION

- *Straw colored fluid* – Radicular cyst
  - Odontogenic cysts
  - Cystic ameloblastoma
  - Warthin tumor
- *Empty cavity* – Solitary bone cyst.
- *Milky white fluid* – Odontogenic keratocyst (protein content >4mg%)
- *Thick yellowish white granular fluid*- Epidermoid cyst, Keratocyst
- *Sebum (Thick yellow fluid)* – Sebaceous cyst
- *Cheesy* – Sebaceous cyst
- *Dark amber fluid* – Thyroglossal duct cyst
- *Cloudy and frothy* – Cystic hygroma, Lymphangioma
- *Viscous clear fluid* – Mucocele, Ranula
- *Greenish blue* – Pseudomonas infection
- *Bright red blood* – AV shunt, Aneurysm
- *Bluish blood-* Hemangioma, Varicositis
- *Air* – Clostridium welchi infection.

CAUSES OF HYPOPIGMENTATION AND DEPIGMENTATION

- Albinism
- Vitiligo
- Pernicious anaemia
- Hormonal disturbances
- Parasitic infection
- Chediak – Higashi syndrome
- Tuberous sclerosis
- Cross syndrome
- Severe burns
- Extensive traumatic injury

SYNDROMES ASSOCIATED WITH GINGIVAL HYPERPLASIA

1. Rutherford
2. Cannon's disease
3. Cross disease
4. Zimmermann – Laband
5. Cowden's syndrome
6. Papillon – Lefevere
7. Tuberous sclerosis
8. Sturge – Weber
9. Melkersson – Rosenthal.

COMPRESSIBLE SOFT TISSUE GROWTH OF ORAL CAVITY

- Eruption cyst
- Mucocele
- Mucous cyst
- Ranula
- Gingival cyst
- Nasoalveolar cyst
- Epidermoid cyst
- Cavernous
- Capillary hemangioma
- Lymphangioma
- Cystic hygroma

SYNDROMES OF HEAD AND NECK

ADRENOGENITAL SYNDROME

- Due to hyperplasia or tumors of renal cortex
- Pseudohermaphroditism, sexual precocity and virilism in women and feminization in men.
- Oral features- premature eruption of teeth if the disease begins in early life.

ALBRIGHT'S SYNDROME

- Also called as *'McCune-Albright syndrome'*
- *Severe* fibrous dysplasia involving nearly all bones of the skeleton.
- Pigmented lesions on skin (café-au-lait spots).
- Hyperfunction of one or more endocrine glands.

ALDRICH'S SYNDROME

- Also called as 'Wiskott-Aldrich' syndrome.
- Characterized by thrombocytopenic purpura, eczema, and increased susceptibility to infection.
- Palatal petechiae can be seen.
- Spontaneous bleeding from gingiva

AMELO-ONYCHO-HYPOHIDROTIC SYNDROME

- Defective nails and hypofunction of the sweat glands and seborrheic dermatitis.
- Severe hypoplastic hypocalcified enamel.

ANDERSON SYNDROME

- Also called as *familial osteodysplasia*
- Skeletal and craniofacial anomalies.
- Hypertension and hyperuricemia.
- Maxillary hypoplasia, reduced ramus height, prognathic mandible and malocclusion.

ANGIO-OSTEOHYPERTROPHY SYNDROME

- Portwine stain on the face, varices.
- Hypertrophy of bone including jawbone.
- *Oral* features—facial asymmetry, malocclusion and altered eruption pattern of teeth.

AORTIC ARCH SYNDROME

- It is also called as *pulseless disease.*
- It is caused by narrowing or obstruction of the major branches of the arch of the aorta.
- *General* features—dizziness, headache, visual disturbance, and anginal pain
- Topic ulceration and pain while chewing.

APERT'S SYNDROME

- It is also called as 'acrocephalosyndactyly'.
- *Skeletal* deformities—there is syndactyly and acrocephaly. The skull is ovoid, brachycephalic and often presents a horizontal supraorbital groove.
- *Facial deformities*—the middle third of face is underdeveloped.
- Oral *features*- High palatal vault and V-shaped maxillary alveolar ridge.
- There is posterior palatal cleft and bifid uvula.
- Retarded eruption and dental malocclusion.

ASCHER'S SYNDROME

- Patients have a double lip.
- Blepharochalasis, i.e.drooping of the tissue between the eyebrow and the edge of upper eyelid.
- Non-toxic thyroid goiter.

AURICULOTEMPORAL (FREY'S) SYNDROME

- It is caused by damage to auriculotemporal nerve.
- Flushing and sweating of the involved side of face, chiefly in temporal area, during eating.
- Gustatory sweating when eating spicy food.

AVELLIS SYNDROME

- Unilateral paralysis of larynx and soft palate.

B-K MOLE SYNDROME

- It is autosornal dominant condition.
- It is characterized by large pigmented nevi.
- There is high-risk of development of melanoma.

BABY BOTTLE SYNDROME

- It is also called as *nursing bottle* caries or *bottle mouth syndrome.*
- It occurs due to habitual use of bottle usually as an aid for sleeping in night.
- There is wide spread carious destruction of deciduous teeth, most commonly the four maxillary incisors followed by the first molars and then the cuspids if habit is prolonged.

BEHCET'S SYNDROME

- *Recurrent oral ulceration*— has similar appearance as aphthous ulcer.
- *Recurring genital* ulceration—ulcer of scrotum and penis in males and ulcers of labia in females.
- *Skin lesions*—large pustular lesions.
- Ocular lesions—uveitis, retinal vasculitis, optic atrophy, recurrent conjunctivitis, and keratitis.

BECKER SYNDROME

- Severe muscular dystrophy that results in progressive weakness of limb and breathing muscles.

BECKWITH'S HYPOGLYCEMIC SYNDROME

- Macroglossia—enlargement of the tongue.
- Other features—neonatal hypoglycemia, mild microcephaly, umbilical hernia, fetal visceromegaly, and postnatal somatic giantism.

BERNARD-SOULIER SYNDROME

- It is transmitted as autosomal dominant trait with variable penetration.
- The membrane receptor on platelets is absent and it accounts for bleeding problems.
- The bleeding time is prolonged.

BIEMOND SYNDROME

- Congenital obesity

- Hypogonadism

BINDER SYNDROME

- Congenital maxillonasal dysplasia
- Absence or hypoplastic frontal sinus

BLEPHAROCHEILODONTIC SYNDROME

- It is transmitted as autosomal dominant inheritance.
- Eye anomalies—it includes lagophthalmos, ectropion of lower eyelid.
- Lip—there is bilateral cleft lip and palate.
- Teeth—oligodontia, microdontia including tiny molars.

BLOCH-SULZBERGER SYNDROME

- Erythematous and vesiculobullous lesions on the trunk and extremities.
- These are replaced by white keratotic, lichenoid, papillary or verrucous lesions.
- Brownish gray macules in a streaked, patchy distribution over the trunk and extremities.
- Oral features—delayed tooth eruption, peg or cone shaped teeth, congenitally missing teeth, malformed teeth and additional cusps.

BLEPHARONASOFACIAL SYNDROME

- It is characterized by mental retardation, joint disorders and craniofacial anomalies.
- Facial features—affected individuals show microcephaly, an anti-mongoloid slant of palpebral fissures.
- Oral features—there is also hypoplastic maxilla, protruding lip and malocclusion resulting form midface hypoplasia.

BLOOM SYNDROME

- Congenital telangiectasia
- Depigmentation
- Short stature

BOOK'S SYNDROME

- Premature whitening of hair.
- Hyperhydrosis of palms and soles.
- Oral features—absence of the premolars and third molars.

BOWEN SYNDROME

- It is also called as cerebrohepatorenal syndrome.
- Craniofacial anomalies, hypotonia, hepatomegaly and renal cortical cysts.
- Oral features—it includes micrognathia, protruding tongue and high arched palate.

- There is increase serum iron level and decrease in serum immunoglobulin levels.

BURNING MOUTH SYNDROME

- Pain and burning sensation in the mouth.
- Altered taste sensation and xerostomia.
- No clinically detectable lesions in the oral cavity

CAFFEY-SILVERMAN SYNDROME

- It is also called as infantile cortical hyperostosis.
- Development of tender deeply placed soft tissue swellings and cortical thickening or hyperostosis involving various bones of the skeleton.
- There is also pain, fever and irritability in infants.
- Increased serum levels of alkaline phosphatase and increased ESR.

CANDIDOSIS ENDOCRINOPATHY SYNDROME

- *Oral* features—chronic oral candidiasis and enamel hypoplasia.
- *Endocrine disorders*—it includes hypoparathyroidism. hypothyroidism, and hypoadrenocortism.
- *Metabolic* disorders—diabetes mellitus.

CEREBROCOSTOMANDIBULAR SYNDROME

- Thoracic deformity with barking cough and mental retardation.
- Oral features—it includes mandibular micro-gnathism, palatal defect and absence of uvula or even soft palate.

CHEDIAK-HIGASHI SYNDROME

- It is transmitted as autosomal dominant trait.
- General—it includes oculocutaneous albinism, photophobia, nystagmus and recurrent infection of respiratory tract and skin.
- Oral—ulceration of the oral mucosa, severe gingivitis and glossitis.

COSTEN'S SYNDROME

- There is impairment of hearing, either continuously or intermittent.
- A stuffy sensation in the ears especially at mealtime.
- Tinnitus, otalgia, dizziness and headache about the vertex, occiput and behind the ears.
- Burning sensations in the throat, tongue and side of nose.

COWDEN'S SYNDROME

- It is autosomal dominant disease characterized by facial trichilemmomas associated with gastrointestinal tract, central nervous system, thyroid and musculosketetal abnormalities
- Papillomatous lesion as well as *'pebbly'* lesions of lip, gingivae, palate and pharynx occurs.

- Fibromas at various sites in the oral cavity.
- Lichenoid and papillomatous lesions of perioral, perinasal and periorbital areas of ear and neck.
- Hematoma of skin, gastrointestinal tract, breast and thyroid.

CRACKED TOOTH SYNDROME

- Development of crack in a restored or unrestored tooth due to excessive occlusal force.
- Sharp pain on biting.

CROSS SYNDROME

- *Oral* features—it include gingival enlargement.
- *Other features—it* includes hypopigmentation, oligophrenia, microophthalmos, and athetosis.

CREST SYNDROME

Associated with Scleroderma

- C—Calcinosis cutis
- R—Raynaud's phenomenon
- E—Esophageal dysfunction
- S—Sclerodactyly
- T—Telangiectasia

CROUZON SYNDROME (*Craniofacial dysostosis*)

Cranial deformities

- Protruberant frontal region with an anteropos-tenor ridge overhanging the frontal eminence and often passing to the roof of nose (triangular frontal defect).
- The cranium is brachycephalic.

Facial malformations

- There is hypoplasia of maxilla with mandibular prognathism.
- The upper lip is short and nose resemble *Parrot's* beak.
- Oral feature includes high arched palate, V-shaped dental arch, peg shaped teeth, partial anodontia.

Eye changes

- Hypertelorism, exophthalmos with diver, strabismus, optic neuritis and choked disc resulting frequently in blindness.

Others

- Spina bifida occulta.

CUSHING'S SYNDROME

- It is characterized by adiposity about the upper portion of the body, mooning of the face and tendency to become round shouldered.
- *Buffalo* hump—it is seen at the base of the neck.
- There is dusky plethoric appearance with formation of purple striae.

- There is also muscular weakness, vascular hyperten-sion, glycosuria and albuminuria.
- Children—there may be osteoporosis and premature cessation of epiphyseal growth.

CURRY-HALL SYNDROME

- Short limbs, polydactyly and nail dysplasia.
- *Oral* features—deciduous teeth are small and conical. Incisors are retained as permanent successors may be congenitally missing.

DEJERINE-ROUSSY SYNDROME

- Tumors of the pons or occlusion of the posterior cerebral artery with sensory or motor abnormality on the contralateral side.
- *Oral* features—orofacial pain and dysgeusia are also present.

DOWN'S SYNDROME

- It is also called as *trisomy 21 syndrome* or *mongolism*.
- Cardiovascular—there is ventricular septal defect. ALV communication, patent ductus arteriosus and mitral valve prolapse.
- Haematological- impaired immunodeficiency, risk of neutropenia, eosinophilia, leukaemia.
- Musculoskeletal- atlantoaxial instability, midface is underdeveloped with relative prognathism, narrow and partially obstructed nasal passage and open bite.
- Nervous- delayed motor function, dementia.
- Oral – Vshaped, high vault palate, soft palate insufficiency, open mouth, macroglossia, malalignment.

EAGLE SYNDROME

- It is characterized by elongation of styloid process or ossification of stylohyoid ligament.
- Features—it includes dysphagia, sore throat, otalgia, glossodynia, headache and vague orofacial pain

EDWARD'S SYNDROME

- It is also called as trisomy *18 syndrome.*
- The affected individuals are mentally retarded and show hypertonicity.
- *Facial* features—there are small eyes and prominent occiput.
- The index finger overlaps the 3rd finger and 5th finger overlaps the 4th finger.
- *Oral features—it* includes micrognathia. High arched palate, cleft palate and bifid uvula.

EHLERS-DANLOS SYNDROME

- It is also called as *rubber man* and is autosomal dominant.
- *General—there* is hyperelasticity of skin, hyper-extensibility of joint and fragility of skin and blood vessels.

- *Oral features*—it includes enamel hypoplasia and periodontal destruction is severe. There is also hyper-mobility of TMJ resulting in repeated dislocation.

ELLIS VAN CREVELD SYNDROME

- *Skeletal* deformities—the affected person is of short stature due to chondrodysplasia. Polydactyly is also reported.
- Cardiac anomalies—congenital heart disease may cause neonatal death.
- *Hair and nails defect—nails* are dystrophic. Eyebrows and pubic hair are often deficient.
- *Oral features*- Fusion of middle portion of the upper lip to maxillary gingival margin eliminating the normal upper labial sulcus, Deciduous teeth show hypoplasia and permanent tooth eruption is delayed, Accessory cusp is common.

EPIDERMIS NEVUS SYNDROME

- Cutaneous nevi extending upto oral mucosa and gingiva.
- Mental deficiency, skeletal abnormality.
- There is also presence of hypoplastic teeth.

FANCONI'S SYNDROME

- Congenital or familial aplastic anemia.
- Bone abnormalities, microcephaly and generalized olive-brown pigmentation of the skin.

FAVRE-RACOUCHOT SYNDROME

- It occurs due to ultraviolet light and excessive smoking habit.
- There is extensive sun damage of the facial skin.
- There are also numerous open, dilated and cystic comedones.
- Dermis show solar elastosis characterized by dilated pilosebaceous opening with distended, horn filled hair follicle.

FIRST ARCH SYNDROME

- Oral features—it includes cleft lip and palate and mandibulofacial dysostosis.
- Hypertelorism and deformities of ear.

FLOPPY INFANT SYNDROME

- Generalized weakness due to hypotonia.
- Inability to sit, stand and walk.
- Hypotonia may involve tongue and facial muscles.

FRAGILE X SYNDROME

- X-linked mental retardation, macro-orchidism and large ears.
- Long narrow face and cleft palate.
- Mitral valve prolapse.

FROEHLICH SYNDROME

- Congenital obesity
- Hypogonadism
- Risk of learning disability
- Open bite

GARDNER'S SYNDROME

- *Systemic* features—multiple polyposis of large intestine and polyp of colon and rectum.
- Tumors—osteomas of bone including long bones, skull and jaws. There may be occasional occurrence of desmoid tumors. Other tumors which can occur are lipoma, leiomyoma and adenocarcinoma of colon.
- Cysts—multiple epidermoid or sebaceous cyst of skin particularly of scalp and back.
- Oral features—hypercementosis, multiple unerupted supernumerary teeth and compound odontoma.

GILES DE LA TOURETTE'S SYNDROME

- Spontaneous erratic behavior of the patients.
- Incoherent facial expressions and verbalization.
- Tendency for self mutilation of oral tissue by use of nails.

GOLTZ GORLIN SYNDROME

- It is also called as focal *dermal* hypoplasia syndrome. It is transmitted as an autosomal dominant trait.
- *General* features- Focal absence of dermis associated with herniation of subcutaneous fat into the defects. There is also skin atrophy, streaky pigmentation and telangiectasia. Multiple papillomas of skin or mucosa. Syndactyly, polydactyly, and adactyly.
- Oral features—papillomas of lip, microdontia lip and cleft palate.

GORLIN-CHAUDHRY-MOSS SYNDROME

- It is characterized by craniofacial dysostosis, ductus arteriosus, hypertrichosis and hypoplasia of labia majora.
- Oral feature of this syndrome is hypodontia.

GOLDENHAR SYNDROME

- Unilateral microstomia, mental retardation, hypoplastic zygomatic arch.
- Facial features—there is downward slanting of palpebral fissures, malformed pinna and iris coloboma
- Oral features- high arched palate, clefts, malocclusion.

GORHAM SYNDROME

- It also called as *massive osteolysis* or *phantom bone.*
- Osteolysis of single or multiple bones followed by replacement with fibrous tissue.
- Pain in the bone and pathological fractures.
- *Oral features*—there may be destruction of mandible or maxilla. Pain and facial asymmetry can be seen.

GRAHAM LITTLE SYNDROME

- It combines small confluent patches of progressive scarring alopecia resembling that of lichen planus follicularis.
- There is also follicular keratosis, and non-cicatrical alopecia of the axilla and pubis.
- Patches on the scalp are atrophic and cicatrical in the center but erythematous and squamous around the edges, where follicular keratosis occurs when the disease is actively progressing.

GRINSPAN SYNDROME

- It is triad of lichen planus, diabetes mellitus and vascular hypertension.

GUILLAIN-BARRE SYNDROME

- Acute infective polyneuritis
- Facial palsy

HAJADU CHENEY SYNDROME

- It is rare autosomal dominant disorder characterized by short stature, disintegration of terminal phalanges of fingers and toes.
- *Facial features*—long nose, low frontal hairline and flared ears.
- *Skeletal feature*—the individual is usually victim of multiple fractures of bones. Sutures are usually open and frontal sinuses are absent.
- *Oral features*—there is premature loss of teeth and abnormal shape of skull.

HANHART'S SYNDROME

- *Digital deformities*—it includes oligodactyly, syndactyly and hypoplastic digits.
- *Oral features*—there is micrognathia, microglossia and hypodontia.

HALLERMANN-STREIFF SYNDROME

- *Skeletal and genital*—it includes syndactyly and hypogenitalism.
- *Facial* features—it includes microphthalmia, long thin tapering nose, strabismus, double cutaneous chin with central furrow, hypotrichosis of the scalp and eyebrows and prominent scalp veins.
- *Oral features*—it includes hypodontia, microstomia, malocclusion, malformed teeth and retained deciduous teeth.

HEERFORDT'S SYNDROME

- Firm painless, bilateral enlargement of parotid gland.
- Inflammation of uveal tract of the eye.
- Facial palsy.

HETCH-BEALS-WILSON SYNDROME

- Limited mandibular opening.
- Shortened leg, hamstring muscles and club foot.

HORNER'S SYNDROME

- Miosis or contraction of pupil of the eye due to paresis of dilators of pupil.
- Ptosis or drooping of eyelid due to paresis of smooth muscle elevators of upper lid.
- Anhidrosis and vasodilatation over the face due to interruption of sudomotor and vasomotor control.

HORTON'S SYNDROME

- It is also called as *sphenopalatine* neuralgia.
- Unilateral paroxysms of intense pain in the eye, maxilla, ear, mastoid region, base of nose and beneath the zygoma.
- Absence of trigger zones and occurrence of pain everyday exactly at the same time for this reasons it is called as alarm *clock headache.*

HURLER'S SYNDROME

- It is disturbance in mucopolysaccharide metabolism.
- *Facial* features—prominent forehead, broad saddle nose, wide nostrils, hypertelorism and puffy eyelids. There is also corneal clouding present.
- There is also nasal congestion with noisy breathing.
- *Claw* hand resulting from flexion contractures.
- Hepatosplenomegaly results in protuberant abdomen. Death usually occurs before the age of 10 years.
- *Oral features—thick* lips, large tongue, open mouth.

HUNTER'S SYNDROME

- Similar feature like Hurler's syndrome but they are mild.
- Corneal clouding is absent.
- Death usually occurs before the age of 15 years.

HUTCHINSON GILFORD SYNDROME

- It is also called as *progeria.* It is transmitted as autosomal dominant trait. There is manifestation of old age features, pro—before, geria—old.

- Alopecia. Pigmented areas of trunk, atrophic skin, prominent vein and loss of subcutaneous fat.
- The individual has high pitched, squeaky voice and beak-like nose.
- Oral *features*—loss of all teeth in very young age, hypoplastic mandible, and delayed eruption of teeth can also occur.

HYPOGLOSSIA-HYPODACTYLIA SYNDROME

- Total or partial absence of the tongue.
- Micrognathia, high arched or cleft palate, glossopalatine ankylosis, defects in the lower lip and hypertrophy of sublingual glands.
- Hypodactylia and hypomelia.

JAW WINKING SYNDROME

- It is also called as *marcus gun phenomenon.*
- Rapid elevation of the ptotic eyelid occurring on movement of the mandible on the contralateral side.
- Congenital unilateral ptosis.

JADASSOHN-LEWANDOWSKY SYNDROME

- Bilateral oral white lesions involving the tongue and buccal mucosa.
- Laminated thickening of fingers and toe nails.

JAW CYST-BASAL CELL NEVUS-BIFID RIB SYNDROME

- It is also called as *Gorlin-Goltz syndrome*
- Cutaneous anomafies—basal cell carcinoma, dermal cysts and tumors, palmar and plantar keratosis and dermal calcinosis.
- Dental abnormalities—odontogenic keratocysts and mild mandibular prognathism.
- Osseous abnormalities—bifid rib, vertebral anomalies and brachymetacarpalism.
- *Ophthalmologic* anomalies—hypertelorism with wide nasal bridge, dystopia canthorum, congenital blindness and internal strabismus.
- *Neurological* anomalies—mental retardation, agenesis of corpus callosum, ductal calcification, congenital hydrocephalus and medulloblastomas.
- Sexual anomalies—hypogonadism, ovarian tumors.

JUGULAR FORAMEN SYNDROME

- Dysphagia, hoarseness of voice, glossopharyngeal neuralgia like pain.
- Palatal weakness and vocal cord paralysis.

KBG SYNDROME

- The affected individual show short stature and mental retardation.
- *Facial* features—flat bridge of nose, round face, long philtrum and abnormal auricle, with or without hearing defect.

- *Oral* features—include macrodontia, oligodontia, hypoplasia of enamel and micrognathia.

KLINEFELTER'S SYNDROME

- It occurs in males whose sex chromosome constitution includes one or more extra chromosomes.
- The patient develops infertility and gynecomastia.
- There may be fatigue, osteoporosis, mitral valve prolapse and varicose veins.
- The patients develop taurodontism.

LARSEN'S SYNDROME

- It is an autosomal dominant disorder.
- There is prominent forehead with frontal bossing, flattened midface, depressed nasal bridge and hypertelorism.
- There is bilateral anterior dislocation of tibia or femur with displaced patella.
- *Oral* features—it includes cleft palate and malocclusion.

LAUGIER-HUNZIKER SYNDROME

- Acquired pigmented macules in the lips, oral cavity and fingers.

MAFFUCCI'S SYNDROME

- Multiple chondromas of the jaw bone.
- Multiple hemangiomas of skin and oral mucosa.
- Phleboliths can also occur.
- In oral mucosa, it occurs on the tongue.

MARFAN'S SYNDROME

- Skeletal—excessive length of tubular bone resulting in disproportionate long thin extremities.
- Craniofacial—skull and face are long and narrow. Ears are large. eyes appear sunken and frontal bossing is seen.
- Ocular—ocular lens subluxation with a defect in the suspensory ligament.
- *Cardiovascular*—aortic aneurysm and regurgitation.
- Oral—temporomandibular joint dysarthrosis, multiple odontogenic cysts of maxilla and mandible, high arched palate and bifid uvula.

MAGIC SYNDROME

- Mouth and genital ulcers with inflamed cartilage.

MARIN-AMAT'S SYNDROME

- It is also called as *inverted marcus gun* phenomenon.
- Eye closes automatically when patient opens his mouth forcefully and fully, tears may also follow.

MELNICK-NEEDLES SYNDROME

- It is autosomal dominant condition characterized by generalized bony dysplasia and abnormal facies.
- There is marked exophthalmos. full cheeks and large ear.
- *Oral features*—micrognathia, *transversely* long mouth and malocclusion.
- Skeletal—delayed closure of anterior fontanelle, defect in clavicles, ribs and vertebrae.

MEDIAN CLEFT FACE SYNDROME

- It is also called as *frontonasal* dysplasia.
- There is nasal clefts and notches, preauricular tags and ocular hypertelorism.
- There is also median cleft of premaxilla and palate and malocclusion.

MELKERSSON-ROSENTHAL SYNDROME

- It is triad of cheilitis granulomatosa. facial paralysis and scrotal tongue.

MIESCHER'S SYNDROME

- It is also called as *cheilitis granulomatosa.* - Diffuse swelling of lip especially lower lip.
- Scarring, fissuring, vesicle or pustule formation on the vermilion border.
- It is associated with Melkersson-Rosenthal syndrome.

MIDDLE FOSSA SYNDROME

- It occurs due to tumor in the region of gasserian ganglion.
- There is hyperesthesia, paresthesia and paralysis of ocular muscles.
- Deviated mandibular opening and unilateral soft palate paralysis.

MOBIUS'S SYNDROME (CONGENITAL FACIAL DIPLEGIA)

- In infancy, failure to close the eyes during sleep.
- Partial/complete facial paralysis results in no change in facial expressions while crying or laughing
- Drooling of saliva and difficulty in mastication.
- There is also external ophthalmoplegia, deformity of external ear, deafness, defect of pectoral muscle, paresis of tongue, soft palate or jaw muscles, clubfoot, mental defects and epilepsy.

MOHR'S SYNDROME

- It is autosomal recessive disorder characterized by several oral, facial and digital defects. The affected individual is moderately short.
- *Digital* deformities—brachydactyly. syndacryly or polydactyly
- *Facial deformities*—midline cleft lip and bifid tip of nose.
- *Oral* feolures—there is high arched palate. lobate tongue, hypoplastic body of the mandible and hypodontia.

MORQUIO'S SYNDROME

- Severe enamel hypoplasia with grey and pitted enamel.
- Severe bone changes, corneal clouding and aortic regurgitation.

MULTIPLE ENDOCRINE NEOPLASIA SYNDROMES

MEN 1

- Tumor or hyperplasia of pituitary: parathyroid gland, adrenal cortex and pancreatic islets. ·
- There is also peptic ulcer and gastric hypersecretion.

MEN 2 (Sipple's Syndrome)

- Parathyroid adenoma or hyperplasia but no tumor of pancreas.
- Pheochromocytomas of adrenal medulla and medullary carcinoma of thyroid gland occurs.

MEN 3

- *Systemic*
- Mucocutaneous neuromas, pheochromocytomas of adrenal medulla and medullary carcinoma of thyroid.
- Marfanoid *habitus*—it refers to a slender body build, with long, thin extremities and increased laxity of joints. The face appears long and thin.
- Oral Neuromas of lip, tongue and buccal mucosa.
- Thick and bumpy lips and infrequent prognathism.

MURRAY PURETIC-DRESHER SYNDROME

- Gingival fibromatosis.
- Multiple hyaline fibromas of head, trunk and extremities.
- Suppurative skin lesions and flexion contractures.

MUCOCUTANEOUS LYMPH NODE SYNDROME

- Bilateral congestion of ocular conjunctive and edema of extremities.
- Dryness and fissuring of the lips.
- Strawberry like redness and swelling of tongue.
- Acute non-purulent swelling of the lymph nodes.

NANCE-HORAN SYNDROME

- X-linked congenital cataract.
- Supernumerary teeth.
- Incisor teeth can resemble Hutchinson's incisor.

NECK-TONGUE SYNDROME

- Unilateral upper nuchal or occipital pain, with or without numbness in the area.

- Simultaneous numbness of the tongue on that side.

NOONAN'S SYNDROME

- Congenital heart disease, chest deformity and mental retardation.
- Short stature, facial bone anomalies and cryptorchidism.

OROFACIAL DIGITAL SYNDROME

- It is X-linked condition which is exclusively found in females.
- Facial *features*—it includes frontal bossing, hypoplasia of alar cartilages, broad nasal root and ocular hypertelorism
- clinodactyly, syndactyly, brachydactyly and polydactyly.
- *Oral features*- Cleft tongue, cleft of alveolar process (mandi-bular) and cleft lip. Thick fibrous bands in the lower rnucobuccal fold eliminating the sulcus, Supernumerary canine and premolars. Malpositioned teeth.

PATAU SYNDROME

- It is also called as *trisomy 13 syndrome.*
- The affected individuals may show polydactyly and heart anomalies.
- *Facial features*—it includes microcephaly, microphthalrnia. ocular hypertelorism and deafness.
- *Oral features*—it includes cleft lip and cleft palate.
- Polydactyly and heart anomalies.

PARRY ROMBERG SYNDROME

- There is also atrophy of skin, subcutaneous tissue, muscle and bone.
- Loss of hair and vitiligo can be seen.
- Contralateral Jacksonian epilepsy and trigeminal neuralgia also occur.
- Oral features—atrophy of half of the tongue and retarded dental eruption on the involved side.

PEUTZ-JEGHERS SYNDROME

- It is also called as *hereditary intestinal polyposis syndrome.*
- There is familial generalized intestinal polyposis.
- Pigmentation of face, oral cavity and sometimes on hands and feet.
- There may gastric, duodenal and colonic adenocarcinoma.

PFEIFFER'S SYNDROME

- Skeletal *deformities*—it includes craniosynostosis with turribrachycephaly, broad thumbs and halluces.
- *Facial* deformities—midface hypoplasia, shallow orbit, hypertelorism. proptosis and antimongoloid obliquity.
- *Oral features*—it includes maxillary underdevelopment resulting in mandibular prognathism,

high arched palate and bifid uvula.

PIERRE ROBIN SYNDROME

- There is U-shaped cleft palate, micrognathia and glossoptosis.
- Occasionally hydrocephaly or microcephaly can be seen.

PLUMMER-VINSON SYNDROME

- Cracks or fissures at the corner of mouth (angular cheilitis).
- Dysphagia due to esophageal webs.
- Atrophy of filiform papillae and koilonychia.

PORTSMOUTH SYNDROME

- Normal ADP-induced platelet aggregation but abnormal or absent collagen induced aggregation.
- It is associated with thrombocytopenia purpura.

RAEDER'S SYNDROME

- It is also called as *paratrigerninal* syndrome.
- Headache or pain in thearea of trigeminal distribution.
- Ocular sympathetic paralysis.

RAMON SYNDROME

- Hypertrichosis, epilepsy and mental retardation.
- Gingival fibromatosis and cherubism.

RALEY DAY SYNDROME

- Congenital absence of tongue papillae.
- Vasomotor dysfunction, loss of reflexes and feeding problems.
- Lack of pain and taste sensation.

RAMSAY HUNT SYNDROME

- Zoster infection of geniculate ganglion with involvement of external ear and oral mucosa.
- Facial paralysis
- Vesicular eruptions.

RUTHERFURD'S SYNDROME

- Congenital enlargement of the gingivae and altered eruption of teeth.
- There is corneal dystrophy, conjunctivitis and mucocutaneous lesion.

RUBINSTEIN-TAYBI SYNDROME

- It is associated with *talon's* cusp.

- Developmental retardation, broad thumb and great toes.
- Delayed or incomplete descent of testes in males.

SANFILIPPO'S SYNDROME

- Severe CNS defect, mild somatic disturbance.
- Enamel hypoplasia and excessive dentinogenesis with obliteration of pulp chambers.

SAETHRE-CHOTZEN SYNDROME

- It is an autosomal dominant trait characterized by short stature and mild mental retardation.
- Facial deformities—it includes ocular hyrpertelorism, ptosis of eyelids, deviated nasal septum and mild conductive deafness.
- Other deformities—finger exhibits cutaneous syndactyly and occasional renal abnormalities can be seen.
- *Oral features*—it includes prognathism, high arched palate and resultant malocclusion.

SCHEIE'S SYNDROME

- Stiff joints, corneal clouding, aortic regurgitation and normal intelligence.

SCHEUTHAUER-MARIE-SAINTON SYNDROME

- It is also called as cleidocranial *dysplasia*.
- Open fontanelle of skull and partial or complete absence of clavicles.
- Underdeveloped maxilla, multiple impacted or unerupted, permanent or supernumerary teeth.

SJOGREN'S SYNDROME

- Primary- Keratoconjunctivitis sicca and xerostomia.
- Secondary- Keratoconjunctivitis sicca and xerostomia with Lupus erythematous, polyarteritis nodosa, scleroderma and rheumatoid arthritis.

STEVENS-JOHNSON SYNDROME

- Oral mucous membrane lesions—severe form of erythema multiforme.
- Eye lesions—photophobia, conjunctivitis. corneal ulceration.
- Genital lesions—nonspecific urethritis, balanitis, or vaginal ulcers.

STURGE-WEBER SYNDROME

- Angiomatosis of face (nevus flamrneus) and leptomeningeal angiomas.
- There is also intracranial calcifications and contralateral hemiplegia.
- Massive growth of gingiva and asymmetrical jaw growth and tooth eruption sequence.

TREACHER COLLINS SYNDROME (MANDIBULOFACIAL DYSOSTOSIS)

- *Facial features*- Downward sloping of palpebral fissures (anti-mongoloid obliquity), underdeveloped cheek bone, receding chin and malformation of external ear,Hypoplasia of facial bone, especially of malar bone and mandible.

- Blind fistulae between angle of mouth and angle of ear.
- Facial clefts and skeletal deformities. ·
- *Oral features*—fish like mouth, macrostomia. high arched palate, malocclusion, pronounced concavity of the undersurface of the mandible and an obtuse mandibular angle.

TROTTER'S SYNDROME

- Carcinoma of nasopharynx often producing trigeminal neuralgia like pain in the mandible, tongue and side of the head.
- There is also middle ear deafness.

TRICHODENTAL SYNDROME

- Inherited dominant condition and is characterized by fine short hair.
- Thinning of lateral end of eyebrows.
- Hypodontia and conical teeth.

TRICHODENTOOSSEOUS SYNDROME

- It is transmitted as an autosomal dominant trait.
- Hair and *nail* deformities—it includes kinky hair and nails show white band and are brittle.
- *Oral features*—it includes hypomaturation type of amelogenesis imperfecta, enamel hypoplasia, unerupted teeth and taurodontism. The mandibular angle is obtuse and the jaw is square.

TRICHONYCHODENTAL SYNDROME

- It is autosomal dominant trait.
- Fine curly hair and thin dysplastic nails.
- *Oral* features—taurodontism and developmental defect of enamel and dentin.

TURNER'S SYNDROME

- Short stature, cabitus vulgus, webbed neck, renal disorders and sexual infantilism.
- *Oral features*—it includes micrognathia, high arched palate and corners of mouth appear pulled down. There is premature eruption of teeth.

TUBEROUS SCLEROSIS SYNDROME

- Oral-gingival lesions and enamel hypoplasia.
- Skin-adenoma sebaceum.
- *Associated* anomalies-epilepsy, mental retardation and hamartomas of brain, heart and kidney.
- Associated malignancy—astrocytoma and glio-blastorna.

VAN DER WOUDE'S SYNDROME

- Occurrence of pits of lower lip
- Presence of deft lip and cleft palate.

VAN BUCHEM'S SYNDROME

- Excessive deposition of endosteal bone throughout the skeleton.
- Facial swelling and occasional facial paralysis.
- Visual acuity and deafness.

VON RECKLINGHAUSEN'S NEURO-FIBROMATOSIS

- Oral lesions—intraoral neurofibromas leading to macroglossia
- *cafe*-au-lait spots, giant nevi and multiple neurofibromas.
- Malignancy—malignant neurilemmoma and pheo-chromocytomas.
- Neurological—CNS tumor, mental retardation.

VON HIPPEL'S SYNDROME

- Hemangioblastomas in retina and cerebellum.
- Pancreatic and renal cyst, renal adenomas and hepatic hemangioma.
- Multiple endocrine neoplasms.

WERNER SYNDROME

- Congenital Alopecia
- Dwarfism
- Senility
- Early Atherosclerosis
- Delayed tooth eruption
- Mandibular hypoplasia

WHISTLING FACE SYNDROME

- It is also called as craniocarpatotarsal dysplasia.
- It is characterized by sunken eyes, true ocular hypertelorism and antimongoloid obliquity of palpebral fissures.
- It also includes small nose, microstomia, high skull and protruding; lips as seen during whistling.
- The palate is high arched and mandible is small and retrognathic.
- There is presence of a fibrous band demarcated by two grooves extending from the midline of the lower lip to the chin, often presenting in 'H' or 'V' shaped.

XXY SYNDROME

- There is hypoplastic midface, short stature, mental retardation, speckled eyes and hypertelorism.
- Oral *features*—it includes taurodontism and bifid uvula.

ZINSSNER SYNDROME

- Oral leukoplakia, dystrophic nails and hyperpigmentation of skin.
- Pancytopenia and aplastic anaemia.

NORMAL VALUE FOR LABORATORY TESTS

I. Hematologic blood values (whole blood [EDTA]

A. Red blood cell values

1. Red blood cell count
    (a) Male-4.5 to 6.0 million/mm^3
    (b) Female-4.0 to 5.5 million/ mm^3
    (c) During pregnancy—greater than 3.6 million/ mm^3
2. Hemoglobin (Hbg) content
    (a) Male-13.5 to 17.5 g/100 ml
    (b) Female- 12 to 16 g/100 ml
3. Packed cell Volume or hematocrit
    (a) Male- 41-53%
    (b) Female- 36-46%
4. Mean corpuscular volume (MCV)
    (a) Male-82.2 to 100.6
    (b) Female-81.9 to 100.7
5. Mean corpuscular hemoglobin (MCH) content
    (a) Male-28.4 to 32.0 pg
    (b) Female-28.3 to 32.1 pg
6. Mean corpuscular hemoglobin concentration (MCHC)
    (a) Male-32.7% to 35.1% (g/100 ml)
    (b) Female-32.5% to 34.7% (g/100 ml)

B. White blood cell values

1. White blood cell count
    (a) Infants-6000 to 17,500/mm^3 (first day of life-9400 to 34,000 mm^3)
    (b) Adolescents-4500 to 13,500/mm^3
    (c) Adults-4500 to 11,000/mm^3
2. Differential white blood cell count
    (a) Neutrophils-35% to 73%; 1680 to 7884/mm^3
    (b) Lymphocytes-23% to 33%; 1500 to 3000/mm^3
    (c) Monocytes-2% to 6%; 100 to 900/mm^3
    (d) Eosinophils-1% to 3%; 50 to 450/mm^3
    (e) Basophils-0% to 1%; 50 to 200/mm^3

C. *Bleeding and clotting abnormalities*

1. Platelets (whole blood [EDTA])-150,000- 400,000/mm^3
2. (Ivy) bleeding time (blood from the skin)-2 to 7 min
3. (Lee-White) clotting time (whole blood [no an-ticoagulant])-5 to 8 min
4. Prothrombin time (one stage) (whole blood [no citrate])-12 to 14 sec
5. Partial thromboplastin time (whole blood [no citrate])-25 to 30 sec
6. Fibrinogen (whole blood [no citrate])-200 to 400 mg/100 ml
7. Specific factor analysis (plasma [no citrate])
   (a) Factor II assay-60% to 150% of normal, or 0.5 to 1.5 U/ml
   (b) Factor V assay-60% to 150% of normal, or 0.5 to 2.0 U/ml
   (c) Factor VII assay-65% to 135% of normal, or 60 to 135 AU
   (d) Factor VIII assay-60% to 2145% of normal 60 to 145 AU
   (e) Factor IX assay-60% to 140% of normal, or 60 to 140 AU
   (f) Factor X assay-60% to 130% of normal, or 60 to 130 AU
8. Prothrombin consumption test (whole blood) no anticoagulant)-greater than 30 sec
9. Thrombin time (whole blood [no citrate])-control time (9 to 10 sec) # 2 sec

II. Serum enzymes (serum)

A. Serum glutamic-oxaloacetic transaminase-15 to 40 U/L
B. Serum glutamic pyruvic transaminase-15 to 35 U/L
C. Lactate dehydrogenase-45 to 90 U/L
D. Creatine phosphokinase-0 to 170 U/L
E. Alkaline phosphatase
   1. Male-62 to 176 U/L
   2. Female-56 to 155 U/L
F. Acid phosphatase
   1. Male-0.01 to 0.56 U/L
   2. Female-0.13 to 0.63 U/L
G. Amylase-80 to 180 (Somogyi) U/d1

III. Blood chemistry (serum)

A. Calcium (total)-8.4 to 10.2 mg/100 ml
B. Phosphorus-2.7 to 4.5 mg/100 ml
C. Glucose
   1. Under 60 years of age-70 to 105 mg/100 ml
   2. Over 60 years of age-81 to115 mg/100 ml
D. Blood urea nitrogen-7 to 18 mg/100 ml
E. Uric acid
   1. Male-3.5 to 7.2 mg/I00 ml
   2. Female-2.6 to 6.0 mg/I00 ml

F. Cholesterol (plasma [no citrate] or serum) (EDTA)

   1. 20 to 29 years of age

     (a) Male-Greater than 194 mg/100 ml

     (b) Female-Greater than 184 mg/100 ml

   2. 30 to 39 years of age

     (a) Male-Greater than 218 mg/100 ml

     (b) Female-Greater than 202 mg/100 ml

   3. 40 to 49 years of age

     (a) Male-Greater than 231 mg/l00 ml

     (b) Female-· greater than 223 mg/100 ml

   4. Over 50 years of age

     (a) Males- greater than 230mg/l00 ml

     (b) Females- greater than 252 mg/100 ml

G. Protein (total) - 6-8.4 g/100 ml

   Albumin -3.5 – 5.0

   Globulin- 2.3- 3.5

QUESTIONS

1. Ectodermal dysplasia is - [AIPG 2005]

   1. Autosomal recessive.

   2. Autosomal dominant.

   3. X-linked dominant.

   4. X-linked recessive.

Ans.   **4**

Ectodermal dysplasia is a triad marked with partial or complete anodontia, decreased sweating and thinning of hair. Manifested in males more frequently than females. However, it may also be transmitted as autosomal dominant or recession trait in some cases.

2. The most reliable criteria in Gustafson's method of identification is - [AIPG 2005]

   1. Cementum apposition.

   2. Transparency of root.

   3. Attrition.

   4. Root resorption.

Ans.   **2**

3. A black line on the gingiva, which follows the contour of the margin, is due to - [AIPG 2005]

   1. Lead.

   2. Argyria.

3. Iron.

4. Mercury.

Ans. **1**

Bismuth pigmentations seen on gingiva and buccal mucosa. It appears as a thin blue-black line in the marginal gingiva, which is sometimes confined, to the gingival papilla. Bismuth lines occur in majority of patients receiving prolonged treatment and are more frequent in unclear mouth.

'Lead lines' are gray or bluish black line similar to 'bismuth line', but more diffuse.

Gingival pigmentation due to mercury is seen only in severe cases. More common manifestations are oral ulceration.

Argyria causes bluish gray pigmentation of oral mucosa, which is diffusely dispersed throughout the oral cavity.

4. **Hair and nails are usually preserved in poisoning from:** [AIPG 2004]

1. Arsenic

2. Phosphorous

3. Barbiturates

4. Carbon monoxide

Ans. **1**

5. **Which of the following elements is known to influence the body's ability to handle oxidative stress?** [AIPG 2004]

1. Calcium

2. Iron

3. Potassium

4. Selenium

Ans. **4**

Selenium is a potent antioxidant.

6. **Patients with Down's syndrome normally have:** [AIPG 2004]

1. IQ score above 80

2. Brachychephalic skull

3. Stiff muscles

4. All of the above

Ans. **2**

IQ score is < 60 and flaccid muscles are seen.

7. **Rumpel - Leede test measures the:** [AIPG 2004]

1. Bleeding time

2. Platelet count

3. Capillary fragility

4. ESR

Ans. **3**

8. **Which of the following areas of the oral cavity are affected by inflammatory papillary hyperplasia?** [AIPG 2004]
   1. Lips
   2. Tongue
   3. Palate
   4. Gingival

Ans. **3**

Due to ill-fitted dentures.

9. **Superimposition is the technique applied to establish the identity of the individual from:** [AIPG 2002]
   1. Skull
   2. Pelvis
   3. Mandible
   4. Long bone

Ans. **1**

This technique is commonly used in forensic science to establish identity.

10. **All are findings in ectodermal dysplasia except:** [AIPG 2002]
    1. Hereditary disorder
    2. Depressed nasal bridge
    3. Lip withdrawn inside
    4. Defective mental development.

Ans. **4**

These is no mental deficit.

11. **Pink tooth is:** [AIPG 2002]
    1. Chronic hyperplastic pulpitis
    2. Internal resorption
    3. Pulpal hyperaemia
    4. Periapical abscess.

Ans. **2**

Due to internal resorption pulp tissue shows through the thin external surface of the tooth giving it a pink appearance.

12. **EB virus is associated with which carcinoma?** [AIPG 2001]
    1. Carcinoma of larynx
    2. Carcinoma of bladder
    3. Nasopharyngeal carcinoma

4. Chronic lymphocytic leukemia

Ans. **3**

13. **Dinesh, a 24-year old male, complains of loose teeth in single quadrant. His radiograph shows irregular bone loss and histopathology reveals eosinophils and histiocytes. The most probable diagnosis is:** [AIPG 2000]
    1. Hand-Schuler-Christian disease.
    2. Parasitic infection
    3. Osteoclastoma
    4. Albright's syndrome.

Ans. **1**

Hand-Schuler-Christian disease is marked by multifocal eosinophilic granuloma. Radiographically, diffuse are as of alveolar bone destruction are seen with tooth displacement. It is characterized by classic triad of single or multiple areas of a 'punched-out' lesions is skull, unilateral or bilateral exophthalmos and diabetes insipidus.

14. **The commonest method of detection of diphtheria carriers is:** [AIPG 99]
    1. Schick test
    2. Dick test
    3. Casonis' test
    4. Charles' test

Ans. **1**

Dick test is for scarlet fever.

15. **Monospot test is diagnostic of:** [AIPG 97]
    1. Infectious mononucleosis
    2. Sarcoidosis
    3. Hodgkin's disease
    4. Lymphoma

Ans. **1**

For sarcoidosis, kevim test is diagnostic. For diagnosis of Hodgkin's disease or lymphoma, FNAC of enlarged lymph nodes or biopsy is needed.

16. **Down's syndrome patients shows:** [AIPG 97]
    1. Early exfoliation of deciduous teeth
    2. Microdontia of teeth over retained teeth
    3. Periodontitis
    4. All of the above

Ans. **4**

Oral manifestations of Down's syndrome include macroglossia with protrusion of the tongue, fissured or pebbly tongue, high arched palate, malformed teeth, enamel hypoplasia, microdontia.

Also the patient is mentally retarded. So due to neglect of oral hygiene, premature exfoliation of primary teeth and periodontitis is seen.

17. Transillumination is used as a diagnostic aid to diagnose: [AIPG 1995]
1. Hydrocele
2. Mucocele
3. Ranula
4. Aneurysmal bone cyst

Ans. **1**

Transillumination is used as a diagnostic aid in
- Hydrocoel
- Cystic hygroma
- Diseases of maxillary sinus

18. Lead intoxication causes: [AIPG 1995]
1. A thin blue line on the alveolar mucosa
2. A blue black patch on the marginal gingiva
3. Burtonian line
4. Blue black line in gingival sulcus

Ans. **4**

Lead intoxication causes:-
- GIT symptoms like nausea, vomiting, colic and constipation
- Peripheral neuritis characterized by wrist drop or fool drop.
- Blood charges- hypochromic anemia with basophilic stippling of RBC's
- Lead line or Burtonian line in gingiva
- Ulcerative stomatitis
- Excessive salivation
- Metallic taste
- Swelling of salivary glands.

19. A 5 cm suspicious looking lesion of oral mucosa should be: [AIPG 94]
1. Incised and sent for biopsy
2. Excised and sent for biopsy
3. Irradiated
4. Offered palliative treatment

Ans. **1**

Incisional biopsy is indicated whenever the size of lesion is > 1 cm. If it is < 1 cm, excisional biopsy is done.

20. Scleroderma involves: [AIPG 94]
1. Tightening of oral mucosa and periodontal involvement

2. Multiple palmar keratosis

3. Raynaud's phenomenon

4. All of the above

Ans. **4**

Other features are diffuse systemic sclerosis of many internal organs like GIT, lungs, cardiovascular, renal, musculoskeletal and central nervous systems, CREST syndrome.

21. **Darier's disease is associated with:**   [AIPG 94]

1. Pernicious anemia

2. Rickets with involvement of teeth and bones

3. Vitamin A deficiency and involvement of oral epithelium and skin

4. Diffuse tender ulceration on the palate predominantly

Ans. **3**

Darier's disease or keratosis follicularies is a genodermatosis, which is transmitted as an autosomal dominant characteristic. It gives a cobblestone appearance to oral mucosa and thought to be related to vitamin A deficiency. Corps, ronds and grains are important histological findings.

22. **Premature exfoliation of teeth is seen in:**   [AIPG 94]

1. Papillon-Le-fevre syndrome

2. Hypophosphatasia

3. Juvenile diabetes

4. All of the above

Ans. **4**

23. **The proper rate of rescue breathing in an adult is:**   [AIPG 92]

1. 4 times per minute

2. 12 times per minute

3. 20 times per minute

4. 28 times per minute

Ans. **2**

24. **A 3-year old child presents with only deciduous canine and molars. The child has light fine hair, light complexion and over all appearance of an older person. The findings suggest:**
                    [AIPG 92]

1. Cleidocranial dysostosis

2. Osteogenesis imperfecta

3. Crouzon's disease

4. Hereditary ectodermal dysplasia

Ans. **4**

Hereditary ectodermal dysplasia is marked by hypodontia, hypohidrosis and hypotrichosis.

25. **Before dental treatment, prophylactic antibiotic coverage is indicated for patients with each the following conditions except:** [AIPG 91]
    1. Coronary artery bypass
    2. Rheumatic heart disease
    3. Prosthetic aortic valve
    4. Kidney damage needing hemodialysis

Ans. **1**

Prophylactic antibiotic coverage is not needed after myocardial infarction, isolated secundum atrial septal defect, coronary artery bypass graft, pacemakers, stents or defibrillatous, mitral valve prolapse without regurgitation, pulmonary stenosis, innocent cardiac murmurs.

26. **Dry socket is a form of:** [AIPG 91]
    1. Osteomyelitis
    2. Osteitis
    3. Osteoma
    4. Periostitis

Ans. **2**

Another name for dry socket is alveolar osteitis.

27. **Inflammatory palatal hyperplasia which is associated with poor oral hygiene and ill fitting dentures is called:** [AIPG 91]
    1. Palatal torus
    2. Denture sore spot
    3. Denture sore mouth
    4. Palatal papillomatosis

Ans. **4**

Palatal papillomatosis is caused by an ill fitted denture associated with poor oral hygiene. It is seen on palate below the "maxillary denture".

Denture sore mouth is chronic atrophic candidial infection.

Denture sore spot is due to trauma by sharp margins of denture.

Torus is a developmental anomaly.

28. **The most likely tissue reaction to gross over-extension of a complete denture that has been worn for a long time is:** [AIPG 1990]
    1. Epulis fissuratum
    2. Giant cell reparative granuloma
    3. Papillary hyperplasia
    4. Denture stomatitis

Ans. **1**

Rolls of tissue are formed in mucobuccal fold.

2- Is due to chronic imitation

3- Due to ill fitted dentures, lesions occur on palate.

4- Due to poor hygiene of denture.

29. **A 24 years old male suffers from loose teeth and gingivitis in one quadrant. Radiographs show extensive bone loss. The blood chemistry is normal. Biopsy reveals proliferation of histiocytes and abundant eosinophilic infiltration. With this limited information, the likely diagnosis is:** [AIPG 1989]

   1. Apical granuloma

   2. Chronic granuloma

   3. Parasitic infestation

   4. Eosinophilic granuloma

Ans. **4**

Teeth appear 'floating in air'.

Non lipid reticuloendotheliosis or histiocytosis X. disease which includes

1. Hand Schuller Christian disease

2. Eosinophilic granuloma

3. Letterer siwe disease

30. **A 3 years old child has only deciduous canines and first molars present. General observation shows the child to have light fine hair, fair complexion and appearance of an older person. This condition suggests:** [AIPG 1989]

   1. Cleidocranial dysostosis

   2. Osteogenesis imperfecta

   3. Crouzon's disease

   4. Hereditary ectodermal dysplasia

Ans. **4**

Hereditary ectodermal dysplasia

- Hypohidrosis – dry skin

- Hypotrichosis- sparsed hair

- Hypodontia

- Pseudorhagades – HED (Rhagades in syphilis)

41 Unsolved Questions

1. **Diascopy is performed in case of:**
   1. Vascular lesions.
   2. Bony hard lesions.
   3. Lymph node examination.
   4. Salivary gland studies

2. **Sialorrhoea can occur as a result of all except:**
   1. Oral cancer.
   2. Familial autonomic dysfunction.
   3. Sarcoidosis.
   4. Teething.

3. **Leontiasis ossea can cause:**
   1. Micrognathia.
   2. Macrognathia.
   3. Cleft palate.
   4. Facial edema.

4. **"Ghost teeth" refer to which condition:**
   1. Treacher Colin syndrome.
   2. Regional odontodysplasia.
   3. Amelogenesis imperfecta.
   4. Dentinogenesis imperfecta.

5. **Diffuse swellings occurring in the lips is a feature of:**
   1. Wegener's granulomatosis.
   2. Meisher's syndrome.
   3. Treacher- Colin syndrome.
   4. Apert syndrome.

6. **The consistency of lymph nodes in lymphoma is described as:**
   1. Soft.
   2. Rubbery.
   3. Stony hard.
   4. Firm.

7. **Chemical substances responsible for halitosis are:**
   1. Hydrogen sulphide and methyl mercaptan.
   2. Hydrogen peroxide and methyl carbide.
   3. Carbon monoxide and hydrocarbons.
   4. Nitrous oxide and sulphur.

8. **Removal of pulp tissue results in the loss of translucency of the teeth because of:**
   1. Dehydration of the tooth.
   2. Loss of enamel.
   3. Resorption of dentin.
   4. Inability of light to penetrate the hard tissue structure.

9. **Among smokers gingival inflammation can occur because:**
   1. Tobacco is an irritant to gingiva.
   2. Physical injury caused by cigarette.
   3. Nicotine from tobacco is an irritant.
   4. Frequent drying and moistening of the gingiva.

10. **Among the following syndromes which is not associated with gingival enlargement:**
    1. Cowden's syndrome.
    2. Cross syndrome.
    3. Reiter's syndrome.
    4. Rutherford syndrome.

11. **Unusual extensibility of the tongue is called:**
    1. Lingual varicosity.
    2. Elastic tongue.
    3. Rubbery tongue.
    4. Gorlin sign.

12. **Jarrisch- herxheimer reaction can occur following treatment of:**
    1. Syphilis.
    2. Leprosy.
    3. Tuberculosis.
    4. Cervicofacial actinomycosis.

13. **"Ray fungus" is a term given for:**
    1. Candida albicans.
    2. Actinomyces israelii.

3. Borrelia vincentii.

4. Treponema pallidum.

14. **A complication of acute necrotizing ulcerative gingivostomatitis is:**

1. Osteomyelitis.

2. Actinomycosis.

3. Cancrum oris.

4. Gingival abscess.

15. **A diagnostic test for the diagnosis of herpetic gingivostomatitis is:**

1. Viral culture.

2. Tzanck smear.

3. Mono spot test.

4. Compliment fixation test.

16. **Diseases associated with aphthous ulcers are the following except:**

1. Behcet's disease.

2. Crohn's disease.

3. Gluten- sensitive enteropathy.

4. Eosinophilic granuloma.

17. **Pebbly appearance of the lower lip is termed:**

1. Cheilitis glandularis.

2. Angular cheilitis.

3. Macrocheilia.

4. Exfoliative cheilitis.

18. **Pigmentation associated with pregnancy is called:**

1. Cholasma.

2. Chloroma.

3. Chlorophylia.

4. Cheilosis.

19. **Among the following which is not associated with endogenous pigmentation:**

1. Whipple's syndrome.

2. Peutz-jegher's syndrome.

3. Hemochromatosis.

4. Heck's disease.

20. **Photophobia is a feature of:**

1. Herpes zoster.

2. Measles.

3. Mumps.

4. Infection mononucleosis.

21. Spontaneous oral bleeding can occur if the platelet count falls below_____ mm³:
    1. 50,000.
    2. 1,00,000.
    3. 2,00,000.
    4. Unaffected by fall in the platelet count.

22. Thrombocytopenia may be associated with all except:
    1. Sjogren's syndrome.
    2. Systemic lupus erythematosus.
    3. Felty's syndrome.
    4. Pemphigus foliaceous.

23. "Leutic tongue" is a feature of:
    1. Tertiary syphilis.
    2. Tuberculosis.
    3. Leprosy.
    4. Leukoplakia.

24. "Split papules" occur in:
    1. Tuberculosis.
    2. Leprosy.
    3. Verrucous carcinoma.
    4. Secondary syphilis.

25. "Wash leather" elevated membrane of the tonsil is a feature of:
    1. Leprosy.
    2. Tuberculosis.
    3. Diphtheria.
    4. Scarlet fever.

26. One of the side-effects of using sanguinaria-containing mouthwash is:
    1. Oral candidiasis.
    2. Leukoplakia-like lesions.
    3. Allergic stomatitis.
    4. Burns.

27. Nitroblue tetrazolium reduction test is:
    1. Caries activity test.
    2. Assessment of functioning of WBCs.
    3. Test for AIDS.
    4. Test for tuberculosis

28. Large lymphangiomas spreading into and distending the neck are called:
    1. Thyroglossal cyst.

2. Cystic hygroma.

3. Brachial cyst.

4. Lymphangiosarcoma.

29. Among the following which is not a hamartoma:

1. Glomous tumour.

2. Lymphangioma.

3. Granular cell tumour of the tongue.

4. Pseudoepitheliomatous hyperplasia.

30. Kaposi's sarcoma may be treated with intralesional use of:

1. Methotrexate.

2. Vincristine.

3. Vinblastine.

4. Bleomycin.

31. A sclerosing agent used to treat hemangioma is:

1. Hot water

2. Absolute alcohol.

3. Sodium thiosulfate.

4. Sodium tetradecyl sulfate.

32. What is the percentage of aqueous solution used in toluidine blue staining?

1. 0.1%.

2. 1.0%.

3. 10.0%.

4. 100.0%.

33. Radiotherapy is not indicated for the treatment of ameloblastoma because:

1. It can cause osteoradionecrosis.

2. It causes anaplastic transformation.

3. It causes radiation induced sarcoma.

4. It reduces the vascularity of the bone.

34. Deposition of various immunoglobulins and C3 in a granular band involving the basement membrane zone on immunofluorescent studies is suggestive of:

1. Oral lupus.

2. Lichen planus.

3. Epidermolysis bullosa.

4. Pemphigus.

35. The finding of six or more macules greater than 1.5 cm in diameter in case of neurofibromatosis is called:

1. Trousseau's sign.

2. Crowe's sign

3. Bull's eye sign.

4. Eagle's sign.

36. **One of the possible etiological factors that is suggested for Paget's disease is:**

1. Bacteria.

2. Virus.

3. Fungus.

4. Endocrine.

37. **What is the action of mithramycin in the treatment of Paget's disease?**

1. Removes secondary infection.

2. Inhibits osteoclastic activity.

3. Reduces bone pain.

4. Reduces alteration of the bone morphology.

38. **Which salt can reduce the bone resorption in case of paget's diseases?**

1. Glucocorticoids.

2. Calcium carbonate.

3. Phosphate.

4. Diphosphonate etidronate.

39. **Computer – assisted analysis of oral brush cytology helps to identify:**

1. Oral candidiasis

2. AIDS

3. Oral submucous fibrosis

4. Abnormal cell morphology and Keratinization

40. **Scorbutic gingivitis is associated with deficiency of which vitamin?**

1. A.

2. B.

3. C.

4. D.

41. **Phenytoin induced gingival hyperplasia is usually seen following intake of the drug more than:**

1. 3 days.

2. 3 weeks

3. 3 months

4. 3 years

42. **Among the following which is not a feature of Rutherford's syndrome?**

1. Epiphora

2. Enlargement of gingiva

3. Delayed tooth eruption

4. Superior corneal opacities

43. **Among the following which is not a feature of Cross syndrome?**
    1. Gingival and alveolar enlargement
    2. Microphthalmia
    3. Facial Paralysis
    4. Athetosis

44. **In order to recognize tumour invasion, which is the most reliable diagnosis modality?**
    1. Immunocytochemistry
    2. Study of lymphatics
    3. Evaluation of blood vessels
    4. Study of perineural spaces

45. **Among the following, which is not an isotope used in brachytherapy?**
    1. Cesium
    2. Helium
    3. Iridium
    4. Gold

46. **Among the following conditions which is associated with parotid gland agenesis.**
    1. Hemifacial microstomia
    2. Mandibulofacial dysostosis
    3. Ectodermal dysplasia
    4. Lacrimoauriculodentodigital syndrome

47. **Which of the following regulates the flow of electric current to the filament of X-ray tube?**
    1. High voltage circuit.
    2. Low voltage circuit.
    3. High voltage transformer.
    4. Low voltage transformer.

48. **Which of the following does not occur when the high voltage circuit is activated?**
    1. The unit produces an audible & visible signal.
    2. Electron produced at the cathodes are activated across the tube to the anode.
    3. X-rays bard from the filament to the target.
    4. Heat is produced.

49. **Which of the following accounts for 70% of all the X-ray energy produced at the anode?**
    1. General radiation.
    2. Characteristic radiation.
    3. Coherent Scatter.
    4. Compton Scatter.

50. **Which of the following type of scatter occurs most often with dental X-rays?**
    1. Compton.
    2. Coherent.

3. Photoelectric
4. None of the above.

51. Identify the KV range for most X-ray machines:
1. 50–60 KV.
2. 60–70 KV.
3. 65–100 KV.
4. > 100 KV.

52. Identify the mAmp range for dental radiology:
1. 1–5 mAmp.
2. 4–10 mAmp.
3. 7–15 mAmp.
4. > 15 mAmp.

53. If Kvp is decreased with no other variations in exposure factors, the resultant film will:
1. Appear lighter.
2. Appear darker.
3. Remain same.
4. Either 1 or 2.

54. Identify the error that causes teeth to appear foreshortened on a radiograph –
1. Excessive vertical angulation.
2. Insufficient vertical angulation.
3. Excessive horizontal angulation.
4. Insufficient horizontal angulation.

5. Identify the film size and vertical angulation required to expose a maxillary occlusal projection on a 5-year old child:
1. Size 2 film; + 60 degrees.
2. Size 4 film; + 60 degrees.
3. Size 2 film; + 90 degrees.
4. Size 4 film; + 90 degrees.

56. A diagnostic film is produced using 10 mAmp & 0.45 sec. what exposure is needed to produce same film at 15 mAmp:
1. 0.25 sec.
2. 0.30 sec.
3. 0.45 sec.
4. 0.50 sec.

57. The length of the PiD is changed from 16 inches to 9 inches the resultant intensity:
1. 4 times as intense.
2. Twice as intense.
3. One half as intense.

    4. One fourth as intense.

58. Roof of the maxillary sinus is visualized better by

    1. PA waters view.

    2. PA Caldwell view.

    3. PA mandible view.

    4. Towne's view.

59. Radiation dose from one dental periapical film is calculated as –

    1. 0.03 mR.

    2. 0.04 mR.

    3. 0.05 mR.

    4. 0.01 mR.

60. MPD for gonads in 1 year is:

    1. 5 rem.

    2. 75 rem.

    3. 15 rem.

    4. 10 rem

61. 'Joint mouse' radiographically seen in:

    1. Internal disc derangement.

    2. Disc perforation.

    3. Osteoarthritis.

    4. Joint effusion

62. In normal dental diagnostic procedures, the principal radiation hazard to the operator is produced by

    1. Gamma radiation

    2. Primary radiation

    3. Secondary radiation

    4. All of the above

63. Crainofacial malformations are seen in all of the following conditions except

    1. Down syndrome

    2. Cleft palate

    3. Myasthenia gravis

    4. Cretinism

64. Clubbing of the fingers is most often seen in

    1. Congenital heart disease

    2. Tuberculosis

    3. Stroke

    4. Hypertensive disease

65. Dental development is delayed in

1. Hyperthyroidism
2. Hypothyroidism
3. Bronchial asthma
4. Bulimia

66. Which of the following would not prompt you to consider a possibility of cancer

1. A sore lip that does not heal
2. Multiple vesicle of short duration
3. Changes in a wart or mole
4. Difficulty in swallowing for a month

67. Someone who is paraplegic

1. Is affected only in the upper body
2. Is affected only on one side of the body
3. Has all four limbs affected
4. Has lower limbs most affected

68. Cleft lip occurs during which part of the fetal development

1. First 2 months
2. Second trimester
3. Third trimester
4. First 2 weeks

69. The term used to describe a specific sensation (usually a sound or smell) preceding a seizure is

1. An aura
2. Oracle
3. A presentiment
4. Drama

70. Which of the following is not a condition considered high risk for the development of subacute infective endocarditis

1. Rheumatic heart disease
2. mitral valve surgery
3. Renal dialysis patient with A-V shunt
4. Indwelling cardiac pacemaker

71. Which of the following is unlikely to cause enamel hypoplasia

1. Fluoride
2. Congenital syphilis
3. Exanthematous disease
4. Cleidocrainal dysostosis

72. **Characteristic dental findings of cleidocrainal dysostosis include**

    1. Increased caries susceptibility
    2. Enamel hypoplasia and lack of enamel formation
    3. Juvenile periodontitis and subsequent premature loss of the teeth
    4. Failure of shedding and eruption, and numerous unerupted supernumerary teeth

73. **An inflammed capillary hemangioma of the oral cavity looks similar microscopically to a(n)**

    1. Nevus
    2. Neurofibroma
    3. Angiosarcoma
    4. Pyogenic granuloma

74. **All the following may have similar radiographic findings except**

    1. Ameloblastoma
    2. Radicular cyst
    3. Complex odontoma
    4. Lateral periodontal cyst

75. **The radioopacity that frequently obliterates the apices of maxillary molars when using the bisecting principle of intraoral radiography is the**

    1. Zygoma and the zygomatic process of the maxilla
    2. Orbital process of the zygomatic bone
    3. Palatine bone and the zygoma
    4. Maxillary sinus

76. **The first consideration in the differential diagnosis of a painless palatal perforation would be**

    1. Syphilis
    2. Histoplasmosis
    3. Actinomycosis
    4. Tuberculosis

77. **Of the following materials used in dentristry, which is most difficult to distinguish radiographically from caries**

    1. Zinc oxide euginol
    2. Silver amalgam
    3. Calcium hydroxide methyl cellulose paste
    4. Zinc phosphate cement

78. **The most reliable single histologic criterion for a diagnosis of squamous cell carcinoma is**

    1. Invasion
    2. Degeneration
    3. Hyperchromatism
    4. Encapsulation

79. **Copper beaten appearance of skull is seen in**
    1. Craniofacial dysostosis
    2. Cleido cranial dysostosis
    3. Multiple myeloma
    4. Marfan's syndrome

80. **Cellulose acetate is no longer used as a film base because:**
    1. It is costly
    2. It is not easily available
    3. It itself casts a shadow
    4. It is highly inflammable

81. **Kerma measures**
    1. Radioactivity
    2. Absorbed dose
    3. Equivalent dose
    4. Exposure

82. **Parma modification aims at**
    1. Reduced surface exposure
    2. Longer FSFD (Focal spot to Film distance)
    3. Easier placement
    4. Blurring of tube side structure

83. **Identify the maximum permissible dose (MPD) of a nonoccupationally exposed person:**
    1. 0.001 Sv/year (0.1 rem/year)
    2. 0.002 Sv/year (0.2 rem/year)
    3. 0.003 Sv/year (0.3 rem/year)
    4. 0.005 Sv/year (0.5 rem/year)

84. **In an intensifying screen, the phosphor layer when struck by photons fluorescence occurs the phosphor used in dentistry & medicine include all except:**
    1. Calcium tungstate
    2. Magnesium bromide
    3. Terbium activated gadolinium oxysulfide
    4. Thullium activated lanthanum oxybromide.

85. **When a patient is asked to keep his mouth open in a P.A. Water's view the _____ is projected on the palate.**
    1. Foramen magnum.
    2. Ethmoid sinus
    3. Nasolacrimal canal
    4. Sphenoid sinus.

86. **Increasing the operating kilovoltage peak (kVp) will cause:**
    1. An increase in density; the film appears darker
    2. An increase in density; the film appears lighter
    3. A decrease in density; the film appears darker
    4. A decrease in density; the film appears lighter

87. **A dental patient has thick soft tissues and dense bones. To compensate for this increase subject thickness and provide a film of diagnostic density, the dental radiographer may:**
    1. Increase the exposure time
    2. Increase the milliamperage
    3. Increase the operating kilovoltage peak
    4. Any of the above

88. **The drug of choice in facial nerve palsy is**
    1. Vitamin B12
    2. Anti – infectious drug
    3. Vitamin A
    4. Corticosteroid

89. **Sodium salicylate is administered in rheumatoid arthritis**
    1. To provide an anticoagulant effect
    2. To provide relief from pain
    3. To provide a sedative effect
    4. As a bactericidal

90. **The treatment for herpangina is**
    1. Application of an antiviral ointment
    2. Supportive and symptomatic
    3. High dosage of acyclovir and idoxuridine
    4. Antibiotics and analgesics

91. **Diminished taste sensation is termed**
    1. Hypogeusia
    2. Hypophrenia
    3. Hyposmia
    4. Hypocapnea

92. **The generalized out break of which of the following diseases is preceded by the appearance of a 'Primary lesion' or 'herald spot'?**
    1. Erythema multiforme
    2. Keratosis follicularis
    3. White sponge nevus
    4. Pityriasis rosea

93. **A diagnostic test where a pustule is formed 24 hrs after a needle puncture, done in Behcet's disease is**
    1. Patch test
    2. Pathergy test
    3. Schilling's test.
    4. Puncture test.

94. **Ulcers of the lingual frenum in neonates caused by abrasion of the tongue by teeth during suckling is called as**
    1. Baked tongue
    2. Parrot tongue
    3. Rigafede disease
    4. Reye's syndrome.

95. **Hot spot on technetium scan is characteristic of**
    1. Pleomorphic adenoma
    2. Adenoid cystic carcinoma
    3. Warthin's tumor
    4. Mucoepidermoid carcinoma

96. **Which of the following L.A. is contraindicated in cardiac patients?**
    1. Lignocaine
    2. Bupivacaine
    3. Procaine
    4. None of the above.

97. **The emotional status of a patient may be a contributing factor in all of the following, except**
    1. Aphthous ulcers
    2. Pain in the tongue
    3. Gingival pigmentation
    4. Necrotizing ulcerative gingivitis

98. **Antihypertensive drugs can lead to**
    1. Xerostomia
    2. Ulceration
    3. Lichenoid reaction
    4. All the above

99. **Dental effects of congenital heart defect can include:**
    1. Cleft palate
    2. Turner's syndrome
    3. Enamel hypoplasia
    4. All the above.

100. **Giant cell lesions of jaw along with congenital heart disease are seen in**

1. Turner's syndrome
2. Williams syndrome
3. Noonan syndrome
4. None of the above.

101. **Risk of bacteremia following extraction in a cardiac patient is**

1. 0 - 25%
2. 25 – 50%
3. 50 – 75%
4. 75 – 90%

102. **Antibiotic prophylaxis may not be needed for:**

1. Coronary artery bypass graft
2. Prosthetic valves
3. Cyanotic congenital heart disease
4. None of the above

103. **Which of the following dental procedures are on indication for antibiotic prophylaxis?**

1. Extraction
2. Sialography
3. Rubber dam placement
4. All the above.

104. **When planning an elective dental extraction, the aspirin should be:**

1. Continued in same dose
2. Stopped 3-7 days prior
3. Dose should be increased
4. Dose should be decreased.

105. **What is not the acceptable INR value of patients on anticoagulant therapy to plan dental treatment?**

1. 1.0
2. 1.5
3. 2.5
4. 4.5

106. **A superficial abscess connected through the sinus to a larger deep abscess is called as**

1. Cold abscess.
2. Collar stud abscess
3. Blind abscess
4. None of the above.

107. **Asthmatic patients using corticosteroid inhalers commonly have:**

1. Adrenal insufficiency

2. Oral thrush
3. Lupoid reaction
4. Pigmentation.

108. Trotter's syndrome is associated with:
1. Auriculotemporal nerve
2. Glossopharyngeal nerve
3. Mandibular nerve
4. Chorda tympani

108. Secondary trigeminal neuralgia can be caused because of all of the following except
1. Carcinoma of maxillary antrum
2. Ischemia at some portion of trigeminal nerve
3. Intracranial vascular anomalies
4. Multiple sclerosis

109. Trotter's syndrome is a result of
1. Metastatic tumor of the pterygopalatine fossae
2. Paralysis of tongue
3. Carcinoma of maxillary antrum
4. Tumor of nasopharynx.

110. Miosis, ptosis and anhidrosis is seen in
1. Horner's syndrome
2. Frey's syndrome
3. Raeder's syndrome
4. Horton's syndrome

111. Which of the following antibiotics is contraindicated in myasthenia gravis?
1. Tetracycline
2. Penicillin
3. Erythromycin
4. Ciprofloxacin

112. Anticonvulsant drugs can cause
1. Xerostomia
2. Gingival hyperplasia
3. Erythema multiforme
4. All the above

113. Mycobacterium avium complex involve:
1. Skin
2. Lungs
3. Lymph nodes
4. All of the above

114. **The most likely cause of necrotizing sialometaplasia is:**
    1. Autoimmune
    2. Viral
    3. Local ischemia
    4. Chronic irritation.

115. **Patients with gastro esophageal reflux disease (GERD) should be treated in:**
    1. Supine position
    2. Semisupine position.
    3. Sitting position.
    4. Any of the above.

116. **Oral manifestation of peptic ulcer disease includes.**
    1. Dental erosion.
    2. Pallor of oral mucosa.
    3. Vascular malformation of liver
    4. All of the above.

117. **Which of the following is contraindicated in gastric ulcers?**
    1. Steroids
    2. Cox-II inhibitors.
    3. Paracetamol
    4. Anti cholinergic drugs

118. **Bleeding in renal disorders is controlled by –**
    1. DDAVP
    2. Cryoprecipitate
    3. Estrogen
    4. Any of the above

119. **Bleeding tendencies in renal disorders is due to**
    1. Platelet defect
    2. Prostacycline activity
    3. Intrinsic coagulation defects
    4. All the above

120. **Dose reduction is indicated for which of the following drugs, in patients on dialysis?**
    1. NSAID's
    2. Ampicillin
    3. Erythromycin
    4. Paracetamol

121. **Which of the following is contraindicated in renal disorders?**
    1. Gentamycin
    2. NSAID's

   3. Amoxycillin

   4. Paracetamol

122. **Fluoride therapy to patients with renal disorders should be given:**

   1. Topically

   2. Systemic

   3. Any of the above

   4. Both are contraindicated

123. **Intraoral changes in uraemia are seen at BUN levels**

   1. < 100 mg/dl

   2. > 150 mg/dl

   3. > 300 mg/dl

   4. > 50 mg/dl

124. **The desired whole blood glucose levels while treating a diabetic patient are:**

   1. < 120 mg/dl

   2. 120-140 mg/dl

   3. 120-180 mg/dl

   4. 150-200 mg/dl

125. **Elective surgery should be deferred if FBS levels are above:**

   1. 120 mg/dl

   2. 150 mg/dl

   3. 200 mg/dl

   4. 250 mg/dl

126. **Triad of diabetes mellitus, lichen planus and hypertension is called:**

   1. Albright syndrome

   2. Grinspan syndrome

   3. Simmonds disease

   4. Nelson syndrome

127. **Circumoral paraesthesia is seen in**

   1. IDDM

   2. NIDDM

   3. Insulin treated diabetes

   4. Patients on hypoglycemic

128. **Which of the following antibiotics is avoided in Crohn's disease?**

   1. Amoxycillin

   2. Erythromycin

   3. Metronidazole.

   4. All the above.

129. **Oral lesions of Crohn's disease includes:**
    1. Cobblestone appearance of oral mucosa
    2. Pustules
    3. Fluid filled vesicles.
    4. All the above

130. **Oral lesions of ulcerative colitis include**
    1. Chronic ulceration
    2. Multiple intraepithelial micro abscess
    3. Hemorrhagic lesions
    4. All the above.

131. **Congenital hyperbilirubinaemia is associated with:**
    1. Gilberts syndrome
    2. Crigler – Najjar syndrome
    3. Rotor syndrome
    4. All the above.

132. **Which of the following is contraindicated in liver disorders?**
    1. Opioids
    2. Paracetamol
    3. Lignocaine
    4. Prilocaine

133. **Pruritis is a common manifestation of:**
    1. Impaired bilirubin metabolism
    2. Impaired bilirubin exertion
    3. Impaired excretion of bile salts
    4. Impaired liver cell metabolism

134. **Which of the following infections does not spread with dental treatment?**
    1. Hepatitis A
    2. Hepatitis B
    3. Hepatitis C
    4. Hepatitis D

135. **Patients with chronic renal failure have –**
    1. Low incidence of dental caries
    2. High incidence of dental caries
    3. Depend upon severity of disease
    4. None of the above

136. **Uraemic stomatitis appears as**
    1. Undermined ulcers
    2. Scrapable white patch

    3.   Erythemo pultaceous lesions

    4.   Fluid filled vesicles

137. **The most appropriate time for elective dental treatment in renal patients is –**

    1.   Day after dialysis

    2.   On the day of dialysis

    3.   One day before dialysis

    4.   None of the above

138. **All are the lab findings seen in AIDS related complex except:**

    1.   Decreased T4:T8.

    2.   Anemia.

    3.   Diarrhoea since four months.

    4.   Increased serum globulin level.

139. **"Lumpy jaw" is a feature of:**

    1.   Actinomycosis.

    2.   Tuberculosis.

    3.   Mucormycosis.

    4.   Osteomyelitis.

140. **"Bull neck" is associated with:**

    1.   Scarlet fever.

    2.   Diptheria.

    3.   Sarcoidosis.

    4.   Tetanus.

141. **Which of the following in not a feature of Eagle's syndrome?**

    1.   Sore throat

    2.   Dysphagia

    3.   Pain on turning head

    4.   Epiphora

142. **Gustatory sweating refer to:**

    1.   Brogorad syndrome

    2.   Sphenopalatine neuralgia

    3.   Frey's syndrome

    4.   Alarm clock headache

143. **Gingival enlargement due to phenytoin:**

    1.   Affects males more than females

    2.   More in edentulous areas

    3.   Dose dependence

    4.   Occurs within 8 – 12 months after beginning of therapy.

144. **"Buffalo hump" in patients with renal transplant is seen due to –**
    1. Swelling of salivary gland
    2. Acquired adiposity
    3. Fungal infection
    4. Hepatic dysfunction

145. **Renal osteodystrophy is manifested in jaws as–**
    1. Loss of lamina dura
    2. Osteoporosis
    3. Giant cell lesions
    4. All the above

146. **Patients who should be considered for antimicrobial prophylaxis prior to extractions include:**
    1. Those with polycystic kidney
    2. Those with kidney transplant
    3. Those receiving peritoneal dialysis
    4. All the above

147. **The screening test for CA prostate is –**
    1. Serum testosterone levels
    2. Serum cortisone levels
    3. Serum acid phosphatase
    4. Serum alkaline phosphatase

148. **Facial flushing is an adverse effect of:**
    1. Chlorpropamide
    2. Metformin
    3. Acarbose
    4. All the above

149. **A patient reports with melanin pigmentation of the lips and oral mucosa present from birth. The patient complains of having frequent episodes of abdominal pain. The most likely diagnosis is**
    1. Addisons' disease
    2. Malignant melanoma
    3. Hodgkin's disease
    4. Hereditary intestinal polyposis

150. **Modification of steroid regimen is required when:**
    1. Patient is currently taking steroid
    2. Taken steroid during previous 12 months.
    3. No steroids were taken in test 12 months
    4. All the above

151. Nelson's syndrome is related to:

1. Adrenal glands
2. Pancreas
3. Thyroid
4. Parathyroid

152. Werner's syndrome refers to:

1. Adenoma of pituitary
2. Hyperplasia of parathyroid
3. Adenoma of adrenals
4. All the above

153. Sipple syndrome includes:

1. Pheochromocytoma
2. Parathyroid hyperplasia
3. Medullary cell CA
4. All the above

154. Which of the following is not a feature of Schmidt syndrome?

1. Pituitary adenoma
2. Oral neuromas
3. Marfanoid features
4. Pheochromocytoma.

155. Lazy leukocyte syndrome is a result of

1. Loss of phagocytic activity of WBC
2. Loss of chemotactic function
3. Loss of bactericidal activities
4. All the above

156. Bing Neel syndrome is marked by

1. Macroglobulinemia
2. Hypoprothrombinemia
3. Hypofibrinogenemia
4. Telangiectasia

157. Treatment of Felty's syndrome is:

1. WBC transfusion
2. Corticosteroids
3. Splenectomy
4. Allogenic bone narrow transplantation

158. Chediak – Higashi syndrome affects all the following except:

1. Nerve cells
2. Lymphocytes

3. Neutrophils
4. Melanocytes

159. **CML is related to all of the following except:**
    1. Exposure to ionizing radiation
    2. Philadelphia chromosome
    3. HTLV – 1 and HTLV – 2
    4. Decreased leukocyte alkaline phosphate

160. **A child with fever and sore throat developed acute cervical lymphadenopathy. Most likely investigation to be done is:**
    1. Open biopsy of node.
    2. Radical neck dissection.
    3. Neck X-ray.
    4. Complete hemogram

161. **Which of the following is true of mumps?**
    1. Salivary gland involvement is limited to the parotids.
    2. Patient is not infectious prior to clinical parotid enlargement
    3. Meningoencephalitis can precede parotitis
    4. Mumps orchitis frequently leads to infertility

162. **Single dose NSAID:**
    1. Aspirin.
    2. Diclofenec.
    3. Naproxen.
    4. Piroxicam

163. **A lesion was excised from the lower lip of a 14 yr old boy.It consisted of a central cavity filled with clear fluid and lined with granulation tissue only.surface epitlelium was extremely thin but intact.A few collections of salivary gland acini and bundles of skeltal muscle fibers were found deep to the lesion.The diagnosis is**
    1. ranula
    2. fibroma
    3. mucocele
    4. pleomorphic adenoma

164. **Leukemic gingivitis, because of spontaneous hemorrhage and necrosis, may be misdiagnosed as**
    1. necrotizing ulcerative gingivitis
    2. thrombocytopenic purpura
    3. desquamative gingivitis
    4. infectious mononucleosis

165. A patient exhibits multiple radiolucent areas in the jaw bones which stimulate both periapical and perodontal lesions .The serum calcium is 13.5mg%. A biopsy from one of the radiolucent areas reveals a giant cell lesion
    1. hyperparathyroidism
    2. multiple myeloma
    3. myxedema
    4. Hand-Schuller-Christian disease

166. Paget's disease is associated with which of the following changes in the blood
    1. Elevated serum amylase
    2. Decreased serum calcium
    3. Elevated serum acid phosphatase
    4. Elevated serum alkaline phosphatase

167. The most benign type of histiocytosis X disease is
    1. Letterer-Siwe disease
    2. Hand-Schuller-Christian disease
    3. Eosinophilic granuloma
    4. Behects syndrome

168. A high titer of serum hetrophile antibody is found in patients with
    1. Herpangina
    2. Actinomycosis
    3. Herpes simplex
    4. Infectious mononucleosis

169. A friable,elevated,bright purplish-red tumour like mass with a raspberry appearence, located most frequently on the gingiva and consisting of granulation tissue with young fibroblast,proliferating capillaries and inflammatory cells is
    1. Fibroma
    2. Pyogenic granuloma
    3. Dilantin hyperplasia
    4. Peripheral gaint cell granuloma

170. Of the following conditions, gingival involvement would be unusual in
    1. Pemphigoid
    2. Primary herpes
    3. Recurrent apthae
    4. Pyogenic granuloma

171. Presence of Heberdens nodes is most characteristic of
    1. Fibrous dysplasia
    2. Osteoarthritis
    3. Rheumatoid arthritis
    4. Albrights syndrome

172. **Raynauds disease or syndrome frequently precedes,or is found in association with, scleroderma. Common findings include all the following except**
    1. Brittle nails
    2. Trophic changes in the skin
    3. Excessive moist skin
    4. Ulceration of the digit and extremities

173. **The malignant tumour of the salivary gland which is seen most often in the posterior palatal area is the**
    1. Papillary cystadenoma lymphomatosum
    2. Mucoepidermoid carcinoma
    3. Malignant mixed carcinoma
    4. Adenoid cystic carcinoma

174. **Pre mature exfoliation of the teeth is seen in**
    1. Papillon-le-Fevre syndrome
    2. Hypophosphatasia
    3. Juvenile diabetics
    4. all of the above

175. **Which of the following bone diseases accompanies callus formation that mimics osteosarcoma**
    1. Osteopetrosis
    2. Caffey's disease
    3. Osteogenisis imperfecta
    4. Cherubism

176. **Abnormal storage of sphingomyelins is characteristic of**
    1. Gauchers disease
    2. Niemann-Pick disease
    3. Tay-Sachs disease
    4. Fabry's disease

177. **If a patient is suspected of being sensitive to acrylic, the test most helpful in diagnosis is the**
    1. Heterophil antibody
    2. Patch test
    3. Scratch tcst
    4. Tourniquet test

178. **Formation of a bulla following stroking of intact skin or mucosa constitute a positive reaction in an attempt to elicit**
    1. Babinski's sign
    2. Chvostek's sign
    3. Nikolsky's sign
    4. Romberg's sign

179. **For how long, the elective dental care should be deferred after an angina attack?**
    1. 9 months
    2. 6 months
    3. 8 months
    4. 1 year

180. **Which surface of teeth is most commonly eroded by gastric acid regurgitation?**
    1. Labial surfaces of maxillary anteriors
    2. Palatal surfaces of maxillary anteriors
    3. Labial surfaces of mandibular anteriors
    4. Lingual surfaces of mandibular anteriors

181. **All are features of multiple myeloma except:**
    1. Punched out bony lesions
    2. Hypergammaglobinemia
    3. Hypercalcemia
    4. Abnormal M proteins

182. **Among the following statements about Herpangina, which is correct:**
    1. Occurs in pregnant woman.
    2. Occurs in the elderly.
    3. Occurs in children under 4 years of age.
    4. Occurs in immunosuppressed individuals.

183. **Morbilli is:**
    1. Zoster infection.
    2. German measles.
    3. Measles.
    4. Mumps.

184. **Lymphogranuloma venerum is caused by:**
    1. Trepenoma palladium.
    2. Donovan granulomatosis.
    3. Chlamydia trachomatis.
    4. Hemophilus ducreyi.

185. **A complication of acute necrotizing ulcerative gingivostomatitis is:**
    1. Osteomyelitis.
    2. Actinomycosis.
    3. Cancrum oris.
    4. Gingival abscess.

186. **Oral hairy leukoplakia mainly affects:**
    1. Tongue.

   2. Buccal mucosa.
   3. Lips.
   4. Palate.

187. Homogeneous viral nuclear inclusions are seen in:
   1. Heck's disease.
   2. Paget's disease.
   3. Oral hairy leukoplakia.
   4. White sponge nevus.

188. Argon laser is used to treat:
   1. Port-wine stains.
   2. Leukoplakia.
   3. Oral submucous fibrosis.
   4. Syphilitic mucous patches.

189. An example for proliferation of vascular channels is:
   1. Thrombasthenia.
   2. Ecchymosis.
   3. Hemangioma.
   4. Bleb.

190. One of the consistent features associated with cherubism is:
   1. Submandibular lymphadenopathy.
   2. Pigmentation.
   3. Blue sclera.
   4. Egg shell crackling of bone during palpation.

191. The oral disease that is prevalent among the inhabitants of Southeast Asia is:
   1. Lichen planus.
   2. Sickle cell disease.
   3. Oral submucous fibrosis.
   4. AIDS.

192. Bowen's disease can resemble:
   1. Leukoplakia.
   2. Erythroplakia.
   3. Papillomatous lesion.
   4. All of the above.

193. Cat-scratch disease is best treated by:
   1. Immunosuppressive medication.
   2. Antibiotics.

3. Analgesic and antipyretic agents.

4. No treatment is required as it is self-limiting.

194. False positive test result with toluidine blue staining can occur in case of:

1. Carcinoma in situ

2. Malignancy

3. Inflammatory areas

4. Leukoplakia

195. The normally salivary gland appearance on a sialogram is described as:

1. Leafless tree appearance

2. Branches fruit – laden appearance

3. Ball – in – hand appearance

4. Cherry blossom appearance

196. Penumbra formation is diagnostically related to:

1. Detail.

2. Density.

3. Fogging.

4. Contrast.

197. Screens are not used intraorally for periapical or occlusal films because:

1. Radiation from dental machines does not require intensification

2. They add to the bulk

3. Intra oral films is not screen sensitive

4. Screen reduce the resolution

198. Cauliflower appearance is seen in:

1. Tonsillolith

2. Chronically inflamed lymph nodes

3. Sialolith

4. Arteriosclerosis

199. 'Ball in hand' radiographic appearance is seen in:

1. Intrinsic parotid mass

2. Sialolith

3. Sialodochitis

4. Sjogren syndrome

200. Which of the following tumors is radiosensitive or is treated by X-ray radiation?

1. Fibrosarcoma

2. Odentogenic myxoma

3. Neurolemmoma

4. Olfactory neuroblastoma

For answers of these questions mail on books@targeteducare.com

NOTES

NOTES